Staff Nurse's Survival Guide

Second Edition

Edited by Elizabeth M. Horne and Tracy Cowan

A collection of articles first published in *Professional Nurse* and here revised and updated for inclusion

Wolfe Publishing Ltd

Published by
Wolfe Publishing Ltd
Brook House
2–16 Torrington Place
London WC1E 7LT

Printed and bound in Great Britain by
BPCC Hazells Ltd
Member of BPCC Ltd

© 1992 Wolfe Publishing Ltd

For full details of all Wolfe Nursing titles please write to Wolfe
Publishing Ltd, Brook House, 2–16 Torrington Place, London
WC1E 7LT, England.

The Professional Developments Series

These eight books provide you with a wealth of insight into all aspects of nursing practice. The series is essential reading for qualified, practising nurses who need to keep up-to-date with new developments, evaluate their clinical practice, and develop and extend their clinical management and teaching skills. Through reading these books, students of nursing will gain an insight into what the essence of nursing is and the wide range of skills which are daily employed in improving patient care. Up-to-date, referenced and appropriately illustrated, The Professional Developments Series brings together the work of well over 200 nurses.

Other titles in The Professional Developments Series:

Dunne **How Many Nurses Do I Need: A Guide** 1 870065 24 7
to Resource Management Issues
This book provides valuable advice and information for all nurses facing the challenge of taking direct responsibility for managing human resources and planning, providing quality assurance and managing financial resources.

Garrett **Healthy Ageing: Some Nursing Perspectives** 1 870065 22 0
This book puts healthy ageing into the context of a growing, healthy elderly population and looks at care aspects of daily living, health problems in old age, and working with older people.

Glasper **Child Care: Some Nursing Perspectives** 1 870065 23 9
In three sections, this book covers many pertinent issues that are associated with caring for babies, young children and adolescents, in hospital and community settings.

Horne and Cowan **Effective Communication: Some Nursing** 07234 1808 X
Perspectives, 2nd edn
This book examines a wide range of communication topics, including counselling, confidentiality, group and team work, compliance and communicating with children.

Horne **Patient Education Plus** 1 870065 11 5
This book helps to develop nurses' teaching roles, and covers an extensive range of clinical topics. Each chapter contains a useful handout which can be freely photocopied or adapted for use with clients.

Horne **Practice Check!** 1 870065 10 7
Each Practice Check presents a brief description of situations which may arise in practice together with open-ended questions and discussion to enable problems to be explored and effective solutions to be found.

Horne and Cowan **Ward Sister's Survival Guide, 2nd edn** 07234 1807 1
This book is essential reading and valuable reference for all nurses with direct clinical management responsibility.

Contents

Issues in Patient Care

Issues in Clinical Management

Introduction

'PREPP', 'quality assurance', 'standard setting', 'resource management' are now key components of nursing practice and play a vital role in every staff nurse's daily routine. Clinical practice is firmly committed to providing holistic care and to meeting individual patient's needs, and staff nurses need to know how to achieve this in practice. They have to be all things to all people: not only must they provide holistic care, but they must also keep up-to-date in their clinical development, remain aware of their legal and ethical responsibilities and be able to make maximum use of sometimes limited resources. This role is clearly dynamic, and staff nurses are taking on new areas of responsibility.

This new edition of the *Staff Nurse's Survival Guide* focuses on the key areas of good nursing practice: professional development, ensuring patients' quality of life, topical issues in patient care and the basic components of effective clinical practice. A chapter on product appraisal offers a useful overview of product assessment. The book offers practical and accessible examples of how the theory of clinical practice can usefully be put into practice.

All the chapters were first published in *Professional Nurse* magazine, and have been revised and updated for this new edition. I hope you and your colleagues will find them useful in your own practice and professional development.

Tracy Cowan
Assistant Editor, *Professional Nurse*
London, March 1992

Your Professional
Development

1

On becoming a staff nurse

Tom Lewis, RGN, RNT, DPNS, BSc (Hons) Nursing, PGCEA
Formerly Staff Nurse, Brighton General Hospital

The excitement of actually passing your exams, even little things like people calling you staff nurse, can be exhilarating. Suddenly everyone wants to talk to you — when people ring up and want to speak to the person in charge, it's you. It's as though you've just been discovered as somebody by all the medical and paramedical staff, the patients too seem to respond to you differently. It's an ego boost, and after all, you've earned it. Haven't you just spent three long years in training? And then it hits you.

Expectations

All of these people want *you*. The patients, the students and pupils, the medical staff, the relatives, the clinical nurse manager – they all have expectations of you. Perhaps the most difficult one to cope with is the feeling that you are expected to know everything. From where every nurse and patient is at any given moment to how to get hold of some outlandish piece of equipment that nobody has used for 10 years on a Sunday afternoon. And then there are the students and pupils. You remember when you felt lost and everybody seemed too busy to help you; you know you didn't get enough supervision or teaching. And the times you didn't understand things – if only somebody could have told you the answer. Well now all that is your job. You are expected to know the appropriate expectations for each level of learner. Now you are suddenly responsible for supervising and teaching them. Why don't you know? You're expected to know. It makes you realise how awful you must have been as a student – you expected those staff nurses to know everything, and were critical when they didn't.

New situations

If you've been diligent during your training, studied hard, and applied yourself, there will be lots of things that you can deal with. Situations that you've met before and people that you've worked with have all helped you to build up a store of knowledge that you can apply to many situations. But now you are learning that every situation you meet is unique. Many of them seem to be totally unrelated to anything you did in your training. Interviewing learners is a good example of this, or supporting junior doctors, or how to get 30 patients into 28 beds. It's at this time you begin to realise just how much you don't know. And somehow all that friendly advice – such as "Realising how much you don't know is the beginning of wisdom", or that classic "You really start learning when you become a staff nurse" — seems a little trite when you're the one carrying the can.

Learning new skills

I think that this is a time of real crisis for the nurse. Confidence can be shattered, and you wonder if you've been trained to be a nurse at all. Or even wonder what nursing is all about. Learning all these new skills of organisation distracts you from what you want to do, what you've trained so hard to do, deliver real care. At this time it really helps to have supportive people around you, colleagues who let you express your distress and understand. It may be something that you should bear in mind when you are choosing your first staffing post. Try to look back over your training and identify the places where the trained staff gave you a lot of help; the chances are that they are well supported and this can be of great benefit to you in those early months in your new role. Getting to grips with the skills involved in organisation can take some time, and like all learning processes there is a lot of trial and error involved. Sometimes you let down people who are depending on you. Organising is about people and to learn to organise we have to learn about people, which can be a painful process. However, you have already mastered lots of skills, and you can master this one.

Applying your knowledge

Then comes the joy of being a staff nurse. When you're no longer distracted by how to do this or that, you can start concentrating on the patients again with a vengeance. Now you really can start to apply all the knowledge that you've acquired during your training, and you realise that it is true, you have learned so much more about the patients' problems since being on the same ward for a while. Somehow you are able to build up expertise. You know about, and look for the kind of things that go wrong. You start to recognise the underlying patterns of disease processes, often masked in their expression because of the unique way people have of displaying their illness. You can prevent problems and save people from unnecessary suffering. You begin to recognise changes in patient status early and intervene to alter the situation. You even start to recognise that it's all right not to know everything, but be glad about the skills you do have and be excited about being able to grow in your knowledge and ability.

But best of all is when you begin to realise the privilege of being a nurse. Recognising just how much trust is vested in you, by so many people, is humbling. The willingness of patients to share a very important part of their lives with you reflects not only the trust they have in your profession but also the gratitude for the care you are able to give. It is this special relationship that you have as a trained, skilled nurse that is the joy of nursing. It is ours to hold and to cherish, to live up to, to fight for, and to be proud of. Recognising the importance of professional nursing to the patient is a major piece of learning for us. When you are learning your practical skills and the tasks that you will have to carry out, and all the theory that at the time doesn't seem to have much real significance, it is difficult to stand back and ponder about the nature of nursing. It is only when you are in the position to order and control the nursing input to a patient or group of patients that you come to understand the vulnerability and dependence of the patient upon the nurse and to recognise the need for the nurse to be totally committed to professional ethics. I hope those of you who have just become, or are about to become, trained nurses find support through your early days and come to enjoy your chosen profession as I have done.

Reference
Department of Health and Social Security (1981) Professional Development in Clinical Nursing – the 1980s. Report of the Harrogate Seminar.

2

Coming down from the ivory tower: putting research into practice

Stephen G. Wright, RGN, RCNT, DipN, RNT, MSc
Consultant Nurse, Nursing Development Unit, Tameside General Hospital

Mark Dolan, RGN
Charge Nurse/Senior Primary Nurse, Nursing Development Unit, Tameside General Hospital

Nursing is renowned for the gaps it endures between theory and practice, and such a gap, it seems, applies as much to nursing research as to any other sector of nursing. Bergman (1986) has argued that "some researchers live in ivory towers, divorced from the reality of daily practice". The researcher, separated in this way, is seen as pursuing esoteric theory which has no bearing on the day-to-day world of nursing practice, instead working for or speaking to fellow like-minded academics. Preaching thus to the converted, the findings of nursing research reach a limited audience and fail to affect the huge mass of nurses engaged at the hard edge of practice.

"Practice can only be as sound as the knowledge on which it is based" (Jacox, 1974).

Some writers have suggested the term 'research' itself alienates many nurses because it is surrounded by mystique, and: "Because nursing is essentially a pragmatic discipline, the usefulness of research endeavours is sometimes equated with practical applicability. Hence, research which is not seen to have an immediate use is often dismissed as a waste of resources with which it is not worth bothering" (Luker, 1986).

Luker goes on to suggest that research may illuminate or bring new insight to what nurses do. It may help to test out and refine methodologies appropriate to nurses, discovering new knowledge which can directly affect practice, such as the work of Norton *et al*, (1962) and their work on pressure sore risk assessment. Given that there are such clear benefits to nursing research, why is it so often ignored and little applied? It is perhaps too simplistic to blame the 'ivory tower' researcher, though this is, no doubt, a contributing factor. Sometimes the language in which a research report is couched is itself counterproductive, simply because it is not described or expressed in such a way that most clinical nurses can comprehend. Sometimes nurses see themselves as too busy with patients to have time for research, and this is reinforced if they regard research as a theoretical issue which has no relevance to practitioners. They are, futhermore: "often unwilling to carry out research through shortage of funds, or lack of awareness of how to go about it, and are put off by the seeming complexities of the ethical issues. On top of this, nurses may simply feel that the 'bosses' (who may not be research minded) would be unsupportive and even hostile" (Wright, 1986).

Bond (1978) believes that nursing research must be 'proletarianised' if it is to have any meaning and relevance to the greatest number of nurses. In other words, thinking about, carrying out, and analysing research need to be commonplace activities accepted by all nurses in their day-to-day practice. The number of research courses available and the trend towards including research awareness in both statutory and continuing education programmes means that, to some extent, this is already underway. A great deal more can be done in the service side of nursing to proletarianise nursing research, and this has been one of the main aims of the Nursing Development Unit (NDU) at Tameside.

Promoting research awareness
Motivated experts at clinical level Benner (1984) argues cogently that clinical experts need to act as role models in promoting research-based practice. While all nursing staff on the NDU have research elements written into their job descriptions, there is no guarantee that this will happen in practice. Other key individuals are needed to be experts in their field, acting as good examples to others, helping them to carry out research and apply findings. A research nurse post was specifically created, and a team of clinical specialists and a consultant nurse also included research in their remit. These nurses can also use informal networks to guide colleagues to others who will assist with information or act as supervisors. This is also seen as a key role for the 'G' grade sister and charge nurse who are the key clinical leaders and innovators. Nurses who have conducted research through research appreciation on graduate courses are in an excellent position to facilitate awareness among others, especially if they work alongside them.

Staff development All the NDU's courses are research-based, and many contain specific education in areas such as research awareness and methodologies. Including research projects as part of course objectives stimulates a spirit of enquiry, while reinforcing the idea that research is 'ordinary'. Staff can be encouraged to attend research courses off site with similar research components or pursue open learning programmes.

Scale Making research 'ordinary' is a key feature in demystifying it. Nurses can be helped to realise that nursing research is simply 'finding out' and choosing the best methods with which to do so. Simple, practical projects related directly to nurses' working experiences (such as the effects of going out of uniform, costing of incontinence devices, evaluating the introduction of pet therapy) were found to be most helpful. Nurses do not need to feel that research should be highly complex in order to discover the meaning of life; setting research projects which are fairly simple, relevant to nurses' day-to-day work and which can be pursued within the time and resources available are good starting points for promoting an acceptance of the relevance of research.

Literature   This includes books, journals and articles on research reports as well as research methods, which need to be made available at ward level and accessible to all staff, day or night. The NDU has set up a small library on site which is open 24 hours a day, and which clearly makes access to literature much easier than relying on the more limited availability in, for example, a more distant school of nursing. Stocks of books and journals can also be kept at ward level. Additional access to literature can be gained by setting up arrangements with local colleges, polytechnics and universities – most will willingly permit external students entry to their libraries. Organisations such as the RCN have extensive library facilities, including assistance with literature searches.

Informal approaches   Introducing a research item to the agenda of a meeting, setting up a research appreciation forum, a journal, club or discussion groups are various methods in which groups of nurses can get together informally and treat research as part of the topic of the day. Nurses at ward level, for example, can introduce a topic of relevance to each ward meeting, while colleagues at all levels can read and précis research reports for discussion, and circulate written summaries to others. Peer group support is essential to successful research awareness. A research interest group can be set up, a quality circle developed or nurses can join in many research interest and development opportunities provided by such professional bodies as the RCN.

Funding and resources   How can we afford to promote research awareness? The real question is how can we afford not to? Nurses, like other professionals, are now being judged in cost-effective terms – a knowledgeable, expert nurse, whose practice is based on sound research, is required to make the best use of resources. Above all, however, patients have a right to a nurse who knows what he or she is doing, and is interested and well-motivated enough to offer skilled, expert care.

Whenever possible, funds and resources have been put to maximum use, for example by using staff training monies on secretarial or word-processing time. In addition a bursary has been set up, derived from various methods of fund raising (Purdy *et al*, 1988), to provide money to support nursing research and staff development which is independent of the limited health authority funds available. Staff can also be encouraged to apply for other sources of funding such as local industry, scholarships, the Nightingale Fund or the Department of Health.

Senior staff need to be prepared to actively support nurses making applications for funding and seeking resources – the latter including not just money, but time. Committed managers will find that releasing staff for study and research, however difficult this might seem in the short term in a hard-pressed service, will be more than rewarded in the long term by the greater energy, motivation and skill of those staff.

The above points have proved helpful to us in developing research awareness in the NDU. One final point is also worth considering: nurses are notorious for not valuing what they do, and much valuable research is lost because no-one is able to read it. The staff's research reports are kept in the NDU library, and summaries can be discussed at meetings or circulated to wards. Letters of appreciation for research projects reinforce researchers' morale and motivation. However small a project, it always provides difficulties which deserve recognition when they are overcome and good work is produced. On a wider scale, the project can be prepared for publication, and many journals will give advice on this. It is a real pleasure for researchers to see their work in print and to know that it has reached a wider audience than their immediate colleagues.

The effects

If research awareness and activity are encouraged, the question has to be asked – is it worth it? The value of nursing research is that it directly benefits both patients and staff. Staff who feel they are learning, trying out new things and improving practice feel better about themselves and

---

- **Uniforms** – trials of going out of uniform were conducted. Some areas remained out of uniform as a result of patient response.

- **Sharing mealtimes** to produce a more therapeutic environment – staff on rehabilitation wards carried out a trial of sharing mealtimes which has now been implemented.

- **Pet therapy** – a research project was completed in the light of earlier evidence of the benefits of pet therapy. A dog is now resident on one ward.

- **Quality circles** – these have been set up and are used as forums to produce change. For example, the night staff formed their own quality circle and examined various problems which affected them. This led to re-examining and changing the way that deceased are removed from the ward.

- **Primary nursing** – the staff have implemented primary nursing throughout the unit, and conducted various surveys to examine patients' and other responses.

- **Self-medication** – evidence of poor compliance with drugs by elderly people after discharge led to designing, implementing and evaluating a patient self-medication programme.

Table 1. Application of research.

more motivated at work, thus contributing to an improved staff morale (with consequent reduction in the costs of high sickness or leaving rates). It cannot be a coincidence that the NDU, with its aroused spirit of enquiry, has a waiting list of staff, while sickness and leaving rates are well below the national average (less than 1 per cent, compared with 18 per cent). Several projects completed in the unit also testify to a further feedback – that 'finding out' stimulates innovation, which in turn stimulates further 'finding out' (Table 1).

Encouraging staff to enquire, innovate and see research as a normal part of nursing practice can change and improve it in many ways. Nursing research achieves its true value in this way, not as an esoteric notion, but a tool to improve the lives of patients and nurses.

References

Benner, P. (1984) From Novice to Expert. Addison Wesley, London

Bergman, R. (1986) Escaping from the ivory tower. *Nursing Times*, **82**, 41, 58-60.

Bond, S. (1978) Dilemmas in Clinical Research. Unpublished paper presented at Northern Regional Health Authority Seminar on Developments in Nursing.

Jacox, A. (1974) Nursing research and the clinician. *Nursing Outlook*, **22**, 82, 16-18.

Luker, K. (1986) Who's for research? *Nursing Times*, **82**, 52, 55-56.

Norton, D., McLaren, R. Exton-Smith, A.N. (1962) An Investigation of Geriatric Nursing Problems in Hospital. National Corporation for the Care of Old People, London.

Purdy, E. and Wright, S.G. (1988) If I were a rich nurse. *Nursing Times*, **84**, 41, 36-38.

Treece, E.W. and Treece, J.W. (1977) Elements of Research in Nursing. Mosby, St Louis.

Wright, S.G. (1986) Building and Using a Model of Nursing. Edward Arnold, London.

3

In service to meet your research needs: the Index of Nursing Research Information Service

Debra Unsworth, BA
Nursing Research Librarian, Department of Health

All nurses involved in research rely on library facilities to undertake literature searches and reviews at whatever level and in whatever field they work. Specialist libraries and organisations make their information available through various means: they may be open to the public, visited by appointment, provide an information service, or make their information available on databases to which many libraries and institutions have access. The Department of Health (DoH) provides an information service to nurses, midwives and health visitors, which is located in the library (serving both Health and Social Security Departments) and is based on the information contained in the Index of Nursing Research (INR). In this context the term 'nursing' also includes midwifery and health visiting.

What is the Index of Nursing Research?

The INR provides an information service to the Nursing Division at the DoH and to the nursing professions, and its main aim is to promote the use of research information in nursing. Begun in 1975 in card form, since 1983 it has been incorporated into DHSS-Data, the online database of the DHSS Library Services, and is managed by the Nursing Research Librarian in the DoH Library.

The INR contains details of UK nursing research. The criteria for inclusion is that the work should be about nurses/nursing or have been done by a nurse, and have implications for the profession, nurse education, practice, organisation and/or management. Research by nurses or where a nurse is a member of a research team is also included. A high proportion of research undertaken by nurses is never published in conventional sources and the INR contains details of this, as well as research currently in progress. While by no means comprehensive, the index aims to list details of research completed and in progress in the UK - a 'grey' area of literature, not normally documented.

Information for inclusion in the INR is gathered by two main methods.

1. The librarian reviews current literature in nursing and related subject areas. Details of books, reports and journal articles are added to the database, and each record contains full bibliographic details (ie, author, title, date, publisher, source) plus keywords or 'index terms' which indicate the subject(s) of the work. Most records also contain a descriptive abstract which summarises the work's content.

2. Details of unpublished completed research and of research in-progress are collected by means of an annual mailing of datasheets to all institutions involved in nursing studies. Researchers submit details of their work on these, along with an abstract for inclusion in the INR.

Who uses the information?

Staff in the DoH Nursing Division rely on the INR to keep them up-to-date with developments in nursing research. Regular bibliographies are produced on topics of current interest, and ad-hoc bibliographies on many different subjects are provided on request. Nursing officers are interested to know what research has been done in a particular subject area and also what is currently being undertaken, not only from the view of professional awareness, but also because they need to feed nursing knowledge and information into health policy discussions. It is, therefore essential that the DoH is made aware what research has been done and is being done in any subject area.

Nurses at all levels use the INR for information, from undergraduate to postdoctoral students, practising nurses to nurse teachers, managers and professional advisers. Many use it to carry out literature searches on a specific subject, or simply to locate details of a particular piece of work, while those embarking on a research project find it useful to see what has previously been done on that subject.

Information on the INR is available through several means. The library database is available online through the database supplier DataStar. Many librarians and institutions have access to online databases for searching - some familiar ones are Medline, Nursing and Allied Health Literature, and DHSS-Data.

The information contained in DHSS-Data, which includes the INR, can be searched in various ways:

• for information on a specific subject, using a keyword search;

• for publications by a certain author/researcher;

• by title, to locate details of a particular work;

• using a 'free text' search which will look for a chosen word in any area of the records, including the abstract.

Librarians usually assist enquirers in conducting these searches, and the combination of the enquirer's subject knowledge and the librarian's professional skills in information retrieval gives the best results in terms of both completeness and relevant coverage.

Prospective enquirers are asked initially to approach their own library for information. Some, however, may not have access to online services and others may have specific queries which cannot be satisfied by initial online searches. The INR is maintained by the Nursing Research Librarian who provides an information and enquiry service to the DoH and to the nursing profession. The librarian can undertake literature searches and produce bibliographies on request and can also answer enquiries regarding details of a particular publication - for example, which issue of a journal a particular article appeared in, and who was the author. This service is provided free of charge and enquiries can be made by telephone or in writing. Personal visits to the INR to undertake searches with the help of the librarian can be arranged for bona fide enquiries and researchers, usually at postgraduate level. Occasional visits are also arranged for formal groups, such as nursing librarians. The INR does not maintain a collection of documents cited and cannot supply loans or photocopies, and these should be obtained by approaching your local library.

Nursing Research Abstracts

Information is continually added to the INR. Recent additions are published quarterly in the journal *Nursing Research Abstracts*, which is the hard copy of the holdings of the index. It contains entries for each record (ie, author/researcher, title, date, publisher, source and abstract), and gives details of the duration, funding, supervisor and institution for research projects where appropriate. Each issue contains author and keyword indexes, with annual cumulated indexes in the final issue of each year.

The journal has been in publication since 1978 and a retrospective volume covering the years 1968-1976 has also been published. It is possible, therefore, to undertake a manual search of current and historical literature using the journal. *Nursing Research Abstracts* is available on subscription from: DSS Leaflets Unit, PO Box 21, Stanmore, Middlesex, HA7 1AY costing £14.00 per annum or £3.50 per single issue for 1992. Details of earlier volumes are available from the librarian.

Researchers are asked to use datasheets produced by the librarian for the submission of details of their work. These are mailed annually to all institutions involved in nursing studies, and are also available in nursing libraries. A copy of the datasheet is also published in the back of each issue of *Nursing Research Abstracts* and can be photocopied, or copies sent on request by the librarian. Any nurse involved in a research study, however local or small-scale, is encouraged to submit details for entry in the INR and published in the online database and the journal.

Other information held on DHSS-Data

After the division of the DHSS into the Department of Health and the Department of Social Security in 1988, the library service continued to provide for the information needs of both Departments. The database is effectively the catalogue of the library, and since 1983 all additions to library stock have been included in the database. Subjects covered include all the social policy issues of concern to the two Departments, such as social policy in general, health and personal social services, social problems, social security and health service administration. The database also extends into less obvious areas, such as safety of medicines, psychology, sociology, public health, education, economics, law and technology, and consists of records of books, pamphlets, reports, journal articles, circulars and other official publications.

The index is contained within this database, to which the Nursing Research Librarian adds entries. Other subject specialists add entries on a range of topics, such as social services and occupational diseases. As well as entering details of nursing research, the librarian also includes entries for articles 'of interest' - those which deal with nursing but are not research, for example nurse education, nursing management, and primary nursing. These entries are given a short description instead of an abstract, and are not included in *Nursing Research Abstracts*, but in bibliographies produced by undertaking literature searches.

A number of specialist organisations provide information services or are open to the public. The Library of the DHSS is included as it is separate from the INR, and it is not open to the public. Always ring the librarian before visiting any specialist library.

Enquiry address
Debra Unsworth,Nursing Research Librarian, Room 105, Hannibal House, Elephant and
    Castle, London SE1 6TE. Tel: 071-972 2551 (direct line).

Information Services
DHSS Main Library, Room 75, Hannibal House, Elephant and Castle, London SE1 6TE. Tel:
    071-972 2609.
ENB Resource and Careers Services, Woodseats House, 764A Chesterfield Road, Sheffield
    S8 OSE. Tel: 0742-551064/65.
Health Visitors Association Library, 50 Southwark Street, London SE1 1UN. Tel: 071-378
    7255.
King's Find Institute Library, 126 Albert Street, London NW1 7NF. Tel: 071-267 6111.
MIDIRS Midwives Information, and Resource Service, Institute of Child Health, Royal
    Hospital for Sick Children, Bristol. Tel: 0272-251791.
Royal College of Midwives Library, 11 Queen Anne Street, London W1N. Tel: 071-580 6523.
Royal College of Nursing Library, 20 Cavendish Square, London W1M OAB. Tel: 071-409
    3333.

4

What are the legal implications of extended nursing roles?

Susannah Derrick, RGN
Senior Staff Nurse, Intensive Care Unit, St Mary's Hospital, London

Recent advances in medical technology have led to constant demands being made on both the knowledge and skills of nurses. This is highlighted in 'high tech' areas of nursing such as intensive care and renal units.

Nurses have a complex role in these areas. It requires not only competence in providing basic care, support and education to patient and family, but also a high level of theoretical knowledge and practical skill to understand and contribute to treatment. The role of the specialist nurse encompasses many procedures which have previously been considered within the medical domain, such as venepuncture and emergency defibrillation.

The legal issues

I would suggest that nurses working in these areas extend their role willingly. However, although they are trained for practice, they may not fully appreciate the legal issues surrounding it.

A research case study carried out using RGNs in an intensive/cardiac care unit as a sample population supports this suggestion and has provided factual information on the degree of knowledge and appreciation of the legal implications of the extended role held by this specific population (Derrick, 1987). The study also presents a reasonable overview of the RGN population as a whole, as it demonstrated the broad background and wide range of hospitals and health authorities in which the sample had previously worked.

What is an extended role?

An extended role can be described as one which is not included in basic training. They have developed for various reasons; the most obvious is development of new technology and treatment. However, economic factors can not be overlooked – nursing manpower may be cheaper than medical.

In the light of the change and extension of the nursing role the DHSS, medical and nursing professional organisations attempted to clarify the situation. The DHSS issued a circular in 1977 explaining the legal implications and training requirements (DHSS, 1977), and this was supported by a publication from the RCN and BMA (1978). These documents set out some clear guidelines for the management of extended roles for nurses, and are summarised by Rowden (1987.)

The guidelines stress the need for joint discussions, mutual trust and respect between professions and state that extension of role must be in the interests of patient care. An opinion often aired is that on a busy ward where staffing levels are low, skilled nurses should not be using precious time administering intravenous drugs.

The circular also states that 'Work which has hitherto been carried out by doctors ought therefore to be delegated to nurses only when:-
a) The nurse has been specifically and adequately trained for the performance of the new task and she agrees to undertake it;
b) this training has been recognised as satisfactory by the employing Authority;
c) the new task has been recognised by the professions and by the employing Authority as a task which may be properly delegated to a nurse;
d) the delegating doctor has been assured of the competence of the individual nurse concerned.'

It also states:- 'In order to be successful and safe such delegation should be in the context of a clearly defined policy . . . and it should be made known in writing to all staff who are likely to be involved.

These points should be considered very carefully and with particular reference to the Department of Health document, the Ministerial Group on Junior Doctors' hours (Department of Health, 1990). Reduction in the hours worked by junior doctors is a subject which rightly gains a great deal of support, and this document presents recommendations to achieve this. However, it is interesting to note one such recommendation in the document. II. Recommendations for Action No. 6 "the UK Health Departments should issue guidelines to health authorities and boards as follows" (d) "in consultation with the UKCC for Nursing, Midwifery and Health Visiting and the Royal Colleges of Nursing and Midwifery, on the need for reviews of local policies concerning activities which appropriately qualified nurses and midwives may reasonably undertake further to improve the quality of patient care. Where such local policies do not exist, arrangements should be made for them to be instituted."

Could this imply transfer of 'activities' or practices from a medical to a nursing responsibility?

It is important that nursing management and individual nurses are flexible to change and are able to respond to the needs of their patients in the light of increasing knowledge and advancing technology. But it is essential they understand the implications of the changes in practice.

Certification

A certificate of competence is issued for some extended role procedures. Unlike the administration of intravenous drugs (Breckenbridge, 1976) many procedures do not require certification in some authorities but do in others. Certification is not a legal requirement, but it does serve a worthwhile purpose.

Each individual nurse has a choice whether or not to extend her or his role. It can be generally accepted that any nurse choosing to work in specialised fields expects, and is willing to undertake an extended role, and with adequate training should be fully aware of the medical and nursing implications of her or his actions. Comment is rarely made, however, about the importance and need for training to enable nurses to appreciate the legal implications of their actions.

Law and the nurse

Accountability "Each registered nurse, midwife and health visitor is accountable for his or her practice" (UKCC, 1984). Accountability means being answerable for work, decisions about work and being professionally responsible for the standard of practice. Nurses are first and foremost legally responsible for each and every nursing action undertaken or omitted, and must practise in accordance with the same standard of care of a reasonably prudent nurse practising under the same or similar circumstances. *Primary liability* is held by the individual nurse for her or his own actions.

It is possible for nurses to be persuaded or pressurised into carrying out treatment or procedures – extending their role – either to be helpful, to save time or 'to keep the peace', particularly when wards are busy or staffing levels are low. In such instances both medical and nursing staff should have the consequences of the unauthorised practise brought to their attention. Protecting one another from primary liability is a duty everyone should adopt, and be thanked for, albeit as an afterthought.

Greater awareness of legal issues surrounding nursing and the extension of the nursing role has developed in recent years. The number of study days and articles published on this subject has undoubtedly increased the level of interest and understanding.

In March 1989 the UKCC for for Nursing, Midwifery and Health Visiting published an Advisory Document 'Exercising Accountability'. It is designed to offer a framework to assist nurses, midwives and health visitors to consider ethical aspects of professional practise and is available free to all on the UKCC's professional register (UKCC, 1989).

Negligence Negligence is divided into three main components (Rea, 1987):
• **The duty of care** The legal duty of care encompasses the professional, moral, ethical and sociological duties of care within which nursing operates. It is what the nurse is required to do under the terms of her

contract of employment. Deviation from this in any way is negligence.
- **The breach of the duty** This is the alleged wrongdoing.
- **The resultant damage** The damage to the patient must be the result of the breach of the duty of care.

The law relating to negligence principally seeks to identify conduct which does not reach an acceptable professional standard. If injury results from such conduct the possibility of an action for damages (compensation) arises. Liability to pay damages may be shouldered by the individual, covered by an insurance company or by membership of a professional organisation which offers legal liability insurance to its members.

Vicarious liability

In the DHSS circular (1977), and in law, it is made clear that any role extension *must* be approved officially by the employing authority. In the United Kingdom (Master-Servant Statutes) "the law takes the view that the master will accept responsibility for the actions of servants, where the servant is working in accordance with the policies agreed by master and servant" (Rowden, 1987). Within the NHS the employing authority is the master and the nurse the servant. It is normally accepted that the senior nurse will act on behalf of the authority.

The health authority will accept responsibility for the actions of nurses when they are working within policies agreed by both parties. It is suggested therefore that it may be good practice for nurses to be certificated for extended role procedures. In the extended role, a certificate not only facilitates education and the maintenance of a high standard of care but is proof of competence and of the authority's knowledge and agreement for the nurse to practise.

If the authority/employer is to accept legal liability for the action of the nurse/employee, it is necessary that the authority should know exactly the role being practised and agree to it. This is known as *vicarious liability* (sometimes called secondary liability). It is essential to confirm in writing any extension of role. It is too easy for confusion to arise where verbal agreements are concerned. How many times has a doctor been heard to say 'I will cover you'? Doctors are *not* permitted by their defence organisations to take responsibility for the actions of nurses. Documenting the extent and boundaries of an extended role may seem tedious and bureaucratic, but it is in the interests of practitioners and patients alike.

Ensuring knowledge

It is essential to ensure nurses have an appreciation and thorough understanding of the implications of the extension of the nursing role. With the ever increasing expectation that all nurses at all levels extend their role further, I would make the following recommendations:

- Individuals and management must be alerted to the need for more education.

- The teaching of the legal aspects of nursing should be incorporated into basic training and all nurses should be encouraged to question their own knowledge and safeguard their own practise.

- Incorporation of the legal implications in the criteria of certification for an extended role procedure would ensure awareness of the policy and requirements of the issuing health authority/employer.

- Attempts should be made to find time and finance to increase the number of study days, teaching sessions, workshops and discussions available.

Each registered nurse, midwife and health visitor is accountable for his or her practice. It is every nurse's individual responsibility to understand the legal implications underlying that accountability. Do you?

References

Department of Health (1990) *Heads of Agreement. Ministerial Group on Junior Doctor's Hours.* December. DoH, London.

Derrick, S.M. (1987) Unpublished case study on nurses' appreciation of the legal implications of taking an extended role.

DHSS (1977) *The extending role of the clinical nurse – legal implications and training requirements.* DHSS, London.

RCN/BMA (1978) *The Duties and Position of the Nurse.* RCN, London.

Rea, K. (1987) Negligence. *Nursing,* **3,** 576.

UKCC (1984) *Code of Professional Conduct for the Nurse, Midwife and Health Visitor.* UKCC, London.

UKCC (1989) *Exercising Accountability.* UKCC, London.

5

A structured way to fulfil ambition: how to make rational career plans

Kevin Teasdale, MA, Cert Ed, RMN
Director of In-Service Training, Pilgrim Hospital, Boston

How many of us can honestly say our career has followed a rational plan which helps us to fulfil our ambitions within the limits of our abilities and circumstances? This article offers some ideas on how nurses can improve their approach to making career choices.

For most of us, career choices are very much a matter of chance. We happen to be reading a nursing journal and see a job that appeals, or meet a tutor, manager or specialist nurse we like and admire, and think "I'd like to have a job like that". Yet the choices and plans we make in such a casual fashion may affect our whole lives, and those of our family and friends. Part of the problem is that our culture gives us unconscious taboos which stop us from making rational career choices, and particularly hinder us from planning for the longer term. One example is the taboo that says, 'Don't think about the future, it's unlucky', another is the little voice that says, 'If I make plans, I'll only end up disappointed'.

Yet what happens if we think about the taboos from a different perspective? Nurses sometimes speak in terms of patient's 'career paths' when in hospital, and work in partnership with them to assess their needs and problems, plan for the future, set goals as milestones along the way, and help evaluate progress towards those goals. We would think it ridiculous if a nurse said, 'It's unlucky to make a nursing care plan', or 'You'll only be disappointed if you set long-term goals'. The taboos have no force when it comes to planning for other people, so why should we let them stop us planning for ourselves?

A rational model

Most people assume all that is required to make rational career choices is to obtain as much information as possible about jobs and career pathways. While information is certainly important, a genuinely rational approach to planning requires attention to four key stages:

Self-awareness Becoming aware of personal wants and values, and also of personal abilities and limitations.

Decision-making   Making a realistic match between self and the opportunities available.

Opportunity awareness   Being able to assess the current range of opportunities and understand the pressures of the job market.

Dealing with stress   Choices are seldom easy: people usually both gain *and* lose something from any change. It is necessary to plan ways of coping with the stresses of transition, and to recognise that the changes may also tax the coping abilities of family and friends.

This model (Figure 1) emphasises the fact that the search for career choices begins within ourselves. It also suggests we need to involve others in our plans, and think beyond the successful appointment.

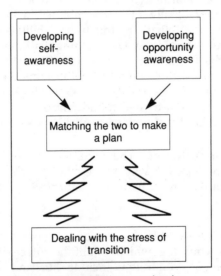

Figure 1. The rational career planning
model (based on Malkin, unpublished).

Developing self-awareness

The challenge here is to answer the following questions, remembering that the answers may change over time. Each question is followed by an exercise designed to help you explore possible answers.

Activity 1: needs and wants   Write down what made you enter nursing in the first place. What were the rewards you hoped for, and the needs within you which you believed a nursing career would satisfy? Then write down the factors keeping you in nursing now. How do the two lists compare? Can you see from them what it is you are really looking for in working as a nurse, and set the factors in priority order?

What do I value in a job?   This involves considering the extent to which work is a means to end (eg, financial success) or an end in itself, and a means of achieving Maslow's idea of self-actualisation.

Activity 2: plus, minus and interesting (de Bono, 1976)   To try to form an objective picture of your own capabilities. Time yourself for 15 minutes, and give five minutes to listing all the 'plus' points you can think of about yourself: they may be aspects of your personality, qualifications or types of experience you have had - write down anything you can think of. Then give five minutes to the 'minus' points about yourself: what do you know about your personality that will limit the type of job in which you could be successful or happy? What are the limits to your qualifications - are they signs of permanent limits to your academic ability or of lack of motivation or concentration? What does your record of work experience so far tell you about areas where you have not been successful or happy? Finally, give five minutes to thinking of what is interesting about you. What are the traits, abilities and experiences which make you different? Jot down anything that comes to mind.

At the end of the 15 minutes, have a cup of tea, then come back and work out what your lists tell you about your capabilities and interests in relation to the types of job you could do, and in which you could be happy. Show the lists to a trusted friend who knows you - or even ask them to make a similar list showing an outsider's view of you.

What are my capabilities?   This involves considering strengths and weaknesses in an objective way by reviewing past experiences, and making sense of them in terms of the information they convey about capability.

Activity 3: outcomes   Make a list of the people and the material circumstances in your life which might be affected by your career choices. For example, you might include husband/wife, boyfriend/ girlfriend, children, parents, salary, house and hobbies. Complete this sentence for each item, 'If I make a career choice, the outcome I want it to have on my (item) is ... '. When you have completed the sentences, put them into priority order running 'most important to me' through to 'least important to me'. Try to be honest with yourself at this stage - the list is for your personal planning and you do not have to show anyone else.

Are limitations imposed by circumstances?   This involves considering personal circumstances such as relationships, geography, finance and disability. To what extent do these factors limit your career choices? Are they permanent or temporary? Are you prepared to make any compromises?

Activity 4: the snake (Priestley *et al*, 1978)   Draw a snake like that in Figure 2; at each twist mark a date in the future, and write by it what you would like to be doing in terms of your career. Many people find this extremely difficult, almost thinking of it as wishing away their lives. It may help if you remember you are not committing yourself to anything by doing this exercise, merely trying to visualise possible future choices and keep the pathways open for as long as possible. If you really want to see if you have overcome the taboo, try writing your age against each year you have marked.

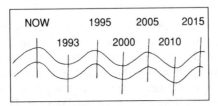

Figure 2. Snake used to plot long-term objectives.

Can I break the taboo over planning for the future? This involves taking what you have discovered about yourself in activities 1-3, and applying the insights not only to your current career choices, but also to those you will have to make in future. This is important, because choices made now can open or close future avenues.

Opportunity awareness

We all tend to make career choices from an unnecessarily narrow range of options. Sometimes it pays to sit back and think of all the possibilities, inside the health service and out. With longer term planning, it is important to build profiles of posts and take into account experiences and qualifications required.

Activity 5: create a career portfolio As a way of becoming aware of a broad range of opportunities, collect articles from the nursing press about different career options. *Professional Nurse* ran a complete series of Career Development articles (Gardner, 1988-89) which could form the basis of a portfolio. Look at job advertisements, as these can help you understand the way supply and demand factors operate in the health service and beyond. Find out which specialties are always being advertised, and which ones rarely become vacant. Which health authorities are repeatedly advertising, and which are not? You may wish to write away for details, even if you are unlikely to follow up the particular posts advertised. The background information accompanying an application form can be particularly informative about the post, and attention should be paid to the qualifications and experience being sought. Your portfolio will need regular updating, but this responsibility could be shared among several people to create a shared resource.

Post profiles   This is a description of the content of a particular job, and an analysis of the kinds of qualification and experience required. It is valuable in short-term planning, when you know a particular post is going to be advertised, and also for longer term career planning, to make sure you build your experience and qualifications along the right lines.

Profiling involves in-depth discussion with people doing jobs which might interest you. Find out from them what they actually do; it may be possible for you to shadow them for a day or two to see for yourself. Find out about the pattern of their career: do not simply ask about qualifications, it is equally important to discover the kind of experience needed to promote eligibility for a particular post. Do not fall into the trap of considering only one type of post. Try profiling one which seems quite uninviting - this will help broaden your awareness, and may give you some further insight into yourself. Do not hesitate to go to the top! If you hope to be a general manager in 10 years, go and talk to your own general manager now. Most will be flattered and impressed by someone who is interested in what they do, and assessing it in a systematic way.

Activity 6 - 5WH (Priestley *et al*, 1978)   This idea can be used when conducting interviews of profiles; 5WH is a simple checklist of questions - Who, What, When, Where, Why and How. Use it to develop your interview questions to ensure you build a full profile for a post. For example, if you were interviewing a theatre sister, you should ask:

- **Who** influenced her decision to work in theatres?
- **What** qualifications and training does she have? What experience did she have before becoming a theatre nurse? What does she think of theatre nursing as a career choice now?
- **When** did she attain her qualifications?
- **Where** has she worked? Did she have to move hospitals to get promotion, or might it be possible to progress in one hospital?
- **Why** did she come into theatre nursing, and why does she stay?
- **How** would she recommend you find out if theatre nursing is for you, and if it is, gain entry to the specialty?

It is not enough to develop self-awareness and a realistic under-standing of the opportunities available to you, as there still remains the hard task of matching the two. If it is any consolation, remember it is probably impossible to stand still in today's health service. If you do not make choices, they will probably be made for you. At the decision-making stage, most people will probably benefit from an interview with a trained career counsellor, but if this option is not available in your district, the following activities may help to clarify matters.

Activity 7: back to the future Look back to the snake in activity 4, and draw another, or extend the existing one, going **backwards in time**. At each turn, place a date and a description of a career choice point. Go back to school days to identify the earliest choices. For each point, complete the following sentences:
'I made this choice because ...' and 'The outcome was ... '

Reviewing the whole pattern, what does it tell you about yourself as a decision-maker? Have you improved over time, or are you still making the same old mistakes? Try to diagnose your own strengths and weaknesses in making career choices. Do you over- or under-estimate you capabilities? Are you cautious or daring? Are you good at profiling posts, or do jobs tend to turn out nothing like you imagined?

Activity 8: you win some, you lose some When considering a particular career choice, go back to activity 3, where desired outcomes were looked at in general terms. If you choose one particular career option, how will it affect each outcome on your list? Will the effect be positive (+), negative (-), or uncertain/neutral (?). It would be unusual to have a complete line of positives, but you will certainly be looking for them against the highest priority items. What about the negatives - can you compromise on any? Are you prepared to live with your decision and its negative as well as positive outcomes?

Dealing with stress
Maslow (1973) suggested that tension exists between safety and growth. This applies particularly to career choices. There will be safe, obvious choices which will not challenge your abilities to any great extent, but will guarantee financial rewards, job security or valued leisure time. Against this, growth choices will be highly demanding and potentially fulfilling - but are frequently risky and may disrupt your personal life. A growth choice for one partner in a marriage can also mean an enforced safety choice for another. Stress can arise from either choice: 'rustout' is the risk from too little stimulus, 'burnout' from excessive demands.

If you have made a career decision, ensure you are aware of its effects on others and for yourself, and identify and use any sources of support either within your family or outside. Keep a check on your lifestyle, as by maintaining good physical health you can place a buffer between yourself and the knocks and bruises of the outside world. Keep in touch with your values, and be aware that they may change over time. Expect stress in transition, notice its effects, and act early to counter or control it.

Activity 9: the mourning cycle   It may help to think of the transition period as one which will involve you and those around you in mourning for the inevitable losses involved in making any major career choice. Everyone involved in a major life transition will go through a mourning process, similar to that in a bereavement; it may be regarded as nature's repair cycle (Southgate, 1989). Figure 3 will probably be most relevant if you are trying to help someone close to you adapt to a change in their life brought about by a choice *you* have made. Work out which point in the cycle the person has reached, and try to find ways of making available the appropriate forms of helping suggested in the table.

Career planning can help you decide exactly what you want from nursing. By assessing your current and potential career opportunities, an extended range of options can be considered, and by relating these to your needs and capabilities, you can devise a rational career plan.

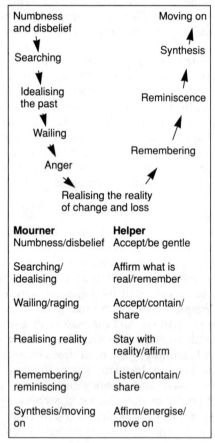

Figure 3. The mourning cycle (based on Southgate, 1989).

References

de Bono, E. (1976) Teaching Thinking. Maurice Temple Smith, London.

Gardner, R. (1988/89) Career Development Plus. (A series of articles published monthly in *Professional Nurse* from October 1988-September 1989).

Maslow, A. (1973) The Farther Reaches of Human Nature. Penguin, Harmondsworth.

Priestley, P. *et al* (1978) Social Skills and Personal Problem Solving. Tavistock, London.

Southgate, J. (1989) On becoming an advocate. *Journal of the Institute for Self Analysis*, **13**, 1, 4-10.

Acknowledgment

Sincere thanks to John Malkin, Principal Lecturer in Careers Guidance at Nottingham Polytechnic, whose basic course on how to offer vocational guidance inspired this article.

6

Applying for a job or course

Jennifer Booth, SRN, SCM, RNT, DipEd, DMS
Was, at the time of writing, Divisional Educational Manager, Bloomsbury College of Nurse Education, London

Applying for a new job or course may be one of the most important activities anyone undertakes during their career. If the steps in this chapter are followed, although it cannot guarantee the application will always be successful, it should ensure you present yourself well on paper and increase your chance of being shortlisted.

Action checklist

Step 1. Ask yourself why you want to change your job or take a course?

Step 2. What jobs/courses are available and where?

- Internal vacancy lists.
- Advertisements in professional journals.
- If you are moving to a new geographical location, a telephone enquiry to the personnel department of a hospital in the area may be helpful.
- Information from the National Boards regarding their approved courses in specialist nursing.

Step 3. Read advertisements and information carefully.

- What does it actually say?
- What experience does the job/course require?
- Is it really what you are looking for?

Step 4. Follow instructions.

Write or telephone for information.
Ask for an informal visit if it is appropriate.
Remember, this is the first contact with your potential employer, so it is important to make a good impression.
When writing:
- print your address;
- state the job or course in which you are interested at the top of the letter;
- give brief information about yourself;

- print your full name and title under your signature.

Keep a copy of this letter and note how soon you receive a reply. The reply should be personalised and may include:
- application form;
- job description/job profile/course details;
- information about the hospital or unit.

The more senior the post, the more detailed will be the information about the hospital unit.

Step 5. Complete the application form.

Photocopy the application form and read all the information carefully, then use the copy to lay out your particulars. Presentation, succinctness and clarity are important. Complete all sections – and sell yourself! Remember if you don't say what your experience and expertise is, the new employer will not know, so may not short list you. As you become more senior and your experience increases it may be more appropriate to attach a curriculum vitae (CV) – but still complete the main part of the form with name, address and other necessary information.

An informal visit
You may wish to go for an informal visit before completing the application form. Remember you will be 'on view' just as much as the people you are visiting.

As a result of the visit you may decide not to proceed, thus saving yourself and the hospital time and money.

Courses
Read the National Board course curriculum. Talk to people doing the course you are interested in, or who have completed it. Write to the referees whose names you are going to use – it is courtesy and prepares them, so that if they are going to be away, arrangements can be made to provide the reference.

Keep a copy of all the papers you return and make sure they arrive before the closing date. Send them first class or recorded delivery.

Short listing
When all the applications have been received, members of the interview panel will shortlist against set criteria for the post or course. These criteria may include academic factors, work experience, and professional qualifications.

The date and times of interview will be notified to candidates. If you have not heard within two weeks of the closing date, check your application was received. Always confirm that you will or will not be attending the interview – there is always someone else who may be able to take your place, particularly for courses, where these are limited.

References will be taken up and health questionnaires may be called for prior to the interview.

Step 6. Prepare for the interview.

Make sure you are up-to-date on:
- professional issues;
- recent papers from the UKCC, National Boards;
- trends in nursing ie, primary nursing, models in nursing;
- trends in nurse education and how they may affect the students in the wards;
- political issues affecting nursing and the provision of care.

Re-read the job description and ask the following questions:

Why are you applying for this post/course and how do you intend to use the experience?

What aspects of the post can you do well and what areas will you need help and the chance to develop?

If this is promotion – how will your role and responsibilities change?

What are your long term career plans?

What do you have to offer in expertise, experience, research and other skills?

If you have not had an interview for some time, ask someone to put you through a 'mock' interview or attend a course on interview skills. Find out as much as possible about the hospital/course and the interviewers' special interests.

Prepare your question list. This may be short if you have been for a visit beforehand.

Plan for the day

Always allow plenty of travelling time, in case of unexpected delays. How would you get there if the car broke down? Plan what you are going to wear. Wear clothes that are smart, comfortable and suitable for the weather, but also remember hospitals are usually very warm.

Collect all the documents you need to take, these will include evidence of your professional, academic and other qualifications or experience.

Finally, try to get a good night's sleep and have something to eat before you go to the interview.

Good luck!

Bibliography

Davey, D.M. and McDonnell, P. (1980) How to be Interviewed. British Institute of Management, London.

Higham, M. (1983) Coping With Interviews. New Opportunity Press, London.

Creamer, M. (1984) How to be interviewed. Modus Publications Ltd., Ampthill, Bedfordshire.

7

Will the minumum become an optimum? PREPP: mandatory study leave for nurses

Ann Shuttleworth, BA
Editor, Professional Nurse

You could be forgiven for heaving a big sigh at the prospect of yet more change in the nursing professions when the document PREPP and You (UKCC, 1991) landed on your doormat. Sent to all practitioners registered with the Council, it solicits your opinions about the recommendations made in Post Registration Education and Practice Project (PREPP: UKCC, 1990). The implications are far reaching and will affect how every practitioner keeps up-to-date, so it is important that people let Council know their opinions. This chapter will raise some of the many issues you will need to think about when making your response, starting with the recommendation that all practitioners complete a minimum of five days study leave every three years.

Ensuring effective practice
There are a number of reasons why you may welcome this recommendation in principle. Most fundamentally, you may think it is essential that nurses keep up-to-date if they are to practise effectively and efficiently and offer their patients the standard of care to which they are entitled. In the past, it has been perfectly possible (at least in theory) for nurses to sail through 40 year careers without undertaking any professional development or updating. While it is unlikely that there have been many instances of this, imagine the effect on patient care if such a nurse was involved in dressing wounds, or in any other field which has developed radically in the past few years? It doesn't bear thinking about, does it?

However, most nurses already see it as essential that they keep up-to-date with developments in their profession in general and their specialty in particular - the wellbeing and even the lives of their patients are at stake. Is this not enough? Do the small proportion of nurses who do not wish to update cause unnecessary stress or suffering to patients as a result? Is that enough to justify a mandatory requirement to update being imposed on everyone? What effect does it have on people when things are made compulsory? Those nurses who do not wish to update may resent being forced to do so. How well can they be expected to learn under those circumstances? And what about nurses who did update before it became mandatory? Will it they resent being 'told', and will this affect the quality of their learning?

What about the managers?

Mandatory updating may, on the other hand, equally be directed at those responsible for sanctioning nurses' attendance at continuing professional education events. Many nurses who have been keen to update themselves have found it far from easy. Delegates to *Professional Nurse* National Study Days, to take one example with which I am familiar, testify to the fact that nurses all too often have to pay their own fees and travel for courses and study days *and* take the day as holiday! While these cases are by no means a majority, they do constitute a significant number of nurses, whose managers appear to to regard clinical updating as a low priority for their staff. Perhaps the introduction of mandatory updating will make these managers more amenable to the idea of supporting their nurses in maintaining and improving their competence.

Why five days?

If nurses are to be compelled to update, should we be talking in terms of days - why not hours? And why specifically five? Surely, as individuals, working in a wide range of fields, some will need more time than others to do the same amount of updating. What about those who need more than five days to maintain their practice at an acceptable standard, either because they work in a rapidly developing specialty or because they simply lose their 'edge' more quickly than others? Should they still be allowed to re-register, simply because they have completed a prescribed number of days? The problem with setting fixed numbers is that, while it makes for ease of administration, it does not take individuality into account. Also, with money as tight as it is currently, could the minimum become the optimum, the prescribed amount of updating employers require their nurses to undertake? Will nurses wishing to undertake more than the five days in three years find it difficult to obtain funds or time away from clinical practice? While it is currently unclear who will be responsible for funding these five days, if the bill has to be picked up by the health authorities, how keen will they be to add to their education costs for qualified staff by paying for extra days study leave? Will nurses too begin to see five days as the target beyond which they need not go?

A diverse enough range?

Since nursing is such a diverse profession, there will need to be a diverse range of updating opportunities to take account of individual, local and specialist needs. Unless this is made clear in the final PREPP legislation, there is a danger that the continuing education opportunities available, rather than growing, will shrink. Would it not be an attractive, cost-effective option for health authorities, if they are expected to fund this, to simply run a standard five day course and compel all nurses to attend? Easy to administer and cheap to run, could it become virtually the only updating available to some nurses?

Whatever final form PREPP's legislation and recommendations take, it is bound to cause difficulties for someone, in terms of cost and administration. It is important, however, that this prospect does not lead to them taking the simplest possible form, because although this may improve the minority of nurses who do not currently take any interest in maintaining their competence, and the minority of employers who see continuing professional education as a low priority for their nurses, it could also have dire consequences for the rest of the profession. Education budgets are all too easy to cut - they don't make the same waves as special care baby units, and if they exceed a minimum standard laid down in law, all the easier to justify cutting them. Nurses are human, and humans are also notoriously adept at seeing the minimum requirement as their goal. Will the setting of a five day rule demotivate nurses who would previously have undertaken much more professional education, once they reach the magic number?

Until PREPP is fully implemented, we cannot answer the questions raised in this chapter. However, none could be described as going into the realms of fantasy. We must hope legislation will take account of such possibilities, and ensure, as far as is feasible, that implementation of PREPP contributes to development , not to stagnation. Perhaps extending individual performance review to cover all nurses, and tying PREPP into this system is a way ahead? It would certainly allow individual needs to be accounted for.

References
UKCC (1990) Post Registration Education and Practice Project, UKCC, London.
UKCC (1991) PREPP and You, UKCC, London.

8

Who pays for PREPP?

Ruth Paton, BA(Hons), RGN, DN Cert
District Nurse, Bath

The report of the Post-Registration Education and Practice Project's (PREPP; UKCC, 1991) aims are twofold: to meet the needs of patients and the health service and to maintain and develop existing standards of nurse education and practice. For the nursing profession as a whole, it heralds widespread change. Indeed, in the words of the chairman of the project, Professor Margaret Green: "The Council does not underestimate the scale and importance of the recommendations contained within this report and how critical they are to the professions and to the future."

The report highlighted nine major recommendations, devised to: "maintain and enhance standards in order to meet the needs of patients, clients and the health services" (UKCC, 1991). Briefly, these recommendations centre on the key issues of providing:
- support for newly qualified staff;
- a written record of maintenance and development of professional skills and knowledge;
- guidelines as to the minimum attendance at study days required to facilitate three yearly re-registration;
- specification for advanced practice;
- guidelines as to eligibility to practice.

For nursing to be regarded as a profession, it is vital that standards of practice are maintained and enhanced. It is also imperative that each practitioner has the implicit knowledge base which patients and clients consider essential for the provision of care. The PREPP proposals will enable nurses to present explicit evidence of their eligibility to practice; indeed, the introduction highlights: "The Council is confident that the final recommendations offer an exciting, workable and cost-effective framework for maintaining and enhancing standards in post-registration education and practice" (UKCC, 1991).

The PREPP document has been offered to the profession for debate, and the nine major recommendations approved for implementation. One central issue was not discussed in the document – that of funding for nurse education, and it is this issue which this article aims to discuss.

Funding

It is clear that post-basic nurse education is under considerable review. As we move into the business orientated health service, characterised by purchasers and providers, the future of nurse education is unclear within

this framework. Various options are available, and funding will come from either:
• the providers of care ie, the health trusts;
• nurses themselves, in the guise of self-funding;
• a combination of the two;
• from possible external sources such as drug companies.

No clear answers have yet emerged as to which of these are the favoured funding option. It is interesting, however, to speculate on the possible implications were one of these options to be adopted.

Funding from the providers of care

If funding were to come from the providers (the health trusts and health authorities), in an effort to keep costs low and to compete with other areas, would this mean that the minimum of five days study in each three year period will become the maximum offered to nurses, and that courses longer than five days will be rendered redundant? If the employers determine that five days study in each three year period is a maximum, what place will there be for provision of courses requiring longer periods of study, such as degree courses, sponsoring for diploma and masters places and the continuing impetus to align nurse training with universities and other centres for higher education? The impetus to promote professional development and enhance nurse status is clearly gaining momentum, but if we allow the links developed with centres for higher education to wither, what effect will this have for the standard and quality of nurse development? Concern over funding is also raised due to the fact that PREPP is competing for finance against other educational changes, such as Project 2000; the projected increase in educational costs facilitated by the introduction of Project 2000 has been calculated by York University to be £140 million (based on 1982-83 prices). In view of this, where will additional finance be found for PREPP?

If employers do finance nurse education, what effect will this have on course provision? At present, it is not uncommon for each area to provide similar or duplicated courses to meet local nursing needs, but as the new health trusts will undoubtedly demand value for money, it can reasonably be assumed that this will cease. As a more cost-effective alternative, course provision may instead be rationalised with regional centres, thus streamlining educational provision. This will have considerable implications for course attendance: if, for example, only one centre provides a particular course which necessitates the participating nurse finding accommodation, who will pay for this? Furthermore as the 'demographic time bomb' increases its impact on nurse recruitment, how will this affect recruitment of mature personnel, who may already have domestic commitments, which preclude either residential courses or self-financing of education? The PREPP report indicates that: "...the professions are already targeting more mature entrants as part of their recruitment drive" (UKCC, 1991), adding that they will bring "...greater expectations of themselves and the organisation they work for". These hidden implications may serve only to dash such expectations and create a new wave of frustration and resentment.

On a positive note, however, if nurses adopt a business orientated approach, health trusts may well have to compete for increasingly scarce and valuable nursing expertise. Why, therefore, work for one health trust, which offers only the minimum period of study leave, when another may fund one for longer periods of study? Similarly, in terms of residential courses, nurses may well use demographic trends to their advantage. In an effort to recruit personnel, funding provision for attendance on courses at regional centres may become important parts of salary and renumeration packages. At present, no clear answer has emerged, but nurses themselves have the power to determine which outcome prevails.

Self-funding

If it is accepted that the financial implications for PREPP are considerable, does this mean we are moving into the area of nurses funding their own professional update? Sylvester (1990) claims: "...it is possible that part of the cost would be met by the employer and part met by the practitioner."

Precedents for this have already been established, the Open Learning Programme being one example. Aimed primarily at enrolled nurses who wish to convert to first level registration, it is also considered suitable for nurses returning to practice and "registered nurses who have had no time to devote to study since they qualified" (Robinson, 1990). Initially, this may seem an ideal way to satisfy recommendations five and six of PREPP pertaining to study leave and return to practice. The cost of the Open Learning Programme, however, is £975 per year, and it is only "hoped that health authorities will help to support students" (Robinson, 1990); for nurses, particularly those at D and E grades, this is not an inconsequential sum. Although most would agree that it is their professional responsibility to ensure their continuing development, will every nurse see that: "putting time and money into study which can move them forward in their careers and ultimately enable them to earn more money can be a good investment?" What will happen to those who cannot afford this? The cost of preparation for first level registration per NHS entrant was £13,090 in 1988 (Bosanquet, 1988). If we rely on staff supplementing their own post-basic education, then the recruit and retrain programme may be seriously affected by the PREPP proposals.

External sources

Drug companies are increasingly realising the influence nurses have in product choice, especially within the community setting. The advent of nurse prescribing, however limited initially, is within sight; the pharmaceutical companies are increasingly promoting their products to nurses, and regional district nurse exhibitions, lunches and lectures are now common. Taking this a step further, what better way of establishing brand awareness than to sponsor educational courses for nurses? As a profession nursing would have to question the ethics of such developments, but it is a scenario with which we may find ourselves dealing.

Professional comparisons

As nursing strives to become recognised as a profession, are we wrong to express concern regarding this new concept of self-funding for post-registration education? How do we answer critics who argue that as individuals nurses should invest in their own future? In an endeavour to answer this question, it is useful to compare the PREPP proposals with systems already in place in the other main professional groups. Having contacted the professional bodies for chartered accountants, solicitors and teachers, it appears that there is no hard and fast rule. The Institute for Chartered Accountants for England and Wales has developed obligatory requirements known as continual professional education (CPE), and to meet these objectives, the Institute recommends "an appropriate mix of structured and unstructured CPE". Meeting these requirements is the individual's own responsibility, but accountants employed by the major practising firms are subsidised by their employers to do this. Accountants in Scotland have voluntary guidelines for continuing education, which amount to a minimum of 100 hours of structured learning, but again, course enrolments come from firms, as opposed to individuals. In the case of solicitors, the Law Society indicates that although responsibility to comply with the society's regulations on updating lies with the individual, most employers fund courses to meet these individuals' training needs.

It is, however, interesting to discuss the position of teachers, perhaps the professional group with which nurses have been most closely identified. In the case of teachers employed in further and higher education, until recently they have had their in-service training paid for by their employing institution, but this situation is now under threat. At present, the situation varies between institutions and individual authorities.

It appears, therefore, with the exception of teachers in further and higher education, that although funding for post-basic education is discretionary, it is unusual for employees to be expected to finance their own education. Although it would not be advisable for nursing to adhere *carte blanche* to the practices of other professional bodies, we should not ignore their example when debating and reviewing the PREPP proposals.

The underlying principle of PREPP is that of maintaining and enhancing standards "in order to meet the needs of patients, clients and the health services" (UKCC, 1991). It has given us an ideal opportunity to enhance our profession by potentially aligning ourselves with institutions of higher education, particularly under the credit accumulation and transfer scheme (CATS). In a purchaser/provider arena, we must be cautious that we do not price ourselves and our skills out of the market. Conversely, it would be a sad indictment of the system, if the positive aspects of PREPP were to be sacrificed as a result of financial insufficiency. As a profession, these are issues we need to be highlighting as we continue to debate the PREPP proposals.

References
Bosanquet, N. (1988) What will it cost? *Nursing Times*, **84**, 31, 34.
Millar, B. (1991) Investing in the future. *Nursing Times*, **87**, 8, 29.
Robinson, K. (1990) Open learning. *Nursing Times*, **86**, 43, 27.
Sylvester, J. (1990) Taking the road ahead. *Nursing Standard*, **4**, 25, 16.
UKCC (1991) The Report of the Post-Registration Education and Practice Project, UKCC, London.

Looking After Yourself

9

Back pain: why bother?

Brenda L. Griffiths, RGN
Senior Nurse, Department of Community Medicine, Royal Free Hospital, London

What is back pain?

This straightforward question has a very unclear answer. A wide spectrum of presentation occurs, ranging from the debilitating and crippling to a vague discomfort. There is no doubt that one person's Radox bath and early night can be to someone else a week off work and a visit to the GP. It is not necessary to emphasise the humanitarian aspects of back pain with its implications for quality of life and patient suffering, but it is of interest to look closely at the problem generally. Broadly, back pain can be divided into four groups:

1. Primary This arises directly from the tissues of the spine; muscle, fascia, ligaments, periosteum, apophyseal joint capsules, adventia of blood vessels, dura and dural root sleeves. All are supplied with sensory nerves which respond to mechanical (and chemical) irritation. Primary back pain can therefore arise through fatigue, a result of trauma, unaccustomed activity, positional stress or local changes (eg, osteoarthritis). It is especially important to note that there is *no* nerve supply to the disc nucleus and cartilage on the vertebral body, therefore the weight-bearing tissues (discs and joints) can be injured without pain at the time of injury.

2. Secondary This arises when nerves have become so irritated — stretched or compressed — that there is interference in the blood and nerve supply. This results in typical persistent chronic backache.

3. Referred This is back pain arising from a structure other than the spine but which has a nerve supply from the same sequestal level, eg, backache arising from the uterus. This pathology must be excluded in every case of back symptoms.

4. Psychosomatic This is often the most difficult to diagnose and treat. Counselling after exclusion of an organic lesion is most important.

In most cases, a definitive diagnosis will never be made. Figure 1 shows that 60 per cent of patients will never know the exact nature of their back pain — it is therefore essential to consider the patient's individual perception of pain.

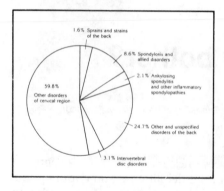

1.6% Sprains and strains
of the back

8.6% Spondylosis and
allied disorders

2.1% Ankylosing
spondylitis
and other inflammatory
spondylopathies

59.8%
Other disorders
of cervical region

24.7% Other and unspecified
disorders of the back

3.1% Intervertebral
disc disorders

Figure 1. Hospital discharges and deaths for back pain; analysis by diagnostic category — Britain 1982.

Source: Back pain: Office of Health Economics, (1985).

NHS cost of back pain

Why do we need to bother about this at all? Figure 2 shows the massive size of this problem, with over 22 million episodes of pain reported each year. This crude approximation shows that only a tiny proportion are actually seen in hospital. What is all this costing? In terms of the NHS, back pain at the primary health care level can be seen as follows:

Back pain accounts for 2.6 per cent of the total GP workload measured by consultation rates, generating an estimated expense of (2.6 per cent of total general practice expenditure)

= £25.7 million

On an assumption (crude estimate) that every consultation with the GP results in a prescription for four weeks' medication, the result is a cost of

= £31.9 million

In addition, a pharmacist's dispensing fee results in a drug bill of

= £38.9 million

Looking at hospital costs, Dixon (1980) reported that problems relating to the spine result in 25 per cent of all outpatients seen in orthopaedic clinics, and that 66 per cent of these are for back pain. Consultations in rheumatology, neurology and other outpatient departments are not known. It is therefore necessary to look at GP referral data for estimate of cost. Fifteen per cent of patients consulting their GP for back pain are referred by the doctor for a consultant opinion, resulting in 330,000 referrals to hospital per year at a cost of

= £25.3 million

A total of 65,572 discharges/deaths for back pain resulted from 783,423 hospital bed days at a cost of

= £58.8 million

However, industrial action by ancillary staff in the year of data collection led to a reduction of inpatient admissions for 1982 and bed days for back pain were 11.3 per cent down on the 1981 figure. A revised figure reveals a new cost of

= £66.2 million

In summary, the cost of back pain to the NHS can be shown as:

	£ (million)
General medical services	25.7
Pharmaceutical services	38.9
Outpatient consultations	25.3
Hospital inpatients	66.2
	£156.1

This sum is equal to 1.15 per cent of total NHS spending in 1982. Looking at this another way, £156.1m is equal to 20 per cent of the amount of money actually spent on hospital development in 1982-83, ie, 18 new hospitals. Another comparison is £156.1m could make possible a 20 per cent reduction in the overall size of hospital waiting lists. The cost of back pain to the NHS is highly significant when seen in these terms.

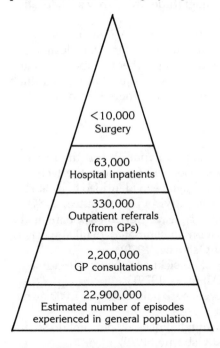

Figure 2. *Estimated impact of back pain on the health services over a 12-month period.*

Source: *Back pain: Office of Health Economics, (1985)*

Non-NHS cost of back pain

The DHSS indicates 622,800 episodes of *certificated* sickness absence due to back pain with an average duration of 14 days off. One in three of these episodes resulted in absence of 25 days or more.

In 1982-83 there were 33.3 million days of certificated incapacity due to back pain. This is a massive amount of lost working time and, indeed, it accounted for 9.2 per cent of all certificated absence. This is more loss than is attributable to coronary heart disease and bronchitis and *six times* the number of days lost due to industrial action.

The lost manufacturing potential is impossible to quantify but:

- £193m was paid in DHSS benefits in respect of certificated absence resulting from back pain.
- £8.6m was paid in industrial injury compensation (18.5 per cent of total) for accidents involving the spine.

In economic terms, then, there is unequivocal evidence that back pain is a major problem which should be tackled appropriately.

Factors associated with back pain

Many factors have been associated with the development of back pain: heavy physical work; lifting and forceful movements; frequent bending and twisting; static work postures; and repetitive work.

All these factors increase the spinal load and are often present at the same time in a given occupation and therefore a single vocational factor is difficult to establish. However, the magnitude, frequency and duration of each factor should be quantified.

Having identified the offending factor(s) a subsequent reduction in exposure to them may reduce the problem; therefore, job design and ergonomics may need full investigation. This is a theory expounded and well supported by the team of investigators at the Manual Handling Research Unit at the University of Surrey, and others (Simpson, 1984; Stubbs et al, 1983).

The nurse at risk

Back pain is rife throughout the general population, but is the nurse at exceptional risk of developing a back disorder? Consider the facts:

- Around 590,000 health care workers have been identified to be at risk; 520,000 are nurses (Health Services Advisory Committee, 1984).
- Nurses have nearly *twice* as much sick leave due to back pain as the rest of the working population, with an estimated 764,000 working days lost each year (Stubbs and Osborne, 1979).
- Almost one sixth (16.2 per cent) of all sickness absence in nurses is due to back pain (Stubbs and Osborne, 1979).
- The hospital admission rate for severe back pain is 4.8 per 1,000 nurses but 1.1 per 1,000 teachers (Cust, 1972).
- Of those leaving the profession through illness, 40 per cent do so due to severe back pain (Stubbs and Osborne, 1979).
- One in six nurses is likely to suffer back injury due to patient handling (Stubbs et al, 1981).
- One fifth (20 per cent) of industrial injury claims in the NHS arise directly from the lifting of patients (Health Services Advisory Committee, 1984).

Stubbs and Osborne (1980) investigated this problem on a wide scale and the findings have enormous implications for nurses — half the profession suffer back pain at least once and most of those people affected can relate the disorder to a specific incident occurring at work. The commonest activity at the time of acquiring the disorder is the handling of a patient, plainly identifying an occupational hazard.

Why is the nurse so at risk?
The exact reason is unknown but many contributory factors can be identified:

Heavy manual load Nursing is not generally considered to be hard manual labour. However, two nurses lifted a total of two and a half tons in one hour while toileting dependent patients in a geriatric hospital (RCN, 1979).

Training This is variable as no firm guidelines are laid down by the English National Board (ENB). A survey revealed that the average nurse learner received one hour of theory and two hours of practical training on lifting with fellow students and that 18 per cent of schools of nursing gave no instruction at all (RCN, 1979). It is to be hoped that this situation has improved since the survey was carried out but no data is presently available.

Equipment The same survey revealed that 83 per cent of schools of nursing possessed no mechanical lifting aids, though 68 per cent claimed that use of the hoist was taught. Use of such equipment in clinical areas is unclear but availability and confidence in handling remain major factors in preventing uptake. There is no requirement for regular refreshers or updates for trained staff.

Environment Nursing is often practised in less than ideal circumstances with cramped, badly maintained, often poorly designed environs — both in the hospital and the community.

Postural stress Most nurses vastly underestimate the postural stress in their workplace. Observational studies showed that nurses spent up to 80 per cent of the working day in a stooped position (Stubbs and Osborne, 1980).

Staffing levels Osborne (1978) found that an increased number of back injuries occurred at times when staff lifted an excessive amount or, worse still, a nurse lifted on her own.

Uniform This is often tight, short and restrictive, ie, less than ideal for physical work.

Ideas for prevention
There is no simple answer to this hazard. However, it is essential that

nurses themselves, and their employing authorities, make some attempts to minimise the risks of developing or further exacerbating a back problem. The following factors have been suggested and should be considered:

Training   *All* staff are at risk and require training, not only those in the school of nursing; adequate refreshers are needed for all grades. Adequate supervision is needed in the workplace to ensure correct techniques are employed *every* time a patient is handled. Ergonomics and job design should be included to minimise postural stress.

Staffing levels   Sufficient staff must be provided to undertake the tasks required, and criteria should be identified to determine staffing requirements for handling tasks.

Mechanical aids   Sufficient aids should be available; they should be regularly maintained; they should be *used;* and perhaps the role of a 'mechanised aids coordinator' should be developed.

Working environment   Space should be available to allow handling tasks to be carried out without restriction; adequate maintenance, eg, even floors and so on; furniture and equipment should be easily movable and adjustable; suitable clothing and footwear should be provided to allow for unrestricted movement.

Information collection/marking   Information should be recorded in accident books and sickness returns which may identify problem areas, eg, areas/grades of staff/type of work generating special risk.

Policy documents and safe procedures   Clear lines of responsibility both for the employee and employer should be defined, perhaps utilising existing local resources, eg, safety representatives, safety committees and the safety policy.

Common sense
None of these suggestions is new and most are common sense. However, the number of back disorders still occurring nationwide surely indicates that provision is not being made for the implementation of any preventative measures in most areas. Even where attempts are being made, constraints on existing resources make improvement slow and difficult to monitor.

References
Cust, G. (1972) The prevalence of low back pain in nurses. *International Nursing Review,* **19,** 2, 169-79.
Dixon, A. St J. (1980) Diagnosis of low back pain – sorting the complainers. In: Jayson, M.I.V. (ed) The Lumbar Spine and Back Pain (2nd ed). Pitman Medical, London.
Health Services Advisory Committee (1984). The lifting of patients in the Health Services. HMSO, London.

Osborne, C.M. (1978) Low back pain in nurses. BSc dissertation, University of Surrey.
Royal College of Nursing of the UK (1979/85). Avoiding low back injury among nurses. Report of RCN working party. RCN, London.
Simpson, G. (1984) Ergonomic problems and solutions. In: Brothwood, J. (ed). Occupational Aspects of Back Disorders. Society of Occupational Medicine.
Stubbs, D.A., Buckel, P.W., Hudson, M.P. and River, P.M. (1983) *Ergonomics*, **26**, 767-79.
Stubbs, D.A. and Osborne, C.M. (1979) How to save your back, *Nursing*, **3**, 116-24.
Stubbs, D.A. and Osborne, C.M. (1980) Materials Handling Research Unit *Nursing*, **3**, 116-24.
Stubbs, D.A., Rivers, P.M., Hudson, M.P. and Waringham, C.J. (1981) Back pain research. *Nursing Times*, 857-58.

Bibliography
A great deal has been written on this subject but the following,from which much of the data presented here is taken, make a short list of essential reading and are highly recommended:

Griffiths, B. L. (1988) Have you ever had a pain in your back? *Professional Nurse*, **3**, 4, 125-30.
Office of Health Economics (1985) Back Pain (No.78). OHE, 12 Whitehall, London SW1A 2DY.
Royal College of Nursing (1979/1985) Avoiding low back injury among nurses. Report of RCN working party. RCN, London.
Royal College of Nursing/Back Pain Association, The Handling of Patients – a guide for nurse managers. RCN, London.

10

Self-help in preventing stress build-up

Rose Evison, BSc, Dip.Ed., C.Psychol, AFBPsS

Organisational Consultant and Counsellor, Sheffield

Your personal diagnostic check

This can be done on your own but it is helpful to discuss the results with colleagues so you can provide each other with extra information and support for change. Collect information over a period of time to try to catch specific symptoms and the situations which evoke them. Why not keep a stress diary for a few weeks in which you:

Destructive coping strategies

Smoking, drinking, over-eating

Destructive drug taking

Denial of problems or feelings

Grumbling, whining, sarcasm

Long-term feelings control, leading to repression and loss of awareness

Seeking arousal, adrenalin highs

Health-enhancing coping strategies

Problem-solving around reducing stress-inducing situations and acquiring skills that can help

Working from strengths

Talking through problems with a safe person, formally or informally

Getting negative feelings off your chest

Relaxation techniques

Satisfying physical recreation

Table 1. Strategies for coping with stress.

1. Note the situations in your life which you find stressful, in work and outside.
2. Note the typical stress symptoms you develop; the descriptions given above may help you here.
3. Note the coping strategies you already use, when you use them, how effective they are, and whether they have destructive effects on you or others. (See Table 1.)

The fact that nursing is a caring profession provides the first source of stress as carers are always at risk of taking on board the distresses of others and of putting their own needs last. Both of these can only be done temporarily without penalty. There are other sources of stress for nurses in the many changes that have taken place in the profession and in the NHS as a whole; change is a source of stress even when it is positive overall — and not all the changes have been. Yet a further source of stress is the ethical dilemmas of modern medicine — to abortion we can add organ transplants, life support and resuscitation, surrogate motherhood, and the choices forced by lack of resources.

Check your ideas with these points:

- **Stress is not a disease.** It arises from our natural responses to threats to our physical and psychological wellbeing. We need our protective responses like anger, grief, disgust, and fear — it is when such responses are unnecessarily prolonged that they become dangerous.
- **Stress is not an all-or-nothing state.** All average normal people will show some symptoms of stress, but the more symptoms, the less efficient the person.
- **Stress is not inevitable even when there are many stressful conditions.** People vary in their responses according to their genetic makeup, their life experiences, and the coping skills they have learned.
- **We may not be aware of suffering stress.** This may be because we can accept many symptoms as a normal part of our personality, or because we have become insensitive to our own bodies and feelings as a way of coping. However, it still takes its toll of our minds and bodies.
- **Stress is like a disease process.** This is in that it decreases our wellbeing, interferes with our skills and problem solving, and its cumulative effects can be debilitating for ourselves and damaging for our professional work.
- **Stress can be reduced in many different ways.** Each time you disrupt a symptom you will be preventing further buildup of stress. However, to reduce the incidence of symptoms you may need to change your ways of reacting which may require a long period of working on them.

Recognising stress symptoms

Inappropriate negative feelings Negative feelings are impulses to act to remove threats and automatically focus our minds and arouse our bodies. Whenever they are inappropriate they interfere and are stressful. They may be basic feelings of anger, fear, grief, disgust. They may be resentment, anxiety, helplessness, depression, which are signals of failure to master some situation and often go along with rigid maladaptive behaviours, destructive of self or others. Because feelings are impulses to action, which we control by controlling the muscles concerned, inappropriate feelings are a source of muscular tension.

Physical symptoms of muscular tension   These may be anywhere in the body but the neck and shoulders are common places. These tensions may progress to fatigue, or focused pain such as headache or backache. Tension is stressful whether caused by feelings control or poor physical skills.

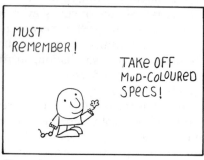

Figure 1.

Repetitive negative thoughts about self or others   These may be aggressive or dismissive, or anxieties about mistakes or disasters. Such repetitive thoughts may be justifying the feelings we have or the actions we take or think should be taken. Thoughts couched in ''oughts'' and ''shoulds'' may create anxiety through guilt, and absolutes such as ''always'' or ''never'' or ''I'm no good at ...'', are to be distrusted.

Sometimes our responses are rigid and repetitive in all three areas and they may be accompanied by compulsive actions. Such a complex of rigid responses can be called a *block* because it blocks us from using our flexible intelligence and learning in that area of our experience.

Strategies for decreasing stress symptoms
Working from strengths   This is a crucial strategy in overcoming stress (and it is useful for helping patients). There are two elements. First, celebrating successes, strengths, skills, positive qualities, things you've learned, difficult things you've done. Celebrating positives you have had a hand in makes your strengths and skills more readily available and less easily masked by negative feelings and thoughts. Remember, all human beings are good at problem solving and learning! Associate your name with your skills; make a list on a postcard to carry around and refer to when you are feeling low.

Second, we are at our most skilled and use our minds most effectively when we are experiencing positive feelings, so working from strengths involves maximizing positive feelings. The practical strategy is focusing our attention on positive experiences as our feelings follow our focus of attention. Successful focus on positives will switch mind and body into positive feelings, unwinding and relaxing us. This can be done through music, or activities that you enjoy. Focusing on positive experiences needs practice: try and find some enjoyable experiences each day and list them, out loud or on paper (see Figure 1). Swop some with a friend or colleague.

Changing situations   Think creatively and use the following strategies to reduce the incidence of situations you find upsetting. Where you have the choice, minimize the number of new or challenging situations you are taking on — at home and work. Consider which situations at work are inevitable and which could be changed. Within working teams discuss the impact of necessary administration and systems that are not under your control and see what ideas there are for minimizing stress produced. In particular this should be done when changes are being implemented.

Find more support from others for yourself and share support with others, among your family and friends or more formally through a colleagues' support group or a women's support group. This will alter the impact of stressful situations for you. Another way of altering the impact of stressful situations is to work on clarifying your personal values. Some useful exercises called "values clarification" can be used with groups or individuals see *Meeting Yourself Halfway*, by Sid Simon).

Dealing with inappropriate negative feelings   The simplest way to unload feelings after upsetting experiences is to talk through them. If you don't talk a lot naturally, try and deliberately increase the amount you do. Talk about what's happened on the wards to friends or family, particularly new experiences. Talk through any particularly negative experiences — several times if you can. Encourage yourself to express any feelings that come up, and be willing to listen to others in return — if you don't take turns you may be increasing someone else's stress level.

To get thoughts and feelings off your chest after you've had to hold them in, express them loudly in uncensored words — when you're alone or with friends who know you are getting rid of unwanted feelings, and not rehearsing for next time you meet the people concerned.

Encourage natural emotional discharge   Laughing, crying, shaking, and storming are all natural healing processes which restore mind and body to alertness and readiness for the next task. When you can let them go, do so. Since we have all been stopped from unloading feelings under the mistaken assumption that it is childish we need to feel safe to let go. When it is inappropriate, save them until later — use positive focusing to help control them and later find someone you can trust to express your feelings to. Letting go is not only immediately freeing, it also helps disrupt blocks (see Figure 2). However, be careful that storming is not destructive. If you are hurting yourself by banging your hands on a hard surface, this is not discharge — try ripping a cardboard box instead. If someone else is being destructive, interrupt them decisively, be supportive and suggest other ways to express anger.

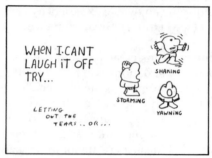

Figure 2.

Dealing with inappropriate negative feelings is working against stress at a fundamental level. This approach may be pursued in counselling and in those growth groups that encourage the expression of feelings; a particularly useful system is co-counselling through peer pairs.

Relaxation   Loosening muscular tension helps reduce stress. Some simple natural methods can often be used on the wards. These are known as "active relaxation" and they directly interrupt muscular tensions.

- **Stretching:** Reach upwards or outwards, make it slow and flowing like a cat.
- **Yawning:** Practise making it long and deep for effective relaxation.
- **Shaking:** Shake any and all parts of your body — this is particularly useful to loosen shoulders when you are feeling tense and anxious.
- **Jaw wobbling:** Let the bottom half of your jaw hang down, then shake your head from side to side so that the jaw wobbles loosely.
- **Neck loosening:** Done in the following way this will untense many other muscles as well. Use when standing still or sitting. Check that you are balanced evenly on both feet or buttocks. Move your arms and legs if necessary so they are not crossed. Loosen the neck muscles by rocking your head *very slightly* back and forth on the top vertebra, where the spinal column enters the skull. Do not tip your chin upwards, but position your head by imagining a gentle tugging on the middle of the top and allowing it to float upwards.

Learning and practising relaxation methods regularly will help you relax anytime you need to by giving yourself an instruction. A very useful relaxation position (see Figure 3) was developed by Alexander (the Alexander technique will be described and discussed in a Factsheet as part of our series on complementary medicine) as was the neck release.

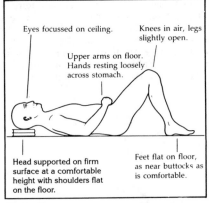

Eyes focussed on ceiling.

Knees in air, legs slightly open.

Upper arms on floor. Hands resting loosely across stomach.

Head supported on firm surface at a comfortable height with shoulders flat on the floor.

Feet flat on floor, as near buttocks as is comfortable.

Figure 3.

Another method is progressive relaxation (Madders (1979)).

Tackle negative thoughts which produce tensions   While focusing on positive experiences can be very helpful, it is often insufficient. A generally useful everyday strategy to reduce stress by discharging tension is the use of humour. Laughter produces relaxation and reduces the likelihood of the negative thoughts being compulsive.

Thoughts or words that are aggressive to others or put-downs of yourself, can be effectively disrupted. The more serious the negative thoughts are the more effective lighthearted disruptors are. Usually laughter will result, but other forms of emotional discharge processes like crying can also occur. There are three types of suitable disruptive phrases:

Contradictions: An opposite or a contradictory phrase, for example "That was really tactful of me" after you've just been tactless.

Parody: Mockery or parody can be used as a disrupter, for instance "I'm the best mess-maker around!"

Celebrate the distress: An exaggerated phrase such as "Whoopee a mistake!" or "Hurrah, a panic!" can disrupt serious negative thoughts. All such phrases work best when you say them loudly and put energy into them. You are not trying to believe the phrases but using them to disrupt unreasonable negatives. Discuss and practise the strategy with colleagues.

Bibliography
Evison, R., and Horobin, R. (1985) How To Change Yourself & Your World: A Manual of Co-counselling Theory and Practice, 2nd edn. Co-Counselling Phoenix, Sheffield.
   This describes the peer support system and includes more information on working from strengths, discharging feelings, and disrupting negative thoughts. For information on basic classes send an sae to Co-Counselling Phoenix, 5 Victoria Road, Sheffield S10 2DJ.
Barker, S. (1978) The Alexander Technique. Bantam Books, New York.
   A practical book about the Alexander technique.
Madders, J. (1979) Stress and Relaxation in Positive Health Guide Series, Martin Dunitz, London.

Covers the practice of progressive relaxation – a method introduced by Jacobsen which concentrates on identifying muscular tension and relaxing deeply.

Meichenbaum, D. (1983) Coping with Stress Century Publishing Co., London.

A short and easily read book, this covers most areas but is short of suggestions for dealing with feelings and blocks – something also apparent in many general texts.

Simon, S. (1974) Meeting Yourself Halfway. Argus Communications, Niles, Illnois.

A series of values clarification exercises for working through individually.

11

What about the carers? The need for staff support in healthcare

Jan Long, SRN, SCM
Staff Support Service Facilitator, Swindon Health Authority

Stress is a normal and necessary part of working in healthcare settings. However, the rising costs of good healthcare are increasing the pressure on all staff to provide the quality of care expected by an informed public.

The issue of who cares for the carers has been disregarded for too long, but the threat of falling recruitment in the 1990s is beginning to occupy the minds of managers. To adequately staff departments in the future, the nursing profession will have to employ at least 50 per cent of all female school leavers with the minimum qualifications of five GCSEs, or their equivalents! The need to conserve staff is, therefore, essential.

Carers' inability
The other major hurdle to looking after the carers is their own inability to accept the need for it. This is particularly true among more senior people, brought up to believe that to be unable to cope is to be a 'failure'.

Many nurses see their role as carer only and that making demands for themselves is a selfish and unnecessary luxury. I consider this to be a 'cop-out', and challenge those who pay lip-service only to both their own needs and those of their staff. Many carers will give defensive answers to the question of staff need:

- "My staff can come and see me any time I am not busy."
- "I don't need support, I can cope."
- "It's not worth it, I'm leaving anyway."
- "We don't have the money."

In response to these and other excuses, many carers have learnt negative, defensive, coping mechanisms to protect themselves. Some use alcohol, smoking, food or even drugs to escape from unacknowledged feelings. Some opt out, become sick, absent themselves on feeble excuses or leave the profession altogether, causing further loss of resources.

What is burnout?
Cherniss (1980) describes burnout as "A process in which a previously committed professional disengages from his/her work in response to the

stress and strain experienced in the job." He lists some of the signs and symptoms of job stress and burnout (Table 1).

Sense of failure.
Absenteeism.
Clockwatching.
Sleep disorders.
Discouragement.
Indifference.
Increased physical illness, coughs, colds, flu etc.
Inability to concentrate and increased marital and family conflict.

Table 1. Symptoms of burnout.

Cherniss explains burnout as being in three stages:
1. Imbalance between demand and resources.
2. Immediate short-term effects – anxiety, tension, fatigue and exhaustion.
3. Changes in attitude and behaviour; becoming detached and cynical – defensive coping.

By becoming cynical and pessimistic carers reduce the guilt and frustration associated with stressful work. Detachment from their patients helps carers psychologically, but the negative effects of staff detachment cause patients to feel more vulnerable and isolated in a situation which for them is already stressful. This can delay their recovery and ultimate release from medical care.

Much research has been undertaken into the measurement of burnout, but little into the effectiveness of interventions. In 1988, I was sponsored by the Artemis Trust to research support services in the USA, to look at models of support and to try to find statistical evidence of their effectiveness. Although our health systems are different, there were many areas where the stresses and strains were identical.

Research

Hare (1988a) compared 10 hospitals, both acute and long-term, to measure the effects of burnout in various settings. During this research only two of the 10 institutions showed any real interest in the results of the study. Those two who did were actively concerned with improving staff morale and awaited the results with interest. They were long-term units, and out of all 10, had the highest level of staff job satisfaction and lowest burnout scores. They also had no staff vacancies.

In another study, Hare compared the needs of trained and untrained nursing staff (Hare, 1988b). On the whole, those who had most direct patient care were the less qualified or junior members of staff. These staff were not expected to deal with the complex emotional needs of their patients, yet were most likely to be faced with these needs. This left them feeling helpless and inadequate.

Hare also noted that those least qualified are much more likely to use negative coping strategies – alcohol, cigarettes or avoidance (sickness, absenteeism) – than to try and deal more effectively with their dilemma, such as by talking, relaxation, using interventions.

Norbeck has completed several studies to measure the effects of burnout using her own measurement tool (Norbeck, 1981; 1982; 1985). She spoke of a short-term study in one coronary care unit which showed that where nurses attended regular support groups, patients made a significantly quicker recovery. This particular survey was too small for publication, but is continued by Dubovsky, in another study of staff at a coronary care unit, where a psychiatrist was employed for both staff and patient support (Dubovsky, 1977). There was a significant drop in patient mortality rate compared to a control unit.

Dubovsky suggests that as staff are less caught up with interpersonal difficulties and distractions, they may be more alert to small changes in their patients. They may also spend more time with the patients, effectively supporting and calming them. The direct result was a shorter hospital stay for patients in this expensive, high-powered unit.

Support models

The American experience offered various support models from support groups, one-to-one counselling, relaxation, self-awareness, professional development and management training, all of which are known to have a direct effect on morale and job satisfaction. From a financial point of view, however, a more effective argument will be that of reducing staff turnover, sickness, absenteeism and the possible effects on patients, thereby reducing mortality and length of stay. When nurses and other health professionals exhibit manifestations of burnout it is not only they who are likely to suffer. Their behaviour plays a major role in affecting the quality of care delivered and the attainment of services by people in need of them.

No-one is a bottomless well of resources. We all need time out, space, rest and recuperation, and we all need to be cared for. If these needs are not satisfied, we become anaesthetised. How can we give of ourselves when we are not in contact with the needs within ourselves? If we continue to try and function without refilling ourselves we will be empty and artificial, mechanically acting out a role and not really caring.

At a national conference of professionals concerned with this issue, held in 1989, it was agreed that a wider network of support was required to encourage the development of services. Accordingly, The National Association of Staff Support (NASS) was launched with the support and sponsorship of The Artemis Trust. We were also made aware of people in the UK who were trying to set up support services in isolation.

One of the first aims of this organisation was to research 'best practices' within the UK to provide information for those districts and hospitals and individuals who are forward thinking enough to want to provide support for all levels of staff. This has already begun. Another major aim was to set up regional groups to provide support and encouragement and to enable a sharing of experiences in the field.

Within three years of its birth, NASS has brought together progressive general managers, tutors, doctors, nurses, qualified counsellors and other healthcare professionals and has shown that successful management can go hand in hand with humanity. Many areas are not so enlightened, however. Some have no positive support programme at all and some have concerned, knowledgeable people thwarted by complacency.

What can we do?

It is time we all made positive moves, not only to be aware of the needs of our patients, but to be more aware of our own! It is time to put our own house in order, to stop expecting a mythical 'them' to come to a mythical 'rescue'. We must realise that *we* are them. We are the health service and we can affect what happens to us.

The following are personal suggestions for a professional action plan:

- Acknowledge your own need for support. Show by example that we do not 'fail' if we find the pressure of caring stressful. Rather, we prove our humanity, the failure is in the accusation.
- Learn to communicate effectively. Attend courses and seminars, and **practise**.
- Do not confuse counselling with support. It is a much abused and overused word and there are other ways of supporting. Skilled counselling is only one way. Counselling is not: advice giving; disciplining; telling; manipulating.
- Learn to love and respect yourself, follow your own self-development and become self-aware.
- Read – anything and everything, know yourself but develop a sound foundation of knowledge too.
- Find like-minded people within your area – they are there. Talk to anyone who will listen. Make a case of need to managers and personnel departments for trained support facilitators.
- If you are trying to set up a service or a group and would like support, get in touch with NASS at the address given left.

You are as valuable and important as any of your patients. Valuing yourself will teach you to value others, colleagues, family or patients.

References

Cherniss, C. (1980) Staff Burnout: Job Stress in The Human Services, Sage, London.
Dubovski, S.L., Getto, C.J., Adams, G.S., Palisy, J.A. (1977) Impact on nursing care and mortality. *Psychiatrist on The Coronary Care Unit, Psychosomatics*, **3**, 18-27.
Hare, J., Pratt, C.C., Andrews, D. (1988a) Predictors of burnout in professional and paraprofessional nurses working in hospitals and nursing homes. *International Journal of Study*, **25**, 105-15.
Hare, J. and Pratt, C.C. (1988b) Burnout: differences between professional and paraprofessional nursing staff in acute care and long-term facilities. *Journal of Applied Gerontology*, **7**, 1, 60-72.

Norbeck, J.S., Lindsay, A.M., Carrieri, V.L. (1981) The development of an instrument to measure social support. *Nursing Research*, **30**, 5, 264-69.

Norbeck, J.S. (1982) The use of social support in clinical practice. *Journal of Psychosocial Nursing and Mental Health Services*, **20**, 12, 22-29.

Norbeck, J.S. (1985) Perceived job stress, job satisfaction and psychological symptoms n critical care nursing. *Research in Nursing and Health*, **8**, 253-95.

For further information about NASS, contact: Grace Owen, NASS Secretary, 9 Caradon Close, Woking, Surrey GU21 3DU.
NASS has regional groups running throughout the UK.

12

Shiftwork can seriously damage your health!

Emma Fossey, MA
Research Assistant, Dept. of Psychiatry, Royal Edinburgh Hospital

The concept of shiftwork is by no means new – in early times the extension of working hours into the night was necessary for security. In today's society the growth of industrialisation has rendered these reasons less cogent but has created new ones. Now, economic gain and continuous availability of public services are the main motivational factors behind the persistence of shiftwork. What is recent however, is the recognition that shiftwork has important implications for both the personal wellbeing of the workers and the safety of the general public both in and out of the work place.

Circadian rhythms

Most biological species are equipped with an inherent endogenous pace-making system known as the biological master clock. This is responsible for synchronising the rhythms of our physiological processes with the 24-hour cyclic changes of the earth, such as the cycle of light and dark. The majority of biochemical, physiological and behavioural processes, ranging from plasma concentration of cortisol and body temperature to the sleep-wake cycle and mood, therefore, have cyclic circadian (approximately 24 hour) rhythms. Each individual rhythm has its own unique and very stable temporal relationship with respect to other internal cycles and to the day-night cycle. For example, body temperature rhythm is dependent upon time of day – it reaches a peak during the late afternoon and falls to a trough during the early hours of the morning.

Any form of shiftwork that intrudes into time normally spent asleep will naturally alter these biological rhythms. It also results in numerous physiological and biochemical changes which include increases during the night of serum glucose, uric acid and levels of urinary excretion of catecholamines. In night workers the cycle of sleep and wakefulness is completely reversed and initially is at odds with other rhythms. For example, secretion of the sleep-dependent growth hormone (hGH) coincides with low levels of time-dependent corticosteroids and adrenaline. The abrupt change in sleep times due to night work means that high levels of corticosteroid and adrenaline secretion still occur at the original clock time – during the day when shift workers are trying to sleep, thus reducing the restorative value of sleep. Conversely, low levels of corticosteroids and adrenaline at night when nightworkers must function at their best cause them to be less efficient (Oswald, 1980).

Resynchronisation is a slow process, and in the case of rotating shiftworkers, readjustment is virtually impossible. Studies of transmeridian air travel have shown that it takes a day for the rhythms to adjust to a one hour shift. The process of resynchronisation to the time shift following air travel is facilitated by the social and environmental cues that help us to adjust to the time change. However, in shiftworkers, adapting to the time shift takes longer because the social and environmental time-cues are inappropriate – everyone around is sleeping and it is dark when shiftworkers are awake and trying to work. Even in non-rotating permanent night workers whose rhythms have time to adjust, the social pressure to conform to regular social sleeping times on days off means they too suffer some circadian disruption.

Consequences of circadian disruption

This physiological disruption, plus the psychological strain of shiftwork can have serious detrimental effects on shiftworkers' health and wellbeing.

Sleep   Shiftworkers regard sleep as the biggest problem in their day-to-day living. Many have great difficulty falling asleep and/or staying awake at appropriate times. When they do sleep, their sleep pattern is altered and tends to be significantly shorter. There is evidence to suggest that for these reasons there is a high consumption of alcohol, tobacco, sleeping pills and tranquillisers among shiftworkers compared to their day working counterparts.

Eating patterns   Eating habits are also upset by irregular sleep-wake hours and the consequences of this are reflected in the high proportion of duodenal ulcers, peptic ulcers and gastroduodenitis in shiftworkers.

Social patterns   Studies have shown that shiftworkers often feel isolated from their family and friends and admit they are less able to fulfil their normal domestic roles, such as spouse and/or parent. This interference with normal family life can adversely affect shiftworkers' mental health, manifesting itself in the form of low self-esteem, anxiety and irritability, which in turn can lead to a deterioration of married and family life, and even divorce. Women in shiftwork are faced with these and other domestic problems. For many, their responsibilities to their family take precedence over their own sleep and as a consequence they suffer to a greater extent.

Circulatory and cardiovascular problems   A study by Knuttson *et al* (1986) found a relative risk of myocardial infarction (MI) associated with shiftwork. This risk increases with length of time involved in shiftwork up to about 11-15 years, and then drops after over 20 years of exposure, which may be because those workers who are able to cope with shiftwork for such a long period are less susceptible to disease. Another study (Alfredsson *et al*, 1982) found evidence that serum cholesterol is higher in shiftworkers leading in turn to a higher incidence of MI, although this is confounded by the fact that the workers in this particular study were also excessive smokers, which may have been the primary reason behind the high rate of cardiovascular disease.

Psychiatric problems High levels of neurotic disorders and depression have recently been indicated in shiftworkers, and those on permanent night shift and men in general appear to be the more susceptible. While researchers are as yet unsure of the specific cause, it appears to be due to a combination of the physiological and psychological stresses of shiftwork upon the individual.

Whether these adverse effects are serious and lasting has been examined in a number of studies of ex-shiftworkers. Overall, the evidence suggests that former shiftworkers may continue to experience disruption of their sleeping and eating patterns, and that depressive disorders, circulatory, respiratory and cardiovascular complaints may also persist. Their health is also likely to deteriorate with age at a much sharper rate than dayshift workers. Unfortunately, these studies do not give an accurate picture of the general effect of circadian disruption because they are dealing with a sample of the population that is self-selected to a large extent and has already proved more capable of adapting to shiftwork. It is likely, however, that the long-term effect of circadian disruption in the average individual is more serious.

Poor work performance

The quality of work performance over a long period does not decline at an even rate, but fluctuates simultaneously with the peaks and troughs of the rhythms of body temperature and arousal. We experience a greater urge to sleep, a poorer ability to perform and an increased likelihood of making errors or having accidents between the early hours of 02.00 and 07.00, and to a lesser extent in the afternoon between about 14.00 and 17.00, regardless of whether or not we have slept. In terms of general performance, the day shift typically yields higher productivity than either the evening or night shifts, the latter being associated with the lowest performance. Some nurses, however, report that the evening shift is the time of their lowest performance. An important factor in this case is the fact that the division of labour for hospital nurses is such that work stress is distributed differentially over the three shifts according to the type and degree of the stress.

Shift schedules for nurses may vary according to the health board or authority, or from hospital to hospital: there may be a two-shift system in operation with an early shift and late shift and a permanent night staff to cover night duty; or there may be a three-shift schedule, such as morning shift from 07.00 to 15.00, afternoon shift from 14.00 to 22.00, and night shift from 21.30 to 07.30. In studies of the effects of shiftwork on nurses, sleep disturbances are mainly connected with evening shifts and fatigue mainly connected with night shifts. Many nurses find rotating shifts in general the hardest in terms of work performance and job-related stress, followed in turn by the afternoon, the night and day shifts. Indeed in one study nurses on rotating shifts were rated lower than fixed shift nurses by their supervisors in terms of job performance, motivation and patient care (Coffey *et al*, 1988).

A number of studies have also considered the performance of junior doctors suffering from varying degrees of sleep deprivation. They have found that in general, interesting tasks that involve relatively simple motor skills are resistant to the desire to sleep for up to 60 hours. The more mundane and monotonous tasks show a serious decline in concentration and an increase in errors after approximately 18 hours of sleep deprivation. Other studies of performance following sleep deprivation have found evidence of impaired retention, concentration, factual recall and manual dexterity, as well as slowed information processing and problem-solving.

Doctors in their first year also experience more psychiatric problems than any other comparable group of young professionals. Again, sleep disruption or deprivation appears to be the major causative factor rather than for example stress of responsibility, anxiety about personal ability or lack of free time. Studies list hyperirritability, less social affection, depersonalisation, feelings of hostility and an increase in alcohol and substance abuse as major problems for junior doctors. Depressive symptoms and in some cases suicidal thoughts have also been reported, and may be partly attributable to sleep loss.

Generating acceptable schedules
Despite numerous and vociferous complaints by those engaged in shiftwork, there is a paradoxical reluctance among employers to change pre-existing systems. However, between 20 and 30 per cent of workers dislike shiftwork so much that they are forced to abandon it – particularly those aged 45 years or more (Minors, 1988), and more employers are beginning to listen to their employees and to scientists. Some are now trying to implement more acceptable work schedules for their employees.

At present there are three main types of schedule: straight, non-rotating shifts; rapid rotating shifts; slow (weekly) rotating shifts. Chronobiologists agree that the best schedules must take into consideration the natural properties of our circadian rhythms. In this respect, two points must be considered – direction of rotation and the length of interval between phase shifts. Studies have shown that extending the 24 hour day/night cycle is more easily adjusted to than shortening the day/night cycle (Czeisler *et al*, 1982), so night workers are able to accommodate sleep disruption more satisfactorily by going to sleep as soon as they finish their shift – after the normal night-time hours, rather than staying up till around midday and going to sleep before normal sleep time. An improved shiftwork schedule would be one in which the shift changes advance in a clockwise direction – from morning shift to afternoon shift to evening shift and so on. It is necessary to take into account the time for adjustment to a change in shift. In most shiftwork systems this is usually one or two days, but the longer the interval the better.

There is still disagreement as to whether rapid shift rotation or slow rotation is better. Disruption of circadian rhythms caused by transmeridian flight is temporary because the rhythms have enough time to readjust to the new time zone. In rotating shiftwork, the rhythms are continually being disrupted. How well they can resynchronise to a new time schedule depends on the rate of rotation: the slower the rotation the longer the time rhythms have to adapt to the change. In slow rotating shifts, the time interval between each shift is generally only long enough for the rhythms to partially adapt – for example, it takes up to 12 days for the temperature rhythm to adjust to a time shift. This partial resynchronisation is potentially harmful to the rhythms which often do not fully adapt.

Arguments in favour of rapid rotation maintain that it avoids the problem of continual partial synchronisation of rhythms and is therefore a more satisfactory alternative. Although this strategy does avoid partial adaption, scientists are faced with the problem that the cumulative effect of rhythms in a continual state of flux may in the long term cause more harm than any short-term good. More importantly for the workers, rapid rotation causes great disruption to their social and domestic life, and this is why many prefer slow rotation. It may be physiologically more harmful to them, but it does accommodate their more immediate need for time for social and domestic pursuits.

Intervention schemes
At present there is no ideal solution to the problem of shiftwork. There are, however, some compensatory behaviours that can ease the disruption.

Napping Many shiftworkers resort to napping before, during or immediately following their shift to supplement their sleep. Employers in a number of Japanese companies are actively encouraging this and provide rooms in which employees may nap during their shift. However there are both positive and negative aspects to napping. On the positive side, it can lower levels of fatigue, increase performance capacity and diminish reduced alertness. On the negative side, it can cause 'sleep inertia' – the inertia felt immediately following a nap (though this is usually quickly overcome by the restorative benefits of the nap). Napping can also disrupt the subsequent main night's sleep and thus reduces its recuperative quality.

According to Akerstedt *et al* (1989) if you are a 'napper' you can benefit by taking naps at specific times according to your shift schedule. If the next main sleep is going to be taken on the following night, it is better not to take a nap. This ensures the main night's sleep is of good restorative quality. However if the following night is a working night it would be advisable to take an afternoon nap, to reduce the inevitable fatigue that accompanies night work.

Exercise A number of studies on women have found that physical exercise can temper some ill effects of shiftwork. Their results have shown that regular, moderate physical training increases physical fitness and subsequently can reduce fatigue and musculoskeletal symptoms. There is also an increase in efficiency on memory-loaded tasks and subjective alertness. Further evidence indicates that the physiological effects of the exercise can speed up the process of resynchronisation of disrupted circadian rhythms, so that adapting to new shiftwork schedules can occur more quickly.

Changing practices for the future

At present, shiftwork is in some respects self-defeating. Instead of benefiting from higher turnover, employers are losing money through increased errors, accidents, sick leave, slower productivity and staff turnover. Employees too are beginning to realise the detrimental effect of shiftwork on their health by far overshadows any pecuniary benefit it may have. By its very nature, shiftwork will always entail physiological and psychological disruption, but the degree of disruption and the resulting threat to the health and safety of both the workers and the public can be tempered. In America, in particular, attempts are being made to achieve this: departments of chronobiology (the study of circadian rhythms) have been established and many concerned employers including the Philadelphia Police Force, the Federal Aviation Administration and various chemical plants are turning to the chronobiologists for advice about improving their shiftwork schedules. In Germany too, companies are beginning to recognise the gravity of the situation and offer their workers general check-ups and the opportunity to normalise their rhythms at regular two or three year intervals at special hospitals. Britain, unfortunately, has been rather slow to follow their example, but changes are beginning to be made. Altering the structure of long-established shiftwork schedules is likely to meet with resistance, but those who have already done so are aware of an increase in productivity and in addition often have a more content work force. While the concept of shiftwork in our society remains necessary, it need no longer be to the detriment of the health and safety of those involved, if only employers take these factors into account when planning their shifts.

References
Akerstedt, T., Torsvail, L., Gillberg, M. (1989) Sleep and Alertness – Chronobiological, Behavioural, and Medical Aspects of Napping. Raven Press, New York.
Alfredsson, L., Karasek, R., Theorell, T. (1982) Myocardial infaction risk and psychosical work environment: an analysis of the male Swedish working force. *Social Science Medicine*, **16**, 463-67.
Coffey, L.C., Skipper, J.K., Jung, F.D. (1988) Nurses and shiftwork: effects on job performance and job-related stress. *Journal of Advanced Nursing*, **13**, 245-54.
Czeisler, C.A., Moore-Ede, M.C., Coleman, R.M. (1982) Rotating shiftwork schedules that disrupt sleep are improved by applying circadian principles. *Science*, **217**, 460-63.
Knuttson, A., Akerstedt, T., Jonsson, B.G., Orth-Gomer, K. (1986) Increased risk of ischaemic heart disease in shift workers. *Lancet*, **2**, 89-91.
Minors, D.S. (1988) Practical applications of circadian rhythms of shiftwork. The Biological Clock – Current Approaches. Inprint (Litho) Ltd, Southampton.
Oswald, I. (1980) Sleep as a restorative process: human clues. *Progress in Brain Research*, **53**, 279-88.
Reinberg, A., Vieux, N., Andlauer, P., Guillet, P., Nicolai, A. (1981) Tolerance of shiftwork, amplitude of circadian rhythms and ageing. Night and Shiftwork: Biological and Social Aspects. Pergamon Press, Oxford.

Bibliography
Haider, M., Koller, M., Cervinka, R. (1986) Night and Shiftwork: Long-Term Effects and their Prevention. Verlag Peter Lang, Frankfurt, Germany.
Monk, T.H. and Folkard, S. (Eds) (1985) Hours of Work. John Wiley, Chichester.
Reinberg, A., Vieux, N., Andlaver, P. (1981) Night and Shiftwork: Biological and Social Aspects. Pergamon Press, Oxford.
These books give a comprehensive account of the negative effects of shiftwork and current ideas on preventive techniques.

Acknowledgements
Thanks to Dr Colin M. Sharpiro for his advice. Emma Fossey is currently supported by a grant from the Asthma Research Council. Further financial support was provided by the Edinburgh Sleep Research Trust.

Ensuring Quality
of Life

13

Returning home with confidence – discharge planning in stoma care: a conceptual framework

Ann Curry, RGN
Senior Ward Sister, St Mark's Hospital, London

The day of discharge is usually an event which people who have just undergone formation of a stoma look forward to a great deal. It may signal the end of the acute phase of their illness, which has required a period of intensive medical and nursing care. However it often raises other concerns for both the patient and their family, such as:

- Will they be able to manage their stoma and appliances?
- What happens if anything goes wrong?
- Will they upset the family routine?

These are all quite normal questions and fears, which will probably arise for the majority of people approaching their discharge date. After all, discharge means they will leave behind the safe confines of the hospital ward, where help and support can always be relied on, and be expected to function with a greater level of independence at home.

In addition to these general concerns, people with newly created stomas, be they ileostomies, colostomies or urostomies, may face additional anxieties about incorporating management of their stoma into their daily routine. It will be the responsibility of the nurse caring for them to ensure they have been taught the necessary practical skills to manage their stoma, have sufficient information to help them overcome any difficulties that may arise and know who to contact for help. As with any planned aspect of patient care, it is essential that it is tailor-made to fit the individual's needs and unique circumstances, and that other professionals are involved as and when necessary. Before planning patient care, it is necessary to make a nursing assessment of the patient's needs, and it may be helpful to use a conceptual framework model for this purpose (Figure 1).

The conceptual framework used (Horsfield-Gardner, 1990) is a tool which enables the nurse to consider the whole patient and his or her environment. It therefore provides more specific information which helps to ensure the planned care is formulated more appropriately .

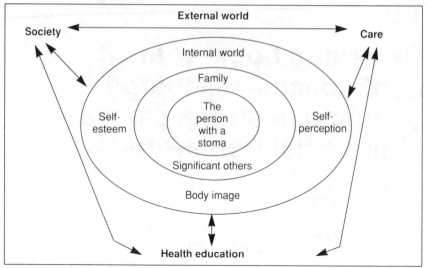

Figure 1. The conceptual framework.

The conceptual framework

At the centre of the framework is the person with a stoma. It is important to remember that this individual has several components to his or her make-up, and many aspects of personality which will not be apparent while in hospital. 'The person with a stoma' is, however, a broad definition, and while this person must remain the focus of attention, he or she cannot be considered in isolation.

Patients are usually part of a family, be it an immediate, closely knit relationship, or a more distant connection. It is necessary, therefore, to consider how a family member having a stoma may affect other members of the family, either directly or indirectly. It is possible that having a stoma will mean the relationship the individual has with members of his or her family may be altered in some way. Will having a stoma affect their expectations of each other?

The person with a stoma will probably have 'significant others' in his or her life - a partner, lover, or close friend for instance. If so, the nursing assessment should involve finding out what type of relationship they hold, and whether they have physical or sexual needs. What implications does having a stoma have for this 'special liaison'? Thoughts of this nature may not necessarily be directly voiced by either nurse or patient, but issues surrounding them can be discussed sensitively.

It is also necessary to consider the person with a stoma in more detail, to assess their personality, as this will also affect their attitude and approach to their newly fashioned stoma, and therefore have important bearings on their individual teaching programme. However prepared for and accepting of a stoma the patient is, it is a change in their body function and having it will necessitate to some extent a modification of their lifestyle.

Internal world Consideration needs to be given to the individual's internal make-up. What makes them 'tick'? What issues do they feel are important to them? How does this person appear to cope with life in general, and how do they manage change or stress? Do they like to feel organised or in control of situations, or are they more 'happy go lucky' in nature? If the individual is having trouble coming to terms with their stoma, they may need referral for counselling. Others find it helpful to meet other people who have a stoma and who have adjusted to it. Looking at a person's character in this way may be helpful when planning care and considering what strategies could be used.

Self-perception This is how people picture themselves and how they hope to come across to others. These two perceptions may be different. It is important to find out what standards they set themselves on a personal, social and professional level. Will having a stoma alter these, particularly considering anxieties about such things as cleanliness, odour and attractiveness.

Body image A person with a stoma does have an altered body image after the operation. The nursing assessment needs to find out how much it will affect them and in what way it will affect them. It will take time for the patient to become familiar with their new body shape and to gradually recognise and accept it as him- or herself. Responses may be varied to a change in body image and the time during which they become apparent differs between individuals. Is appearance important to the patient, and is it important how attractive they feel they are to others? (Salter, 1988).

Self-esteem This is individuals' opinions of themselves, whether they value themselves, and like what they perceive themselves to be. A stoma can affect this, and the assessment should find out whether it does or potentially could, and if so, how it affects the patient's self-esteem. This may be dependent on their type of personality and outlook on life generally. It may also vary according to the circumstances in which they have a stoma. If a person can clearly identify a stoma as improving their quality of life it may be considerably easier for them to incorporate it into their lifestyle than if they were feeling well before the operation. For example:

• Recurrent episodes of acute ulcerative colitis will have made the individual's life revolve around the nearest lavatory and left them generally weak and unwell.

- People troubled by faecal incontinence find it embarrassing and that it limits their social life and sexual relationships.

- Those who have had curative surgery for malignancy can view it as life saving.

If, however, a stoma is performed as an emergency procedure, the individual may have little anticipation of or preparation for the expected outcome. They may not be clear why a stoma should be necessary, and during the recovery period, they may dwell more on the stoma than on why it had to be formed. This can make their belief in themselves become negative.

The components discussed which contribute to an individual's personality are very much intertwined, and therefore cannot be considered in isolation. In turn, they may alter or develop with various events that take place in the individual's external environment.

External world

Once an assessment of the person with a stoma has been made, consideration needs to be given to their external world, and the environment in which he or she will be living following discharge from hospital. Some people may require an element of nursing care when they leave hospital to return to the community. This may be of a supportive or practical nature, ranging from a visit from the community nurse, health visitor or GP, while some patients with newly formed stomas may require terminal care, either at home or in a hospice. It is necessary to consider how much care an individual will need in the community and who is the most appropriate person to provide it. In some circumstances, it may be appropriate for a member of the family to provide the necessary care, while other professionals, such as social workers or occupational therapists may be needed. Whoever has been identified to give assistance to the person will need comprehensive information with the referral, and they should have the necessary knowledge to perform the care. This needs to be incorporated into the discharge planning.

Thought also needs to be given to the type of society to which the person with a stoma belongs, as this may have implications for their teaching programme in preparation for discharge. For example, some people's cultural background makes it more difficult to accept a stoma than others. The primary aim is to return the individual to the position they held in society prior to having their stoma. Consideration should be given to their home surroundings, the type of accommodation they live in and their financial status, to ensure they are fully supported and have the necessary facilities to manage their stoma. The type of social life the individual leads, and their general expectations of life on a personal and professional level are also important.

Everybody is subjected to various health education messages through the media, mainly on environmental, dietary and smoking issues. It may be helpful to clarify any beliefs the patient has relating to health and his or her body, to establish baselines to build on. Patients with newly formed stomas will require some specific health education advice, mainly concerning diet and hygiene, but some may also need advice about travelling, or participating in sport, for example. The type of information given will vary according to the individual, and it is vital that the nursing assessment uncovers all areas in which education is likely to be needed. Education given must also be tailored to suit the individual's level of comprehension, and may need breaking into chunks or repeated on several occasions. Provision of written information to back up these sessions is also helpful, and can be developed by the nurse, or obtained from manufacturers or voluntary organisations.

All the areas of the conceptual framework relating to both the individual and his or her external environment are interlinked, so information gained must be seen within the whole perspective. Many of the topics described appear to pose questions, and these should be seen as guidelines only when speaking to patients and becoming familiar with their situations. The framework should be used as a tool, to maybe act as a prompt for the nurse in assessing the patient. It will not be possible to gain all the information required to make a satisfactory discharge plan during one meeting with the patient. A picture of his or her circumstances and needs will grow over several interviews, particularly as the nurse gains the patient's trust and confidence.

Framework as a tool

Throughout the assessment, it is important to ensure referrals are made to other professionals, such as social worker, health visitor, GP and community nurse where appropriate. The voluntary organisations are able to provide a range of help and advice for people with stomas, and patients should be told how to contact the relevant one.

The support new ostomists receive before discharge, both in practical aspects of management and in the emotional aspects of coming to terms with their stoma is vital in planning for their successful discharge. When they leave hospital, people with stomas should be confident that an appropriate network of support is in place, that they know how to obtain their supplies, and that they have someone they can turn to if they have any problems, whether practical or emotional. Using the conceptual framework should help nurses ensure all these things are in place by the time the patient is discharged.

References
Horsefield-Gardner, J. (1990) A conceptual framework for discharge planning in stoma care (unpublished). College of Nursing and Midwifery, St Bartholomew's Hospital, London.

The Royal Marsden Hospital Manual of Clinical Nursing Procedures - preoperative preparation for stoma surgery.
Salter, M. (1988) Altered Body Image, the Nurse's Role. Scutari Press, London.

Useful addresses

British Colostomy Association, 15 Station Road, Reading RG1 1LG. Tel: 0734 391537.
Illeostomy Association, Amblehurst House. Black Scotch Lane, Mansfield, Notts NG18 4PF. Tel: 0623 28099.
Urostomy Association, Buckland, Beaumont Park, Danbury, Essex CM3 4DE. Tel: 024-541 4294.

14

The shock of the new: altered body image after creation of a stoma

Susan E. Morrall, SRN, RSCN, NNEB, ENB 216
Stoma Care Nurse, Royal Devon and Exeter Hospital

There are four main factors which influence the effect a change of body image has on patients following surgery. These are:
1. The speed with which the change occurs.
2. How visible that change is to others.
3. How much the change will affect the patient's lifestyle.
4. The amount of help and support the patient receives.

   I will discuss these aspects of body image, referring to my own experience of living with a chronic disease and the resulting surgery for the construction of a stoma.

   Body image is the way we see ourselves, and if this image is suddenly altered, it can cause psychological disturbances. Body image is not something we are born with, but is acquired as we grow up. "Imagine a tiny baby. He has no idea of his separate identity from the rest of the world. He responds only to sensations such as hunger or discomfort. He has no 'body image'. Gradually however, as he becomes more mobile, he increases his knowledge of his body through his sense of touch, hearing and smell. He begins to play with objects around him, and to recognise that he is separate from his mother – in other words, he develops an awareness of himself and his body image" (Pettit, 1980). Children find it easier to adapt and adjust to sudden changes in their body image because it is only just developing and is not a fixed state in their minds. This can be seen when young children undergo major mutilating surgery – they may react adversely for a short while, but quickly adjust and continue with their life.

   "A child who has not fully developed his body image would probably suffer little, as he could incorporate the change into his developing image. In adolescence the individual is most preoccupied with attractiveness and normality and a change in body image at this age would be very psychologically traumatic. In the older age group, although appearances and normality have ceased to be of paramount importance the individual's body image has been established for a longer period of time, and so adjustment may be very difficult" (Elcoat, 1986).

Adjusting to an altered image

The attitude of others with whom we are in contact also influences our body image, and if peer groups or parents reject the patient following surgery, this will obviously have a detrimental effect. Conversely, if support is given at the time of surgery, many obstacles can be overcome – both physical and psychological.

Apart from the patient's age, the speed with which surgery occurs also influences how it will be accepted. Someone who has time to consider the change a stoma will bring and adjust mentally to the idea before surgery, is much more likely to accept it. Patients who are given adequate information and preoperative counselling cope much better postoperatively than those who are ill-informed and not counselled.

Unfortunately, many people have their stomas created during emergency surgery, when there is little time for explanation and mental preparation. Psychological adjustment is then disturbed and invariably the patient is too ill to comprehend the impending operation, while fear and the strangeness of unfamiliar hospital surroundings add to their anxiety and vulnerability. These people may totally reject their stoma, denying its existence or withdrawing into themselves. They may erect a barrier between themselves and the outside world, isolating themselves socially even from their closest relatives, and feeling that even their partner could not possibly cope with seeing their stoma. This can obviously be hurtful for their partner and may result in deteriorating sexual relations. At this stage the patient is likely to have lost self-esteem, and feel unclean and inferior; he or she will need much reassurance, encouragement and acceptance as well as the opportunity to talk over their feelings.

Visibility

Other factors which affect body image following surgery are how visible the change is, and how much it will change the patient's lifestyle and encroach upon his or her activities. We all have different interpretations of what we perceive to be 'normal' and 'acceptable'. I have found that the public generally copes fairly well with visible disability or handicap. It has become much more acceptable to see disabled people out and about as opposed to the old idea of keeping them shut away out of sight.

Having spent some time wearing a cervical collar and in a wheelchair (although initially slightly self-conscious about using the chair), I found people accepted me, and were eager to help. The handicap was obvious and most people could cope with this; it was also aesthetically acceptable. The psychological effects were more insidious, since the transition from being 'able' to 'disabled' was gradual. Occasionally I would suffer the 'does he take sugar?' phenomenon, or people would pat me on the head. I would be tempted to bark at them, but I found no real problem in adjusting to this situation – or so I thought! I saw my wheelchair as a means of facilitating a fuller lifestyle impossible to achieve without it, and having seen so many people totally consumed by multiple sclerosis, I was determined that it would only be a small part of my life – not the dominant feature.

One day, however, I saw a photograph of myself in a wheelchair, and suddenly the reality of being disabled hit me – I was shocked at my image. I don't know whether this indicated that I had been denying reality, or a recognition of the severity of my situation. Goffman (1984) quotes a patient saying "when I got up at last and had learned to walk again, one day I took a hand glass and went to a long mirror to look at myself, and I went alone. I didn't want anyone to know how I felt when I saw myself for the first time . . . but there was no noise, no outcry, I didn't scream with rage when I saw myself, I just felt numb. The person in the mirror couldn't be me". That certainly was my experience on seeing myself in a photograph. However, once over the initial shock and with the help of relatives and friends who accepted me, I came to terms with being 'disabled'.

Psychological responses to surgery

One of the first fears new ostomists will raise is "how noticeable is my stoma to other people?". This, in turn, raises the problem of "who do I tell about my surgery?", and "how will they react?". If ostomists try to pass as 'normal' by not disclosing that they have a stoma, the fear that it may leak, or the bag suddenly fill and become obvious will be ever present. This desire to pass as 'normal' can be a significant phase in the adjustment of body image, suggesting a denial of the stoma and providing a means to protect ostomists from facing the facts. With encouragement and the support of family and trusted friends, they may find it beneficial to talk openly about their stoma, coming to accept it and so removing the tension of denial. In the long term, it may mean the subject will eventually become acceptable for open discussion.

I had time to both think and talk about my own surgery for some time before the operation, and was thankful for this. Because of my circumstances – deteriorating health and recurrent urinary infections – the thought of a stoma became more and more acceptable to me as time passed, and I felt I was psychologically well-prepared, having discussed it fully with my parents and closest friends. I was highly motivated to learn to cope with this new addition to my life. However on the first postoperative night the bag leaked on at least three occasions, and bag, bed and nightie were all changed. In my mind I remembered the misery of children with spina bifida who had had urinary diversions when I was a student nurse, and how their constant cry was "I am leaking nurse!". But for the sedation of powerful analgesics, I am sure I would have been very depressed at this stage. The following morning a staff nurse came to attend to me, and once again the bag needed changing. Thankfully she immediately assessed the problem and, using a protective wafer, secured the bag adequately. This appliance stayed in position for almost a week, which did much to boost my moral and regain my self-confidence, though whenever a leak did occur that confidence took a nose dive!

When I came home from hospital, I was very conscious of my stoma and thought everyone else was too. I soon realised some of my clothes were no longer suitable because if the bag suddenly filled, an embarrassing bulge would show beneath my skirt. I felt quite happy to tell certain people about my stoma, but wanted their knowledge of it to come from me, not from their noticing a peculiar bump under my clothes or that the appliance had suddenly leaked. I soon readjusted my style of clothes, and in time selected styles which would camouflage my bag. Kelly (1986) in an autobiographical account of his stoma surgery says, "I only began to feel better about the equipment when I became master rather than its servant, and I learned to relax and trust it. This was a gradual process involving the acquisition of knowledge and the crucial turning point where I realised I could be independent of the ostomy-fitter, and therefore enjoy some autonomy over my own body functions".

When first discharged from hospital, I felt very vulnerable. The realisation that I had a stoma for life and would have to cope with it was almost overwhelming, despite the fact that I could adequately change the bag at this stage. I needed a great deal of support, which I received from my stoma care nurse, district nurse, GP, parents and friends (my parents' acceptance of my surgery was a great help in my own acceptance of it).

Accepting the benefits

The extent of a change in an ostomists' lifestyle depends largely on how ill the patient was before surgery. Patients who felt well before surgery will find the adjustment to their new body image much harder than will those who were ill for a prolonged period beforehand. They may regret having had surgery and resent their stoma and its encroachment upon their lifestyle, and these feelings may result in social isolation. For patients whose surgery brought about an immediate improvement in their quality of life, the effect on body image may be positive.

I had had an indwelling catheter and leg bag for two years before surgery, and found the catheter preferable to constantly being wet. I knew surgery was a possible solution to the problem, but felt, as did the surgeon, that if an alternative solution proved successful, then I certainly didn't want an operation. A stoma seemed all too final, and a step which I wasn't ready to take. However, after two years of deteriorating health and frequent infections, my ideas changed and I decided a stoma could only improve my life. Also, as a Christian, I had prayerfully considered surgery, and felt the right time had come to go ahead with the operation.

Although initially I had to adjust to the stoma, I was quickly aware that my body image had improved. Somehow the stoma, an integral part of me, seemed much more acceptable than a catheter and leg bag, which definitely were not. A change in body image following stoma surgery does not, therefore, have to be a negative thing.

Much is written about the grieving stage following this type of operation, but I was expecting life to improve and I knew little of this stage. However, grief for the loss of a part of themselves is a very real experience for many ostomists, but while totally overwhelming at first, the loss is gradually replaced by a positive approach to the improvements the stoma has brought: the surgery comes into perspective.

The grieving process must be worked through, however, and the tears allowed to flow. It is important for nurses to encourage patients to express their feelings so that they can begin to heal. Once this has begun, gratitude for the gift of life emerges, and a sense of humour returns.

A patient once said to be, "My life had come to a full stop, but my surgeon made it a semi-colon!" This expresses not only gratitude for life, but the realisation of the benefits surgery has brought. When ostomists have accepted their stoma, they may want to meet other people in a similar situation to discuss problems and ideas. Information should be given about the relevant voluntary organisations, and the patient encouraged to attend one of the group meetings.

> "To define postoperative life in positive terms was relatively easy. I began to notice within about three weeks of the operation, that I was experiencing a sense of physical wellbeing which I had not felt for many years. Whatever the objective source of these feelings, I concluded that they were because of the absence of the disease. These feelings continued noticeably for several months, and I genuinely felt as well as I had ever done or could remember. The ileostomy seemed to be a relatively small price to pay for these experiences. I gradually joined in the normal round of social life and activities" (Kelly, 1987).

Unfortunately, Kelly's experience and my own are not always true for people who have emergency surgery for a condition which had been almost symptomless. Postoperatively things seem bleak and compare unfavourably with life before the stoma. The effects on body image will almost always be more devastating, and acceptance harder for these people. The postoperative lifestyle is more likely to be adversely affected and withdrawal, fear of rejection and social isolation can result. These people, while denying their stoma, would probably not want to meet others in the same situation, as they would not identify with them.

As my condition generally improved after surgery, I was able to resume a fuller lifestyle than before. The stoma stopped being a dominant thought in my life, and became a small part of the whole. Providing 'Topsy' behaved I could forget about it, but when it didn't behave it was 'Topsy Turvey'!

Help and support

"The concept of body image is fluid and fragile" (Elcoat, 1986), and I experienced just how fragile it is. Twenty-two months after surgery, I was temporarily back in a wheelchair, when the crisis came. Being in a wheelchair and having a stoma seemed more than I could cope with.

I felt that I looked awful no matter what I wore, and my body image was in a poor state, but thankfully this was a short-lived phase. A good friend, recognising the problem took me shopping, and despite my protests and disinterest, scoured the shops for a suitably styled expensive suit which I needed for an interview – my first hope of work for eight years. I was persuaded to try one on, and finding it ideal, by a generous gift, was enabled to buy it. I looked and felt good in it – the crisis was over and my confidence restored sufficiently for me to wear it to the interview and not feel conscious of my stoma. Mullen and McGinn (1980) say "Clothes that look good are an important bridge back to the world– one way of mending a bruised body image and moving ahead from patient to person . . . In one way or another, though, clothes are a useful shorthand, telling the world an ostomy is okay – and so am I". This has been my experience.

Help and support are vital for ostomists; if I had not had the understanding of that friend to help me cope with the situation, my body image may have become broken rather than just bruised. New ostomists need a great deal of help, encouragement and understanding from both the professionals and the non-professionals involved with their care and rehabilitation into the community. The stoma care nurse has a large role to play here, but so do friends and relatives. Obviously each individual is going to react differently to their new situation, but much can be done to help people to cope with their altered body image.

The quality of life with a stoma will vary from one person to another enormously, but much will depend on the way they perceive themselves, and everything that can be done to improve their body image should be actively encouraged. It is also important to remember that this image is not always affected in a detrimental way but can, on occasions, be a positive improvement for the patient with a stoma.

References
Elcoat, C. (1986) Stoma Care Nursing. Baillière-Tindall, London.
Goffman, E. (1984) Stigma. Pelican Books, London.
Kelly, M.P. (1987) Managing radical surgery from the patient's viewpoint; notes from the patient's viewpoint. *Gut*, **28**, 1, 81-87.
Mullen, B. and McGinn, K. (1980) The Ostomy Book. Ball Publishing, USA.
Pettitt, E. (1980) Body Image. *Nursing*, **16**, 690-92.

Bibliography
Price, B. (1990) Body Image – Nursing Concepts and Care. Prentice Hall, London.
   A comprehensive guide for nurses and tutors working with people with an altered body image.

Useful addresses
British Colostomy Association, 15 Station Road, Reading, Berkshire RG1 1LG. Tel. 0734 391537.

Ileostomy Association (IA), Amblehurst Road, Black Scotch Lane, Mansfield, Notts NG18 4PF. Tel. 0623 28099.
Urostomy Association (UA), Buckland, Beaumont Park, Danbury, Essex CM3 4DE. Tel. 0245 414294.

15

An open approach to minimise the effect: sexuality and renal patients

Gillian Janes, RGN, DipN, BSc(Hons)
Practice Nurse, Hartlepool

End-stage renal disease (ESRD) involves irreversible kidney damage to the extent that life can no longer be maintained without repeated haemodialysis, continuous ambulatory peritoneal dialysis (CAPD) or kidney transplantation. The fate of people with terminal renal failure has changed dramatically in two decades - previously there was no alternative to death by uraemia, while today, even without a transplant, they can live for years on dialysis.

Research and nephrology nursing
Dialysis was initially an exclusively medical procedure (Fuller, 1984), but improved technology has made the management of such patients almost exclusively a nursing procedure, with doctors playing a largely supervisory role. This increased responsibility and accountability has led nurses to evaluate their practice, resulting in a rapid increase in nephrology nursing knowledge and a dramatic effect on clinical practice. Nursing theory, practice and research are all mutually related and interdependent: nursing theory should be born in practice, refined through research and returned to practice as the basis for nursing assessment, diagnosis and intervention.

Patient sexuality
Nurses must help patients react to and cope with the long-term, non-acute effects of renal failure. It was not until the 1970s that discussion of sexuality entered the nursing curriculum in force, and only a few individuals and specialised areas regarded sexuality as an important area of nursing research (Webb, 1985). Bullough and Seidl (1987) suggest that "...there is no other group of professionals better prepared in the psychosocial, biological and cultural aspects of sex than nurses and they have a lot to contribute...". Since nurses are involved in determining patient needs, it is important they understand their patients' sexuality and how to deal with it in a manner beneficial to all involved. Acknowledgement of our own and our patients' sexuality and provision of care for this basic physiological human need is, therefore, vital.

Sexual healthcare is a relatively new domain for nurses. Although the profession claims to treat the whole person, sexuality has seldom been seen as an integral part of treatment. Disabling chronic illness is both physically and psychologically disruptive, and has major implications for sexual wellbeing (Hine and Daines, 1987). Complex life-saving procedures require more technically orientated nurses, so it is not surprising that the effects of these procedures on sexuality are often overlooked.

Human sexuality is a complex phenomenon encompassing the biological being, self-concept and relationships with others. It does not just relate to sexual performance, but also to the influence of illness and disability on self-concept, body image, self-esteem and social roles (Webb, 1985). A sexual problem may be defined as "...a malfunction of any part of an individual organism or life in such a way as to cause his or her sexual life to appear to him or her as unrewarding or inadequate or to be potentially harmful to another individual" (Ulrich, 1987).

Sexuality problems of renal patients
Until recently, scientific data about the nature of human sexual response and the effects of illness on sexuality were limited (Zalar, 1982). Before 1970, knowledge about the sexual dysfunctions of haemodialysis patients was restricted to case histories, and was usually concerned exclusively with male impotence (Comfort, 1978). Abram *et al* (1975) studied dialysis and transplant patients to determine their level of sexual functioning after the onset of kidney disease, institution of dialysis and renal transplant, and although poor sexual performance did not universally accompany renal failure, dialysis or transplantation, reduced potency occurred in 45 per cent of patients before onset of dialysis.

Although Abram *et al*'s findings show a lower incidence of sexual problems than other authors', it must be remembered sexuality involves more than frequency of intercourse - the variable measured in the study. Later authors (Glover, 1985; Solomon, 1986) report much higher figures, and while this may reflect society's more open attitude towards discussing sexuality, it may also be attributable to the authors considering difficulties other than frequency of intercourse (such as loss of interest and reduced libido). The researchers' definition of sexual dysfunction must, therefore, be considered when comparing results.

It is now well-documented that sexual difficulties form part of the complications of ESRD. All people suffering from chronic illness face similar potential disruptions to their sexuality (Hine and Daines, 1987).

End-stage renal disease is a chronic, debilitating disease with potential for causing disruption of sexuality. Diet, drugs, dialysis and transplantation have profound implications for sexuality, and specific effects include loss of libido in both sexes and reduced fertility due to testicular atrophy or irregular/absent ovulation. Men may have difficulty in having or maintaining an adequate erection, and capacity for orgasm is decreased in both sexes. Drugs such as antihistamines, antihypertensives and steroids often exacerbate the situation, and investigations into the biochemistry of sexual dysfunction in people with ESRD indicate that parathyroid hormone and zinc play a causal role. However, women have completed normal pregnancies and some men do father children despite abnormal spermatogenesis.

Major organ failure may result in a negative view of the whole body (Hine and Daines, 1987), while fistulae may be seen as unattractive, especially by women who may feel restricted in dress by the need to keep them covered. Dependence on the dialysis machine and on other people can also be undermining.

The renal nurse's role

Nurses cannot and should not be sex therapists; however, they should be able to identify problems, intervene appropriately within the limits of their knowledge and refer people to specialist practitioners when necessary. There is a growing literature on this topic, and Webb (1985) and Bancroft (1983) provide extensive practical guidelines. One thing is vital though - nurses should be willing and able to consider sexuality issues within the nursing assessment and to identify problems. Solomon (1986) emphasises that discussion of sexuality related problems should take place in a private and quiet setting. It is often the nurse who has to sensitively broach the subject, as many people find it difficult to discuss.

Webb (1985) advises nurses on how to take a nursing history of a patient's sexuality, emphasising the need to begin with general topics and gradually focusing in more detail on particular aspects of sexuality to help build rapport. Questions should be clearly related to health problems so their relevance is made obvious, with no suggestion that intrusive information is being unnecessarily sought. If problems are identified, nurses must then decide whether they are able to assist the patient or if referral is required. Nursing can provide a legitimate theoretical base to the complex area of sexual functioning when counselling is required (Schuster *et al*, 1982).

The ability to use counselling skills in the day-to-day interaction with patients is an important part of the nurse's role. Bancroft (1983) outlines a useful approach, adding that nurses are most often required simply to act as teachers, giving information about sexual response, correcting misconceptions caused by misinformation and facilitating comm- unication between nurse, patient and partner.

Nurses must also be willing to act as a referral agent (Webb, 1985), and be aware of the many self-help groups and voluntary organisations which offer assistance as well as the local procedure for referral to a specialist sex therapist.

Although nursing research on sexual counselling is limited, studies do show examples of sex counselling undertaken by nurses - but those taking on the task must be adequately knowledgeable (Zolar, 1982).

Nurses' knowledge of sexuality issues

Ulrich (1987) investigated the possibility that the lack of emphasis on sexuality issues may result from limited knowledge of sexuality by nephrology personnel. This implies that nursing care pertaining to patients' sexuality cannot be undertaken successfully until nephrology units incorporate sexuality information in their staff orientation and continuing education programmes. Further recommendations were that sexuality assessment should be integrated with other admission and ongoing assessments, and be included in nursing care plans. However, Ulrich's findings have methodological and reliability problems, so care is required when considering them.

Few renal units have a member of staff with special responsibility for providing counselling and other psychological support, and even fewer have a psychologist available to oversee the psychological care of their patients. There is a real need for staff training programmes to be provided to address this topic.

Kreger (1977) used a pre- and post-test design to examine the effects of a three day training programme on sexual counselling upon the knowledge, attitudes and counselling approach of 51 volunteer trainees. Health practitioners from a range of disciplines, including nursing were shown to lack knowledge about sexual adjustment to disability and of human sexuality in general, indicating a serious need for more education and training. Although the results indicated training had been useful, difficulties were encountered when attempting to put it into practice, and this may be an appropriate avenue for future investigation.

Replication of this study using a larger sample is required before generalisations can reliably be made. That the study was undertaken at all shows that health personnel realise they must help people deal with sexual adjustment to chronic illness if they are to provide holistic care.

Patients and their partners

Qualitative research is concerned with individual situations, and does not attempt to count or quantify, aiming to use detail to explain the object of the study. In one such study, a wife of a haemodialysis patient gives a harrowing account of her husband's and her own life before, during and after chronic dialysis (Nichols, 1984), and her account shows that an understanding of patients' feelings is important when care planning. There are very few similar studies available, and this again points to a promising prospect for future research.

Nurses caring for people undergoing chronic haemodialysis must be aware of the potential sexual difficulties they often face, and ensure they enjoy the best possible quality of life. Renal nurses must be sensitive to their patients' sexuality needs, which are affected by the chronic nature of the illness, restrictive treatment regimes, chronic anaemia and potentially problematic drug therapy. Further research is required on the effects on sexuality sufferers of ESRD experience, and how they feel.

There is, however, a growing literature which nurses can use when planning nursing interventions regarding sexuality. Nevertheless, the success of such interventions still needs to be evaluated by research studies, to investigate when, where, how and by whom such interventions are utilised, and whether or not they are successful. Further research on sexuality is also required to help nurses know exactly what they are attempting to deal with, and to form a sound basis for nursing interventions and experimental research.

References

Abram, H.S., Hester, L.R., Sheridan, W.F., Epstein, G.M. (1975) Sexual functioning in patients with chronic renal failure. *Journal of Nervous and Mental Diseases*, **160**, 3, 220-26.

Bancroft, J. (1983) Human Sexuality and its Problems. Churchill Livingstone, Edinburgh.

Bullough, V.L. and Seidl, A. (1987) Attitudes on sexuality in nursing texts and yesterday. *Holistic Nursing Practice*, **1**, 4, 84-91.

Comfort, M.B. (Ed) (1978) Sexual Consequences of Disability. Stickley, Philadelphia.

Fuller, C. (1984) Staffing a dialysis unit. *Nursing Times*, **80**, 38, 59-61.

Glover, J. (1985) Human Sexuality in Nursing Care. Croom Helm, Kent.

Hine, J. and Daines, B. (1977) Sexuality and the renal patient. *Nursing Times*, **83**, 38, 59-61.

Kreger, S.M. (1977) Sexuality and disability. *Journal of Association of Rehabilitation Nurses*, **2**, Jan/Feb., 8-14.

Nichols, K.A. (1984) Psychological Care in Physical Illness. Croom Helm, Kent.

Schuster, E.A., Unsain, I.C., Goodwin, M.H. (1982) Nursing practice in human sexuality. *Nursing Clinics of North America*, **17**, 3, 345-49.

Solomon, J. (1986) Does renal failure mean sexual failure? *RN*, August, 41-43.

Tieze, M. (1983) Human sexuality - female nurses' responses to their male haemodialysis patients. *AAANT Journal*, **10**, 4,19-22.

Ulrich, B.T. (1987) Sexual knowledge of nephrology personnel. *AAANT Journal*, **14**, 3, 179-83, 230.

Webb, C. (1985) Sexuality, Nursing and Health. Wiley, Chichester.

Whitson, S.E. (1982) Nursing care of the chronic renal failure patient with sexual dysfunction. *AAANT Journal*, **9**, 5, 48-58.

Woods, N.F. (1987) Towards a holistic perspective of human sexuality. *Holistic Nursing Practice*, **1**, 4, 1.

Zalar, M.K. (1982) Role preparation for nurses in human sexual functioning. *Nursing clinics of North America*, **17**, 3, 351-63.

Useful address

Association to Aid the Sexual and Personal Relationships of People with a Disability (SPOD), 286 Camden Road, London N7 0BJ. Tel: 071-607 8851.

16

A better life than before: quality of life in people with renal failure

Gillian Janes, RGN, DipN, BSc (Hons)
Practice Nurse, Hartlepool

Quality of life has become an important concern in healthcare and social policy, but problems are encountered in defining and measuring it because people have different values (Ferrans and Powers, 1985). Various definitions are, however, to be found, such as " ... the degree to which one has self-esteem, a purpose in life and minimum anxiety" (Padilla and Grant, 1985). Although many determinants and indicators have been suggested as standards for quality of life, definitions are subjective (Thompson *et al*, 1983) and an agreed definition is lacking. This leads to inconsistencies in interpreting what actually constitutes quality of life.

The Quality of Life Index (QALI) (Ferrans and Powers, 1985) is a comprehensive measure of quality of life, overcoming some of the problems encountered when measuring this phenomenon. It has been demonstrated to be reliable and valid for both healthy individuals and dialysis patients (after modification), and may be used in the future in both nursing research and practice aimed at improving quality of life. This is particularly important in people with chronic illness, such as renal patients, who have to endure unpleasant treatments and strict diet, usually for long periods, and often for life. It is essential, therefore, that nurses do all they can to ensure their quality of life is the best possible.

Using the nursing process

Padilla and Grant (1985) indicated that patients' quality of life is affected by many factors, some over which nurses have little or no control, such as medical treatment, and others over which they may have significant control, such as personal, environmental and informational variables and nursing treatment.

The quality of a patient's survival may also be associated with his or her inherent personal strength, and with how well nurses are able to help with the necessary adjustments and changes (Padilla and Grant, 1985). To help patients achieve the best possible quality of life, nurses must first consider each patient's individual needs. The nursing process is one way of achieving this; it is a systematic, problem-solving approach to nursing, involving interaction with the patient and assessment of individual needs, followed by planning, implementation and evaluation of nursing interventions 'tailor-made' to suit individual requirements (Kratz, 1979). Expert nurses do not rigidly perform routines without reference to the personality, concerns and desires of individual patients; they work with their patients in a partnership that encourages individuality and sense of control (Thompson and Grant, 1985).

Everyone has physical, social and psychological needs, and ill people experience both physiological and psychological imbalances. The needs these create must be considered together for successful nursing care. A holistic approach to disease recognises the importance of the inter-relationship of mind and body (Sorensen and Luckmann, 1980), and there is increasing interest in the feasibility and benefit of offering a more holistic approach to patient care (Holmes, 1986).

Quality of life among people with renal failure
In view of the difficulty of arriving at a definition of quality of life and the diverse needs of individual patients, it was decided to look in more detail at a group of patients suffering chronic, end-stage renal failure. Chronic renal failure is a progressive reduction of functioning renal tissue resulting in the inability of the remaining tissue to maintain the body's environment. The end result is uraemia and death, unless the person receives dialysis either for the rest of his or her life, or transplantation. Renal patients have been described as people who are neither dying nor cured, but still 'in limbo' (Sorensen and Luckmann, 1980). A diagnosis of chronic renal failure, therefore, indicates a lifelong process for patients and their families and friends.

A small-scale survey of eight patients was undertaken to examine more closely their quality of life. All suffer chronic renal failure and are on regular dialysis - five have haemodialysis three times weekly in hospital and three undertake continuous ambulatory peritoneal dialysis (CAPD) daily at home. Each completed a short questionnaire (Table 1).

Results of the survey
In describing what they understood by the term quality of life, three patients considered physical fitness alone. The remaining five indicated a combination of factors, with three saying mental peace and fulfilment at home were just as important as physical fitness; the remaining two valued fulfilment at home and physical fitness alone.

Not surprisingly, these results illustrate great variations in individual definitions of quality of life. When asked to rate their quality of life on a scale of 1-5 at three different times during and before their illness, four patients indicated their quality of life was exceptionally good before the onset of their illness. When they were ill and not receiving regular treatment, quality of life was rated as very poor, but once established on regular dialysis, the ratings rose, becoming almost as high as before the

Please tick the relevant answer(s)

1. What type of dialysis are you on?
    (a) Haemodialysis.
    (b) CAPD.

2. Have you been offered an alternative?
    (a) Haemodialysis.
    (b) CAPD.

3. What do you understand by the term 'quality of life'?
    (a) Feeling physically well.
    (b) Feeling mentally at peace.
    (c) Fulfilled at home.
    (d) Fulfilled at work.
    (e) Combination of the above.
(Please indicate which combination)

4. How would you rate your quality of life on a scale of 1-5 (1 = poor; 2 = below average; 3 = average; 4 = good; 5 = very high quality)
    (a) Before you were first taken ill.
    (b) When you were ill but not on regular dialysis.
    (c) Now you are on regular dialysis.

5. Is there any other factor, so far not stated, that would add to your quality of life?
YES   NO
If yes please state in what way:-

6. Do you feel the nursing staff involved have in any way improved your quality of life?
YES   NO
If yes please state in what way:-

7. Can you suggest any further ways in which the nursing staff could improve your quality of life?

Table 1. Quality of life questionnaire.

illness began. This indicates that quality of life is improved by regular dialysis, a process in which nurses are heavily involved.

These results are perhaps surprising, since they show these patients rate their quality of life as very high, despite having to spend a third of each week in hospital and follow a strict dietary regime - factors which may, to healthy individuals, indicate a severely reduced quality of life. One respondent felt dialysis made her quality of life the same as it was before her illness, but this may be because she suffered no symptoms of uraemia, and her renal failure was discovered purely by accident following a routine blood check. Another actually considered his quality of life to be better since receiving dialysis than before he became ill, because he had been ill for so long before dialysis, he could not remember when his quality of life had been so good.

Asked if their quality of life could be improved, five patients said it could not. Three, however, indicated it could be bettered: one suggested control of pruritis and two longed for a transplant. Again, these results may be surprising, as it could be expected that most patients would cite transplantation as the means of further improving their quality of life. However, the sample consisted predominantly of patients who felt well on dialysis and were mainly satisfied with their present quality of life.

All respondents said the nursing care they received had improved their quality of life. Two indicated the high standard of physical care was the reason for this, whereas others emphasised the following points: treating the patient as an individual; taking time to listen; a kindly attitude; a sense of humour. These results are supported by research involving four groups of patients in acute wards which found they were more concerned with attitudes and interpersonal relationships than with the practical aspects of their care (Buckmann, 1986).

In an attempt to ascertain how dialysis nurses can improve the care they give, participants were asked to suggest ways in which nursing staff could further improve their quality of life. Only two of the eight suggested ideas, and these were that patients should be treated on a more individual basis, nursing staff should communicate more with relatives at visiting times and better communication between doctors and nurses would help improve matters.

It is possible that the six patients who did not suggest ways of improving their quality of life were afraid that these could be seen as complaints against current nursing practice. In an attempt to avoid this, participants were assured their replies would be received in strict confidence and not be interpreted as disloyalty to the nursing staff. In retrospect, however, perhaps this area of the exercise could have been handled more effectively.

Evaluation

The results of this very small, and therefore limited study, seem to indicate that nurses can significantly improve and maintain the quality of life of dialysis patients, since the important factors identified by the patients fall within the remit of nursing practice. Although nursing is, in part, dependent on medical practice, there are also areas in which nurses act independently of doctors, such as in dealing with patients' comfort and social and psychological wellbeing (Thompson *et al*, 1983).

Since dialysis became available to everyone, it has become much more difficult for dialysis teams to justify denying it to anyone with renal failure. There are, however, doubts as to whether dialysis is appropriate for all patients. If not all patients with end-stage renal failure are to receive dialysis, there must be a process by which selection takes place (Davis and Aroskar, 1983).

Kubler-Ross (1970) stated that, when referring someone to a hospice, the aim is to augment the quality, rather than the quantity, of life remaining. This is equally applicable when considering patients with renal failure. Thompson, Melia and Boyd (1983) describe the nurse's role as saving life and alleviating suffering, but practising nurses may experience a conflict between these two aspects. For example, in saving life by initiating dialysis, we may create more suffering for the patient through operations and severe dietary restrictions.

Perhaps medical technology has moved so far that we are prevented from seeing patients as human beings, seeing them instead as machines to be kept going at all costs (Peck, 1986). We must remember patients have feelings, wishes and opinions as well as the right to be heard (Kubler-Ross, 1970); they also have the right to refuse treatment, although this is not absolute because a doctor may legally give treatment against a patient's wishes if it is considered to be in that patient's best interest (Thompson *et al*, 1983).

Problems over quality of life arise for many people having dialysis and awaiting transplant. Life can become an endless cycle of treatments, surgery and rejection of the transplanted organ, while the patient continues a "chronic form of dying"' (Davis and Aroskar, 1983).

When death occurs, questions arise for nurses concerning quality of life versus the sanctity of life and the individual's right to die with dignity (Davis and Aroskar, 1983). The process of dying is controlled, to some extent, by the use of technology, and the question arises whether life ceases to be worth living when it becomes prolonged dying, rather than meaningful life. We now have the ability to prolong life long after any semblance of humanity has gone (Fenner, 1980) and, therefore, the quality of life we can offer to our patients must be a major concern.

Nursing care can undoubtedly significantly improve and maintain dialysis patients' quality of life, and the results of this survey suggest there are ways in which we can further improve the quality of our patients' lives. It is important then, that we, as nurses, do not take this responsibility lightly, or underestimate our ability in this sphere. Miller (1985) compared the nursing care given by the traditional task-allocation methods with individualised patient care delivered using the nursing process, in improving patients' quality of life, and the latter was found to be demonstrably more successful.

The most effective way nurses can enable each renal patient to achieve his or her greatest potential in terms of quality of life, appears to be through delivery of individualised care through use of the nursing process. While the optimum quality of life for patients should always be the aim for nurses, it is doubly important for those whose condition means they depend on us for the rest of their lives.

References
Buckmann, M. (1986) Patients' point of view. *Senior Nurse*, 4, 3, 26-27.
Davis, A.J. and Aroskar, M.A. (1983) Ethical Dilemmas in Nursing Practice. Appleton-Century-Crofts, London.
Fenner, K.M. (1980) Ethics and Law in Nursing. Van Nostrand Reinhold, New York.
Ferrans, C.E. and Powers, M.J. (1985) Quality of life index. *Advances in Nursing Science*, 8, 1, 15-21.
Holmes, P. (1986) Taking the strain. *Nursing Times* , **82**, 8, 28-29.
Kratz, C.R. (1979) The Nursing Process. Bailliere Tindall, London.

Kubler-Ross, E. (1970) On Death and Dying. Tavistock, London.
Padilla, G.V .and Grant, M.M. (1985) Quality of life as a cancer nursing outcome. *Advances in Nursing Science*, **8**, 1, 45-57.
Sorensen, K.C. and Luckmann, J. (1980) Medical-Surgical Nursing. Saunders, London.
Thompson, I.E., Melia, K.M., Boyd, K.M. (1983) Nursing Ethics. Churchill Livingstone, Edinburgh.
Peck, V. (1986) How can we achieve 'successful death'? *Nursing Times*, **82**, 17, 12.

17

A new kind of loving? The effect of continence problems on sexuality

Veronica Wheeler, RGN, RCNT
Clinical General Manager, Physical Rehabilitation Service, Aylesbury Vale Health Authority

Sexuality is not just concerned with sexual activity. Although this is a natural and important form of sexual expression, sexuality is also connected with the projection of sexual image and formation and maintenance of warm, loving relationships.

Recently, more recognition has been given to individual sexuality, indeed, the World Health Organisation (1983) proposed that "sexual health is the integration of the somatic, emotional, intellectual and social aspects of a sexual being, in ways that are positively enriching and that enhance personality, communication and love". While sexuality and sexual needs were identified, the report concluded that little relevant teaching on sexuality was offered in schools of medicine or nursing.

In 1974, Jacobson said nursing was behind in dealing with sexuality in patient and client care, and this is often still the case. She found few nurses or doctors gave patients information on how illness, drugs or procedures may affect their sexuality. Lack of education in this area, or the fact that young nurses and doctors may not yet have come to terms with their own sexuality were suggested as reasons for this. It is important, therefore, that nurses understand the development of their own self-image, as well as those of their patients.

According to Henderson (1969), an individual's health status cannot be fully understood without an awareness of their sexual identity. Without this, individuals' total needs cannot be met, so good healthcare should encourage healthy sexual expression. This is important for people who have to change or relearn their sexual behaviour following illness.

For many, continence problems will mean some modification of their original behaviour. While the principal nursing aim is continence promotion, there are times when this is not possible, and instead, nurses have to rely on bladder training to obtain controlled continence, teach intermittent self-catheterisation or rely on pants and pads for protection.

Since many people experiencing continence problems are over 40, some professionals may not discuss sexual implications of their condition because they think it is not relevant or may not be welcome. In fact many people - women as well as men - continue to engage in sexual activity well into their old age, so the subject should at least be raised with all clients, to give them a chance to ask for advice.

Many couples enjoy a warm, loving and active sexual relationship until late in life. For many, the period between 50 years and retirement is a time in which they face many changes in lifestyle and different demands, many of which are associated with relationships and sexuality (Duval, 1971). Even those with terminal illness, facing a permanent end to a relationship, may need sexual activity to show support and love. Illness, disability and incontinence can interfere with this.

The effects of continence problems

Interviewing women attending an incontinence clinic, Suthurst and Brown (1980) found 73 out of 208 said intercourse took place less frequently since they had developed continence problems, while 17 said it had stopped altogether. Reasons given for reduced frequency were dyspareunia (difficult or painful intercourse in women), wetness at night, embarrassment, depression, leakage during coitus, marital discord and the need for separate beds. Dyspareunia was the most commonly cited reason, because the women were constantly wet and sore.

Knowledge   Nurses need to develop an understanding of the development of sexuality; human sexual response; the relationship between age, illness, disability, treatments and sexual activity; and awareness of the variety of sexual behaviour.
Own values   Nurses need to be able to accept their own sexuality and be comfortable with their own behaviour to enable their clients to feel the same way. This will help nurses assess and identify clients' problems with sexuality.
Communication skills   Many people are reluctant to discuss sexuality, and it is important to be able to pick up non-verbal cues, interpret hidden questions and encourage further communication. It should be said, however, that without proper support and training, nurses are likely to find it just as difficult as others to discuss sexuality. However, it is important to be alert to the problem, so they can refer their clients on to someone who can help.

Table 1. Requirements for successful counselling of sexual problems.

Norton (1981), studied the emotional effects of urinary incontinence, using a sample of 55 women aged 22-78, with a mean age of 50. Nine women had no partner, and of the remaining 46, 26 said their incontinence had affected their relationship. If nurses are to deliver sexual healthcare as part of their holistic approach to patient care, there are three main areas of preparation to consider (Table 1).

The possibility of problems with sexuality can best be ascertained at the initial nursing assessment. The amount of information that can be collected depends very much on the client's feelings about sexuality and on the nurse's communication skills, but assessment should be a continuing process, so further information can be gathered later, when a closer relationship has been established. The initial assessment should identify how the client projects him- or herself as a sexual being (in appearance and dress), whether there is a regular partner (not necessarily opposite sex) and, for females, menstrual history.

Further assessments should identify whether clients' present condition affects their sexual life, concerns about future relationships and specific problem areas. For many people, the fact that someone mentions sexuality to them is enough to encourage them to talk about their concerns. Clients are also being asked to talk about their continence problems – another taboo subject, so the step from continence to sexuality should not be too difficult for most people.

The nurse's role

Nurses should not try to play the role of psychosexual counsellor, but they do need to be able to identify whether clients need this type of help. The real nursing role is to help clients and their partners overcome the problems brought about by their condition. This should include advice on other agencies who may be able to help, including psychosexual counsellors, family planning clinics and the Association to Aid the Sexual and Personal Relationships of People with Disabilities (SPOD). There are a number of areas about which patients may feel concerned when they suffer from incontinence.

Odour Careful hygiene will eliminate the problem of odour, which only occurs when urine is exposed to the air for a time. If there is any leakage of urine, the genital area should be washed frequently. The most convenient way for women is to sit on the toilet and squeeze water from a sponge over the genital area, although this will not be adequate if there has been heavy incontinence or a heavy void, when a proper wash is necessary. If the void happened while the client was sitting down, urine will have travelled up the back, so this area will also need washing. Careful drying, with talcum powder kept to a minimum, should prevent soreness. Pads should be changed every three to four hours to avoid odour, which can also be minimised by the use of neutralising deodorant.

For men, drip pouches or external collecting devices need to be changed regularly, and the skin washed and dried well, while leaving the penis free of appliances for some time each day will help keep the skin intact and healthy. Reusable appliances should be dismantled and rinsed under cold running water to remove all traces of urine before being washed in hot soapy water, rinsed and dried well. Proper care of appliances reduces odour and prolongs their life.

Pants and pads If it is decided a woman needs to wear pads or pants, their effect on sexuality should be considered when they are being selected. Obviously pants must be functional, but nurses should try to avoid the large asexual ones in favour of closer-fitting, more feminine designs, which look similar to normal pants when worn.

Pads should be carefully considered. They must be suitable for the amount of leakage, and comfortable and unobstrusive. For women who like to wear trousers, the bulk of the pad needs to be positioned at the back.

Male devices Couples in a sexual relationship can find appliances quite off-putting. Men may not feel they have a strong, masculine image if they wear a collecting device, while women may find them a 'turn-off'. Although the type of appliance to be used should be assessed carefully, the couple should also have the chance to examine it before it is applied, as this may help them come to terms with its use. Removal at night will help the penile skin to remain healthy and intact, and should also prevent the appliance interfering with the couple's sexual activity.

During the day, urinary devices can be unobtrusive, with the leg bag attached securely to the inner leg. For men who use wheelchairs, longer trousers will ensure the bag and tap are covered.

Sexual activity
While there are hygiene considerations associated with sexual activity and incontinence, the main problems tend to be aesthetic – it is not 'nice' to be incontinent. Other problems include fear of leakage, soreness and embarrassment. Communication is most important in relationships, and clients should be encouraged to discuss their problem with their partner. It is far better to discuss the possibility that leakage may occur than letting it happen without warning. Discussion also means preparations can be made, such as protecting the bed or emptying the bladder. Both partners must be made aware that leakage of urine during intercourse is not harmful unless the urine is heavily infected.

Women with unstable bladders may find intercourse causes bladder spasm leading to leakage. This can be minimised by keeping fluid intake to a minimum and emptying the bladder before intercourse. If the couple normally make love in the missionary position, a change of position may also help reduce leakage, putting less pressure on the woman's abdomen.

Men must also be encouraged to discuss appliances with their partners. If penile vaginal intercourse is not being attempted, there is no reason why the appliance should not be left in place, provided both partners are happy about this. If vaginal intercourse is going to occur and one partner uses an appliance, hygiene is vitally important, but this preparation can become part of the lovemaking.

While leakage is less likely when the penis is erect, the bladder should be emptied prior to intercourse (although men who find it difficult to get and maintain erections may find a partially distended bladder a good stimulation – in these cases clients must be made aware of the problems of going into retention). Dyspareunia is a common problem in women with continence problems, and may be avoided by strict hygiene and frequent pad changes. In these cases, lubrication may also be required, and this should be water soluble, like KY-Jelly; Vaseline should not be used, as it can harbour bacteria in the vagina.

Communication between partners is essential to overcome potential and existing sexual problems. Nurses should ensure both partners are present when they give advice of a sexual nature, and must impress upon them that a satisfactory sexual relationship is still possible.

Long-term catheterisation

For some people, the only satisfactory way to deal with urinary elimination is long-term catheterisation. This will improve the quality of life for many people, such as women who have mobility problems and must rely on others for toileting. The pros and cons of catheterisation should be explained to both partners, encouraging them to play a part in the decision-making process. All aspects of catheterisation should be discussed, and samples of leg bags and catheters shown. The care and hygiene associated with long-term catheters must be explained carefully and the area of sexuality broached early, assuring the partners this does not mean an end to sexual activity.

Any kind of appliance can make clients feel unattractive and unappealing, and careful consideration must be given to positioning of the leg bag to make it unobtrusive but still fully functional. It may be worth giving some clients a bag they can empty themselves.

It is vital that nurses appreciate the problems clients can experience with their sexuality if they are not fully continent, and that they also appreciate that sexual activity is not confined to the under 40s. Unless they come to terms with their own sexuality and become comfortable discussing issues of sexuality with others, nurses cannot give total care to their clients with continence problems.

References
Duvall, E.M. (1971) Family Development (4th Edn). Lippincott and Co., Philadelphia, USA.
Henderson, V. (1969) Basic Principles of Nursing Care. Karger, Basle.
Jacobson, L., (1974) Illness and human sexuality. *Nursing Outlook*, **22**, 1.
Norton, C. (1982) The effects of urinary incontinence in women. *International Rehabilitation Medicine*, **4**, 1.
Suthurst, J.R. and Brown, M. (1980) Sexual dysfunction associated with urinary incontinence. *Nursing Clinician North America*, **10**, 3.
WHO (1975) Education and Treatment in Sexuality. The Training of Health Professionals.

Report of WHO Meeting. Technical Report Series No. 572. World Health Organisation, Geneva.

Useful address

SPOD (Association to Promote the Sexual and Personal Relationships of People with Disabilities), 286 Camden Road, London N7 0BJ. Tel: 071-607 8851.

18

Happy to be home? A discharge planning package for elderly people

Jo Booth, BA, BSc (Hons), RGN
Lecturer, Department of Nursing, University of Manchester; and Clinical Developments Nurse, Nursing Development Unit, Manchester Royal Infirmary.

Cath Davies, MSc, BSc (Hons), RGN, RNT
Senior Nurse, Ellen Badger Community Hospital, Shipston-on-Stour

Adequate provision for discharge of patients from hospital is now regarded as a priority by all healthcare professionals concerned with the quality of care offered to elderly people. This has arisen as a result of extensive research conducted over the past 25 years which has highlighted the numerous and varied areas where deficiency occurs.

The impetus for such research comes not only from the desire to improve care and outcomes of care, but also from the need to minimise readmission due to inadequate aftercare which tends to be both expensive and, in many cases, unnecessary. Improvements in practice have also been instigated at government level with the publication of documents such as the Department of Health circular HC/89/5 which bemoaned the lack of recent guidance on discharge arrangements from health authorities. There has, therefore, been a double stimulus to review the discharge procedures - a bottom up and a top down approach.

Planning discharge goals

Members of the multidisciplinary team must agree on the clear definition of terms before improvements in preparing for discharge can be put into practice. The term 'discharge', for example, may best be viewed as a process rather than a single event. "Discharge is regarded as a stage in patient care which has both a period of preparation and from which there are consequences. It cannot be examined in isolation from what has gone before or separated from what follows after the event when the patient leaves hospital" (Armitage, 1981).

This definition emphasises the complexity of the process, and raises two important issues for healthcare professionals responsible for planning discharges: successful discharge should reflect the care given throughout the hospital stay, and our role as coordinators of discharge extends beyond the hospital into the patient's home life. The ability to assess and meet needs accurately will mean the difference between success and failure for many patients. Embarrassing though a break-down in arrangements may be for the multidisciplinary team, it can be devastating for elderly clients who depend on these arrangements for their health, safety and ability to remain independent in the community.

'Discharge planning' according to Armitage (1981) refers to the 'period of preparation' necessary for arrangements to be made. Four key elements comprise discharge planning (Victor and Vetter, 1988):

- adequate notice of discharge;
- discussion of arrangements for aftercare;
- arrangements for aftercare;
- liaison with primary care services.

A fifth element could usefully be added to this, concerning the education of patients and carers on needs and arrangements.

Preparing a discharge package
The term 'aftercare' was first used by Roberts in 1975 as an outcome measure. She stated that aftercare is successful if it: "counteracts the disabling effects of any current stage of illness or disability, that is, it should make good any deficiency in an individual's ability to care for himself". Recent research, however, has indicated that an increased level of aftercare services is essential for many elderly people following discharge, as their level of independence in activities of living tends to be lower than it was before admission (Bowling and Betts, 1984; Waters, 1987; Victor and Vetter, 1988).

The nursing development unit at Manchester Royal Infirmary has developed a discharge package, based on research findings (Table 1). This will be discussed using Victor and Vetter's key elements as a framework.

Adequate notice of discharge
Skeet (1970) conducted a survey of 1,550 structured interviews with elderly people following discharge, and found that 12 per cent had less than 24 hours warning that they were to be discharged. A survey in 1979 (NCCOP, 1979) found that most elderly patients had two days or less notice of discharge, which is inadequate considering the range of needs which may have to be met. A small study carried out by Bowling and Betts (1984) suggests the situation may have worsened since the '70s, especially in the light of the move towards early discharge. The results showed that 42 per cent of patients were given two or more days notice of discharge, 34 per cent were told the day before and 24 per cent had no prior notice at all. Short notice may, therefore, be a major reason for the lack of accurate assessment of potential post-discharge needs, and subsequent poor planning and coordination of the discharge process, with the almost inevitable consequences of inadequate aftercare.

Discussion of aftercare arrangements

This involves accurate and thorough assessment of each individual's present home circumstances and healthcare needs to maintain or improve on their current health status and reduce levels of dependence. It is pointless investing effort and resources into patient care if discharge proves unsuccessful because nobody bothered to accurately assess and address the patient's homecare needs. Skeet (1970) showed that nurses are often not aware of the home situation of many of their patients and therefore unable to accurately determine special needs and requirements. Reports also suggest that elderly people are likely to require a greater level of aftercare support after discharge than they did before admission (Walters, 1987; Victor and Vetter, 1984; Bowling and Betts, 1984). This is true for both personal needs such as washing and dressing and household needs such as shopping, cleaning and cooking. Many health professionals are unaware of this, believing rehabilitation leads to a lowered dependency at home with less reliance on formal and informal community facilities. Skeet (1970), however, found almost half of the people interviewed had to cope with unmet needs after discharge; these included the need for equipment, advice, help with personal care, domestic support and treatment.

1. Core care plan
2. Health educational needs assessment checklist
3. Patient discharge booklet
4. Multidisciplinary team checklist
5. Information file

Table 1. Components of the discharge package.

Hockey (1968) suggested that greater anticipation by ward staff of needs for domestic assistance could allay many elderly patients' anxieties about going home. This is of vital importance given anxiety's negative effects on consequent recovery (Hayward, 1975; Seyle, 1974).

To achieve both adequate notice of discharge and discussion of aftercare arrangements, parts one and two of the discharge package are used (Table 1). A discharge planning core care plan is incorporated into each patient's complete care plan on admission, and any individual needs are documented as they arise. This usually follows discussion between primary nurse, patients and carers about healthcare needs following discharge, using the health educational needs assessment checklist to ensure that potential problem areas are not missed (Table 2).

Arrangements for aftercare

There has been little interest, until recently, in the plight of elderly people in the community following discharge, even though it was recognised as a problem as early as 1966 (Brocklehurst and Shergold, 1968). This situation has remained fairly static - evidence was available to justify major improvements in the types and quality of arrangements made, but

Activities of living
Mobility around the house
Getting up in the morning
Dressing/undressing; going to bed
Washing and bathing
Footcare
Eating, drinking; preparation of meals
Shopping
Maintenance of continence
Sexuality
Stress management/relaxation
Communication eg, care of hearing aids
Comfort needs and keeping warm

Social needs
Support of carers eg, lifting techniques
    and how to prevent pressure sores
Relief for carers (respite care)
Companionship
Advice on financial needs
Advice on how to obtain information
Self-help groups
Security needs
Worship needs

Nursing/medical needs
Understanding of diagnosis
Understanding of medication
Nursing procedures eg dressings
Arrangements for emergencies
Medical and nursing follow-up

Table 2. Health educational needs assessment checklist.

change tended to be limited to isolated examples. In 1989, however, two powerful documents were published which may have permanent and positive effects on discharge preparation. The first was the British Geriatric Society/Director of Social Services joint statement, Discharge from Hospital/Readmission to the Community, and the second the Department of Health circular HC(89)5, issued in response to the findings of the Select Committee on the Parliamentary Commissioner for Administration.

One guideline common to both documents is that planning for discharge should begin as early as possible - in cases of booked admissions, before the patient is even admitted to hospital. Another important guideline is that patients and carers should be at the centre of the planning, and written information be provided on medication, diet, treatment, lifestyle and symptoms to look for and where to obtain help if needed. These guidelines have been welcomed by professionals as they formalise the basic principles underpinning individualised, patient-centred preparation for home. In the nursing development unit, once the healthcare needs have been elicited, the primary nurse and patient complete the patient's discharge booklet. This is the patient's property and is retained by her or him from admission to hospital on into the community. It contains all the relevant information on discharge and aftercare, including the names of all professionals involved with the patient's case, what the patient should or should not do after discharge, symptoms and treatment to expect and information regarding medication. The booklet serves as a reference source for patients and their families and carers. It includes, when relevant, all the aspects highlighted for inclusion by the DoH and BGS/DSS documents.

Liaison with primary healthcare services

Nurses should coordinate discharge arrangements with the patient. It must be stressed, however, that research has found a number of potential problem areas for people holding this role. Waters (1987) and Roberts (1975) indicate that discharge planning for elderly people is not a high priority, which is reflected in the nature of the communication between hospital and the community.

Skeet (1970) suggests there is a distinct lack of communication between multidisciplinary team members and patients regarding discharge arrangements. The coordinator of the discharge procedure, therefore, faces the often onerous task of ensuring a breakdown in communication does not occur. Bowling and Betts (1984) suggest the answer lies with structured planning and documentation of each arrangement in such a way that is obvious and available to everyone involved in the care and discharge of clients. This recommendation is in keeping with the DoH circular and the BGS/DSS document, which propose that written discharge procedures be agreed and made available to all concerned with the discharge process in hospital and the community.

A multidisciplinary team checklist was therefore devised for use in the unit (Table 2), containing information on specific arrangements relating to discharge which may be of use to the team but not necessarily to the patient (for example, who booked the ambulance and when). This document is kept in a central point, rather than with the patient, so that it is easily accessible to all team members. Completion is the responsibility of the primary nurse, although all team members may make entries where appropriate. This focus of responsibility is in line with the DoH document which recommends that responsibility for coordinating discharge planning should be given to one member of staff caring for that patient.

The discharge package devised by the staff of the nursing development unit in Manchester Royal Infirmary attempts to rectify the problems that can lead to inadequate discharge planning. It has been designed to facilitate a comprehensive and systematic approach towards the process of adequately preparing patients for discharge.

References

Armitage, S. (1981) Negotiating the discharge of medical patients. *Journal of Advanced Nursing*, **6**, 385–89.

Bowling, A. and Betts, G. (1984) Communication on discharge. *Nursing Times*, **80**, 32, 31–33.

British Geriatric Society/Association of Directors of Social Services (1989) Discharge to the community of elderly patients in hospital. BGS/ADSS, London.

Brocklehurst, J. and Shergold, M. (1986) What happens when geriatric patients leave hospital? *The Lancet*, **2**, 1135–35.

Department of Health (1989) Discharge of Patients from Hospital. DoH Circular HC/89/5, London.

Hayward, J. (1975) Information: A Prescription Against Pain. RCN, London.

Hockey, L. (1968) Care in the Balance. Queen's Institute of District Nursing, London.

National Corporation for the Care of Old People (1979) Organising Aftercare: Continuing Care Project. NCCOP, London.

Roberts, I. (1975) Discharge From Hospital. RCN, London.

Royal Commission on the NHS (1978) Patients Attitudes to the Hospital Services, Research Paper 5. HMSO, London.

Selye, H. (1974) Stress without Distress. New American Library, New York.

Skeet, M. (1970) Home from Hospital. Dan Mason, Nursing Research Committee, Macmillan, London.

Victor, C. and Vetter, N. (1988) Preparing the elderly for discharge from hospital: a neglected aspect of care? *Age and Ageing*, **17**, 155–63.

Waters, K. (1987) Discharge planning: an exploratory study of the process of discharge planning on geriatric wards. *Journal of Advanced Nursing*, **12**, 71–83.

Waters, K. (1987) Outcomes of discharge from hospital for elderly people. *Journal of Advanced Nursing*, **12**, 347–55.

19

How is life treating you? Quality of life: a model for cancer care

Sheila Payne, RGN, DipN, BA, PhD
Lecturer in Psychology and Health, Department of Psychology, University of Southampton

Nurses use a number of models to guide their planning and evaluation of care. Each has its advocates, but they are largely based upon theoretical rather than empirical data (Fawcett, 1989). Nursing models are not usually rigorously tested, and nursing retains many ritualised and traditional practices (Walsh and Ford, 1989). Quality of life studies in cancer patients (eg, Padilla and Grant, 1985; Holmes and Dickerson, 1987) provide an alternative research-based body of knowledge from which nurses may derive guidelines for planning care. This paper aims to present a specific model derived from research into the quality of life of women with advanced cancer, undertaken by Payne (1989).

- Psychological state (eg, anxiety, depression)
- Physical function (eg, activities, self-care behaviours)
- Symptoms (these may be due to the disease, such as pain, or side-effects of treatment, such as nausea and vomiting)
- Social relationships (eg, marital and family relationships)
- Social roles (eg, employment, mothering, being a spouse)

Table 1. Principal factors constituting quality of life.

Quality of life is a multidimensional concept. It is useful to nursing because it extends the outcome criteria from merely biomedical aspects of patients' welfare, such as survival and morbidity, to include psychological, social and functional aspects of life. Although there has been a lack of consensus on exactly what would be included in quality of life assessments, recent research (Payne, 1989) suggests that the areas listed in Table 1 are important.

Psychological state

Numerous studies have indicated that a significant minority (25-33 per cent) of cancer patients experience psychological distress. Sadly, much of this goes unrecognised and untreated because health professionals lack the necessary skills to discover, or deal with the distress (Maguire, 1984). Anxiety and depression were found to be the most important predictors of quality of life in a sample of women with advanced breast or ovarian cancer treated by palliative chemotherapy (Payne, 1989).

Anxiety and depression are the psychological states which most commonly inhibit people from being satisfied with their quality of life. Anxiety is an unpleasant feeling of tension, which readers may recall from being new on a ward or from taking examinations. Many people experience anxiety on every outpatient clinic visit. These feelings may be transient and quickly fade on return home, but for some, anxiety remains dominant, making it difficult to relax and preventing them concentrating on everyday tasks or pleasures such as reading or watching television.

Depression, on the other hand, involves gloomy thoughts and feelings, and prevents people deriving pleasure from their normal pursuits. Though it may come and go, when depression settles like a dark cloud over someone, they find it difficult to enjoy anything. It is associated with lethargy and a lack of motivation to do anything. At times, cancer patients may be tired and lethargic because they are too ill to do anything, and feelings of depression may accompany this state.

In assessing patients, nurses can look for behavioural signs of anxiety (eg, clenched hands, tense facial muscles) and depression (eg, failure to smile or laugh). Most patients will be able to describe how they feel 'in themselves', although some people assume nurses are only interested in their physical condition. It is helpful to specifically ask if they have felt 'down', 'sad' or 'uptight' recently and what triggered these feelings.

An alternative method of assessing a psychological state is to use a questionnaire. The Hospital Anxiety and Depression (HAD) scale (Zig-

---

Anxiety question
I feel tense or 'wound up':
  Most of the time
  A lot of the time
  Time to time, occasionally
  Not at all

Depression question
I still enjoy the things I used to enjoy:
  Definitely as much
  Not quite so much
  Only a little
  Hardly at all

Table 2. Examples from the Hospital Anxiety and Depression scale.

mond and Snaith, 1983) is eminently suitable; examples of the questions used are shown in Table 2. The scale contains no questions about physical problems such as anorexia, as these may confuse the results because they can be attributed to the disease. Most people suffering from cancer can answer this questionnaire in about five minutes. Use of the HAD scale could help show which patients need further care to deal with their emotional difficulties.

Helping patients to cope with emotional distress should begin with offering them a comfortable place and plenty of time to disclose their feelings, in privacy. Skills in counselling and active listening are essential to hearing what distressed people are saying. The opportunity to express thoughts and feelings in an accepting therapeutic relationship may be sufficient to promote the patient's own coping resources, but it may be appropriate to refer some patients, with their agreement, to specialist professionals such as social workers or clinical psychologists.

The way nurses interact with patients may contribute to, or alleviate psychological distress. Evidence from a study of women with primary breast cancer suggests the provision of treatment choices and open communication promoted adjustment and reduced the incidence of anxiety and depression in the women and their partners (Morris and Royle, 1988). People differ in the amount and type of information they can deal with at specific time, however, so it is important to ensure that patients and relatives receive as little or as much information as they desire at each stage of their illness.

Physical function

At a basic level, physical function can be assessed by the ability to get out of bed and perform self-care behaviours such as washing and dressing. People with cancer may experience dramatic fluctuations in physical function, for example, related to chemotherapy. The days immediately following a drug cycle may be functionally restricted, perhaps spent lying down, due to severe nausea. A week later, however, the same person may be able to return to work. Functional deficit may be a constant feature of the lives of others, perhaps due to surgery such as loss of the voice after laryngectomy, or the extreme tiredness which may accompany advanced disease.

In assessing physical function of people in hospital, it is helpful to ask people what they can do at home. Many people still anticipate that when they are in hospital, they are expected to become fairly inactive. Patients may appreciate being asked what they would like to do for themselves such as washing in the bathroom instead of by the bed.

Once identified, needs for increased mobility can be negotiated with patients. This may involve identifying and dealing with the factors inhibiting movement, such as metastatic bone pain (give analgesia), fear of falling (offer to accompany the patient or provide a stick), or the fact that there is nowhere interesting to walk to (suggest a trip to the hospital shop or cafe).

Symptoms

Nurses are generally skilled at assessing people's responses to their illness and treatment, but at times, it is difficult to separate the effects of these two factors in contributing to a specific symptom. For example, tiredness may be due to the effects of chemotherapy, radiotherapy, or the cancer itself. This confusion may mean the patient wrongly attributes the symptoms to worsening disease, when in reality, there might be considerable improvement after recovery from therapy. Clear explanation of potential side-effects will help prevent such unnecessary anxiety.

Personal characteristics, such as age and personality, will determine how people perceive symptoms and what those symptoms mean to them. People strive to make sense of their world, especially in the presence of ambiguous information. Women with advanced breast cancer have been shown to attempt to monitor the progress of their cancer and chemotherapy by interpreting their symptoms (Payne, 1989). One woman thought pain indicated the drugs were causing her cancer to shrink. Another was concerned when a drug cycle made her less nauseated than usual, thinking the degree of nausea was directly related to the effectiveness of the drugs. Both women tolerated physical symptoms that could have been relieved because they mistakenly believed they were an essential part of therapy. Unnecessary suffering can be prevented by eliciting patients' understandings of their disease and treatment, and modifying these beliefs if necessary.

Evidence indicates that for most patients, pain continues to be poorly assessed and under-treated (Noyles, 1981), although there have been impressive improvements in palliative care. Only patients can know the true nature and extent of their pain, and since language to describe pain is often inadequate, pain measurement scales can be useful. The visual analogue scale (VAS) consists of a straight line labelled "no pain" at one end and "worst pain ever" at the other (Table 3). The patient is asked to place a mark on the line corresponding to the intensity of his or her pain.

Place a mark on the line where you feel your pain is now
No pain ————————————————————— worst pain ever

Table 3. Pain measurement scale.

A quick and easy method of measuring the effectiveness of analgesia, the VAS can be used regularly as a record of pain, and means patients do not have to rely on nurses' interpretation of their verbal description of pain. It is also suitable for monitoring other subjective symptoms, such as nausea and fatigue.

The body chart is an alternative measure which requires patients to indicate the location, intensity, duration and nature of their pain on outline drawings of the body. It is useful for providing detailed information about pain, particularly when monitoring the effectiveness of analgesic drugs or interventions. The disadvantage to these measures is that they assume patients will respond honestly, and take no account of situational and cultural meanings of pain or analgesic use, while not everyone can understand how to use these techniques and some may prefer to use verbal descriptions.

Social relationships

Cancer affects whole families, not just sufferers. Most people with cancer will have social concerns about their jobs, marriages, and children's welfare, which are influenced by treatment characteristics such as frequency and duration of hospitalisation. Likewise, the type and stage of cancer will make different demands on both the patient's and family's coping resources.

There is considerable, although not unequivocal evidence (Peters-Golden, 1982), that social support (a range of emotional and practical help from family and friends) contributes to a better quality of life, possibly because people who feel they have or can obtain help from others are better able to withstand the stress of life-threatening disease. Social support involves practical assistance, such as doing housework or caring for children, but also in making sufferers believe they are cared for, loved and accepted in a relationship. This helps build up self-esteem.

Social support may also be provided by fulfilling informational needs. People with cancer are often bombarded by advice from many people, and this appears to be appraised in terms of its credibility (Payne, 1989). Women with breast cancer developed a ranking of credible information sources, headed by the oncologist. Since they had little access to him they sought information from their GPs and nurses. Interestingly, nurses were perceived to know little about cancer and its treatment, except for the ward sister. There appears to be an important connection between the perception of informational needs and the ability to provide for them.

A recognition that social support is a contributor to quality of life will raise awareness of the vital role played by families and spouses, who can work with nurses as participants in promoting optimal quality of life. This may mean nurses have to spend time helping them to understand the disease and treatment, or offering support to the spouse who may wish to talk about concerns and feelings away from the patient. Contact can be maintained after patients die, to help relatives to grieve, perhaps by arranging bereavement counselling if this is needed.

Social roles

We all perform a number of social roles, such as spouse, parent, son or daughter, employee, and these provide us with our identity, income, and feelings of self-worth. It is generally disturbing to relinquish a role, even when we do so voluntarily, as in retirement. When it is forced upon us, it can be doubly distressing.

Women with advanced breast cancer used aspects of their roles to monitor their progress (Payne, 1989), defining recovery in terms of their ability to regain control of a task. For example, housewives normally control the family budget, making decisions about choosing and buying food, and prioritising domestic tasks. This provides some women with power, as well as making them feel needed and valued. One woman maintained her control by making the shopping list even when her husband had to buy the food. Another carefully supervised the sorting of the laundry and loading of the washing machine from her chair. Some of the women rejected offers of help once they were physically able to perform domestic chores, because these tasks helped to give their lives meaning. In others paid employment served a similar function.

The learned helplessness theory (Seligman, 1975) suggests that if nurses do too much for patients it teaches them to become passive and helpless. Promoting self-care and facilitating the performance of social roles, however limited, can contribute to people's sense of wellbeing.

People who develop cancer also acquire, sometimes reluctantly, the role of 'cancer patient', and all roles produce expectations about how the person should behave. Not everyone with cancer wishes to affiliate with other sufferers or even accepts the identity and behaviours implicit in the role, and it is important to guard against seeing and reacting to the stereotypical 'cancer patient', rather than the individual who happens to have cancer.

Limitation of quality of life

There are certain problems associated with the quality of life model. The lack of clarity in the concept of quality of life produces an unacceptable degree of methodological confusion. This might mean the model cannot generate clinically useful outcomes in nursing practice. Payne asserts that quality of life should be self-evaluation, but this excludes its use with people who lack insight, such as unconscious or mentally confused people. Decisions are made for these people based on assumed or projected quality of life considerations. Indeed, even patients who are cognitively capable of making quality of life evaluations may produce biased responses, due to coping strategies such as denial, or compliance with authority.

Quality of life is a descriptive construct, and as such provides labels but not explanations of behaviour. Although the model was derived from empirical work with cancer patients, the small sample size may limit its validity for other groups of patients, but this will only tell if nurses evaluate the model in their practice. Only rigorous independent testing will determine the model's value and indicate the modifications that are necessary before it can be advocated for general use.

Quality of life data enable nursing care to be directed toward patients' salient concerns, which are likely to change over time and with changes in treatment. Quality of life assessments therefore indicate which issues are salient and when. They focus on the predictors of illness adjustment, so nursing care plans can be designed for, and targeted to encompass a wide range of psychological, physical and social outcomes. The use of research-based evidence allows nurses to offer optimal quality of care, which is derived from more than simply traditional practices and intuitive assumptions.

References

Fawcett, J. (1989) Analysis and Evaluation of Conceptual Models of Nursing (2nd Ed.). Quest-Meridien Ltd., Beckenham.

Holmes, S. and Dickerson, J.W.T. (1987) The quality of life: design and evaluation of a self-assessment instrument for use with cancer patients. *International Journal of Nursing Studies*, **24**, 1, 15-24.

Maguire, P. (1984) Communication Skills and Patient Care. In: Steptoe, A. and Mathews, A. (Eds) Heath Care and Human Behaviour. Academic Press, London.

Morris, J. and Royle, G.T. (1988) Offering patients a choice of surgery for early breast cancer. *Social Science and Medicine*, **26**, 6, 583-85.

Noyes, R. (1981) Treatment of cancer pain. *Psychosomatic Medicine*, **43**, 1, 57-70.

Padilla, G.V. and Grant, M.M. (1985) Quality of life as a cancer nursing outcome variable. *Advances in Nursing Science*, **8**, 1, 45-60.

Payne, S. (1989) Quality of Life in Women with Advanced Cancer. Unpublished PhD thesis. University of Exeter.

Peters-Golden, H. (1982) Breast cancer: varied perceptions of social support in the illness experience. *Social Science and Medicine*, **16**, 438-91.

Seligman, M.E.P. (1975) Helplessness: on Depression, Development and Death. W.H.Freeman, San Francisco.

Walsh, M. and Ford, P. (1989) Rituals in Nursing. *Nursing Times*, **85**, 41, 26-35.

Zigmond, A.S. and Snaith, R.P. (1983) The hospital anxiety and depression scale. *Acta Psychiatrica Scandinavia*, **67**, 361-70.

Issues in Patient Care

20
Confidentiality

Elizabeth M. Horne, MA
Managing Director, Professional Nurse

The Code of Professional Conduct (UKCC, 1984) states that: registered nurses, midwives and health visitors shall: "Respect confidential information obtained in the course of professional practice and refrain from disclosing such information without the consent of the patient/client, or a person entitled to act on his/her behalf, except where disclosure is required by law or by the order of a court, or is necessary in the public interest."

Conflicts in practice

Isolated from practice, this statement may seem reasonable, but practitioners are daily faced with decisions based on the application of these principles in situations which may contain inherent conflicts of interest. They need confident, working definitions of the elements involved, and to establish clear priorities between the expectations of their patients and those of a wider public. Not so easy when, for example, a sister in a psychiatric day hospital finds a patient in possession of large quantities of controlled drugs that he cannot have obtained legally, or an occupational health nurse is asked by her manager for information about an employee. These examples are cited by the UKCC in an advisory paper on confidentiality (UKCC, 1987), which suggests that the most difficult problem for practitioners is identifying and establishing the boundary between clients' expectations that information will not be disclosed, and the expectations of the public that they will not be unreasonably put at risk.

Confidentiality is important for effective communication

The knowledge that confidentiality will be respected is important for effective communication. There is much information people would not discuss with anyone unless they knew the recipient was completely trustworthy in their offer of confidentiality. Without this trust they may choose to keep quiet, which could affect their health.

Standards of confidentiality should be made clear to clients

It is not practicable to obtain clients' consent every time information needs to be shared with other health professionals, so it should be made known to all clients what standards of confidentiality are maintained.

The practitioner who holds the information must ensure, as far as possible, that it is imparted in strict professional confidence and for a specific purpose serving interests of the client. An individual practitioner is responsible for deciding when it is necessary to obtain the explicit consent of a patient or client.

Practitioners must be familiar with how record systems are used, who has access to them and what are the risks to confidentiality associated with their use. Where students, or those involved in research, require access to records, the same principles of confidentiality apply, and the patient's consent must be sought where appropriate, and the use of the records closely supervised.

Breaches of confidentiality

The principle of confidentiality must be the rule, and breaches of it exceptional; the practitioner must be sure that the best interests of theclient, or thoseof confidential information. The interests of the community may, occasionally, take precedence over those of an individual.

The withholding or disclosing of confidential information may have serious consequences, and the practitioner's decision can be extremely difficult. However, the responsibility cannot be delegated. The individual practitioner must make the decision, and must be able to justify it. It may be helpful to make a written note of the decision and reasons for it on the file for future reference. Situations of this nature can be very stressful, and if other practitioners are aware of them, it may be helpful to discuss the problems. However it is still the responsibility of the individual practitioner, and he or she must ultimately make their own decision.

The UKCC Advisory Paper on Confidentiality is available from: UKCC, 23 Portland Place, London W1N 3AF (send a S.A.E.). It discusses the responsibility of individual practitioners for confidentiality, and the everyday implications for practice, the ownership and care of information, and some of the issues which arise when confidentiality is deliberately breached.

References
United Kingdom Central Council for Nursing, Midwifery and Health Visiting, (1984). Code of Professional Conduct for the Nurse, Midwife and Health Visitor. Second Edition. UKCC, London.
United Kingdom Central Council for Nursing, Midwifery and Health Visiting, (1987). Confidentiality: A UKCC Advisory Paper, UKCC, London.

21

Who needs nursing philosophies?

Dominic Mawdsley, BA, RGN
Charge Nurse, Urology, Hammersmith Hospital, London

Much has been said about philosophies for care, but little literature on the subject has been written for guidance. Most nurses know they are expected to have philosophies of care for their areas, but few know their purpose and how to go about writing them. The English National Board (ENB, 1988) states that all areas involved in nurse training must have a philosophy, while the other national boards also have similar requirements. The mention of national board directives makes most nurses roll their eyes upwards and start muttering profanities under their breath. However, if the boards say so, then that word tends to become law. Everyone rushes off, hurriedly writes a philosophy for care, breathes a sigh of relief when the visit is over and then puts the philosophy in the top drawer of sister's desk until the next visit.

The inclination is, therefore, to mention such directives as an afterthought in order to discourage the view that this is a time-wasting exercise devised to keep nurses busy. Encouragement and motivation are far more likely to get a philosophy written.

A philosophy is an invaluable tool which directs and influences patient care. It is a series of beliefs, feelings, values and outlooks that can be developed in any area concerned with patient care, with the purpose of demonstrating what nurses feel their particular specialty should be achieving both for patients and nursing staff. This will only be the case, however, if nurses have a true understanding of what a philosophy is and how to go about developing one.

How to write a philosophy

Various methods have been used for developing philosophies, such as being presented with one from management and asked to comment on it (the 'top down' approach), questionnaires, or a 'cascade' method. The disadvantage of these methods is that philosophies generated in these ways will all ultimately reflect the preconceived ideas of the initiator. More successful, however, is a 'bottom-up' approach, involving all the staff of the relevant area (Figure 1).

Time should be allocated for study days and fact finding so that all staff become familiar with the process of writing a philosophy and can obtain any relevant research or information required. A nurse specialist or facilitator should be included if one is available, to act as an objective party who can support and advise from the outside. However, if no nurse specialist is available, a facilitator usually emerges from within the group.

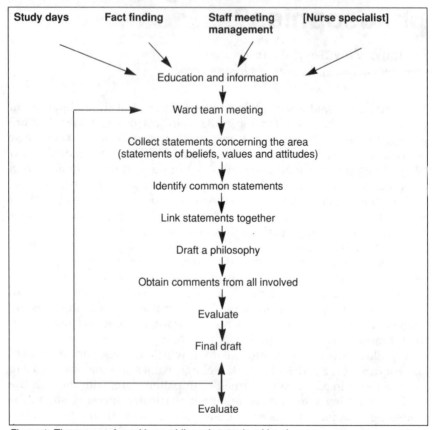

Figure 1. The process for writing a philosophy at a local level.

This initial ground work and organisation means there is a wealth of information and education which is pooled at the ward team meeting. By 'brainstorming', and sharing ideas, common beliefs and values will emerge which ultimately reflect philosophy, purpose and objectives. There are no strict rules and no set length, although a philosophy of three lines will provide little direction, and one several pages long will deter potential readers. What is desirable, however, is that nursing jargon and clichés are avoided. Moore (1971) wrote: "This tendency to make use of pot-boiler statements culled from the folklore of nursing does serve a purpose of sorts: it protects nurses from looking at the realities of their jobs and evaluating their own activities." This can also make a philosophy incomprehensible and indigestible to non-nurses.

Why bother?

Are there any benefits to be gained from having a philosophy, or is it yet another piece of paper produced by nurses who have nothing better to do with their time? If a philosophy is truly a statement of belief and intent, then it must have practical applications (Romhanyi, 1990). A written philosophy provides a chance to reflect on practice: the process of writing it necessitates examining and justifying nursing practice. This leads practitioners to question whether practices are carried out on a traditional basis "because we've always done it this way", or whether they truly benefit patient care, so not only will individual practice be questioned, but also the beliefs and practices of the team.

Philosophies translate practice into writing. Nurses as a group are good at 'feeling and intuition', but are sometimes hard-pushed to clarify these in black and white. This may be one of the most difficult aspects of formulating a philosophy, but once practice is committed to writing, it will direct a group in the achievement of a purpose and therefore promote continuity of care. This must be preferable to a situation where nurses deliver erratic care because they are following a 'gut feeling'.

This continuity will go on to develop a team and promote a harmonious relationship with clinicians from other disciplines. Philosophies need not be solely for nursing; if members of the multidisciplinary team are involved in writing them, a truly holistic approach can be adopted. For instance, physiotherapists in intensive care units play a crucial role in the care of critically ill patients and should therefore have their values and beliefs reflected in their unit's philosophy. It must also be remembered that a philosophy serves to clarify the nurse's role to other members of the team.

A philosophy can also be used as a justification of quality of service. Proof can be given to managers that quality care is being delivered – an extremely important aspect in the light of the proposals contained within Working for Patients (DoH, 1989). Leading on from this, it can also provide a base for the development of standards of care. Either problem areas will be identified when writing the philosophy, or standards will be developed as measuring tools for the quality service being guaranteed in the philosophy.

An appropriate model of nursing may also be developed from a philosophy; once beliefs and practices have been questioned, it may become apparent that care delivery is inappropriate. This, in turn, will lead nurses to question whether the framework being used within the nursing process for delivering care is meeting patients' needs, or whether it can be improved upon. Would the application of an alternative nursing model or the development of one's own enhance nursing care?

Patient expectations

A philosophy can increase the awareness of patients/clients about what they can expect during their period under care if it is displayed in a prominent position. In many ways this is a brave thing to do, as nurses are laying themselves open to potential criticism and complaint, but patients would be quite within their rights to challenge staff and ask why they are not doing what is laid down within the philosophy. However, it has been observed that patients have read philosophies and commented to staff that their care truly reflects them. Medical staff may also find it interesting to read a ward philosophy, as it may clarify the aims and objectives of nursing practices in the clinical area and help them understand the need for the nursing process and individualised patient care at a time when nurses are moving away from the traditional image of 'ministering angels'.

Ward philosophies can also provide invaluable information for student nurses, particularly if they are sent out in an orientation package prior to the start of their allocation. How many of us started on a ward as students and spent the first week hiding in the sluice room trying to work out sister's likes and dislikes – a phenomenon supported by research by Fretwell (1982) and Pembrey (1980)? The ward philosophy can provide insight into the workings and the personalities of the ward.

By the same token, philosophies can be used for recruitment purposes when sent out with job descriptions and application forms. Candidates can then decide whether the unit is compatible with their particular ethos or whether it would be a waste of time for both parties to continue with the application. Should they decide to continue with the application, philosophies can be useful at interview; candidates may question the philosophy and ask for elaboration, and interviewers may be able to ascertain if the candidate is right for the environment.

Taking this one step further, philosophies may then be used to aid nurse appraisal on both sides. If care appears inconsistent and of a poor quality, managers can use the philosophy to redirect care and serve the nurse a reminder of what has previously been guaranteed. On the other hand, nurses may actually use it to demonstrate that the objectives outlined are not being achieved, possibly due to lack of staff or equipment, and that patient care is being compromised.

Finally, philosophies provide tools for teaching. The process of writing a philosophy means all those concerned will have to have access to relevant education and information. This may well involve fact finding and study days, and thus lead on to other areas of interest. Should the need to examine standards of care or nursing models become apparent, that in itself is a different aspect of the trained nurse's education, so philosophies can play a significant part in continuing education.

Evaluation

A philosophy, therefore, is a useful tool with a variety of applications. Table 1 is an extract from one of the ward philosophies at Westminster Hospital, which demonstrates the values and intentions of the nursing staff on a dermatology ward.

It is important, however, to evaluate the philosophy of care regularly, and this should take into account staff changes or change of the clinical specialty; otherwise it should be done at least yearly. Even if the philosophy remains unchanged, the process will serve as a reminder and ensure that it continues to reflect the beliefs of the clinical area.

"We feel that it is important to welcome patients warmly to the ward. We recognise that hospital is not home, but by being friendly and approachable we hope to portray a relaxed environment and also reduce some of the patients' fears and anxieties.

"Any disfiguring disease can cause a distorted body image and also lower a person's morale and confidence. Therefore, it is important for us to promote patients' self-confidence in their appearance and in their personal value, and to be particularly sensitive to their needs and feelings.

"An important part of our work is the education of patients and their relatives. We encourage them to participate in their care and we teach them how to apply any treatments that are to be continued at home. By educating patients and relatives we hope to increase their understanding and awareness of their conditions and also help to maximise the potential of individuals to adapt and to cope with any physical/psychological disorder."

Table 1. Extract from a dermatology ward philosophy.

Nursing philosophies, as well as providing nurses with an opportunity to reflect on ward practice, may also help them harmonise their working relationships; provide written proof that quality of care is being given; and lead to development of an appropriate model of nursing for their clinical environment. As such, they are a resource not to be underused.

References

DoH (1989) Working for Patients. HMSO, London.

ENB (1988) Institution and Course Approval/Reapproval Process: Information required, criteria and guidelines (1983/39/APS). ENB, London.

Fretwell, J.G. (1982) Ward Teaching and Learning. Royal College of Nursing, London.

Moore, M. (1971) Philosophy, purpose and objectives: why do we need them? *Journal of Nursing Administration*, **1**, 3, 9-14.

Pembrey, S. (1980) The Ward Sister: Key to Nursing. Royal College of Nursing, London.

Romhanyi, A. (1990) A time to reflect. *Nursing Times*, **86**, 21, 33-34.

22

The Stirling model of nursing audit: its relationship to standard setting and quality assurance

Moya J. Morison, BSc, MSc, BA, RGN

Clinical Audit Co-ordinator, Stirling Royal Infirmary

Every organisation has a responsibility to monitor the quality of its activities, to identify areas where quality is below an agreed standard and take appropriate remedial action to guarantee the customer a specified degree of excellence of a product or service. This is quality assurance. Quality control is the means by which quality is assured (Table 1). Nurses have long been concerned with assuring their patients a high quality of care, and have employed many methods of quality control including informal peer review, standard setting, monitoring and evaluating practice, and systematic audit using generic tools such as Monitor (Goldstone *et al*, 1983) and Qualpacs (Wandelt and Ager, 1974).

Quality control is the means by which quality is assured
• Informal peer review
• Standard setting, monitoring and evaluation
• Audit

Table 1. Quality control.

Pressures on healthcare professionals to introduce audit are coming from the government, royal colleges and hospital management as well as from within the professions themselves. 'Working for Patients' (DoH, 1989) recognises the most effective studies are likely to be internally generated with local peer group review of the data under analysis. It advocates a 'bottom-up' rather than 'top-down' approach, but with the proviso that management can initiate an independent professional audit, for example where there is cause to question the quality or cost-effectiveness of the service.

Redfern and Norman (1990) argue that a preoccupation with cost-effectiveness threatens to swamp nurses' traditional concern with quality of care and underline the importance of clinical nurses becoming familiar with the concepts and complexities of measuring quality. This chapter aims to explore the nature of nursing audit and its relationship to standard setting and quality assurance, and to describe how one Scottish Unit is developing a philosophy of, and a method for, nursing audit which builds upon the standard setting and quality assurance initiatives already underway.

Chart audit

What is audit? In its oldest sense auditing means: "an examination of accounts by an authorised person or persons" (Chambers 20th Century Dictionary). Churchill's Illustrated Medical Dictionary (1989) defines medical audit as: "Detailed retrospective review and evaluation of medical records by skilled staff to assess the care that was provided". Unless the notes are highly structured, this is a time consuming exercise because of the difficulties in retrieving information, yet review of practice by reference to records is now an established system for medical audit in the USA (Hopkins, 1990), and is the basis of several generic nursing audit tools such as Phaneuf's Nursing Audit (1976).

The assumption with all audits of records is that the quality of care and the quality of documentation are related. This is not always so (Mayers *et al*, 1977). A nurse may give competent technical care in a compassionate manner and have excellent interpersonal skills, but may be poor at documenting the care given. Conversely, several studies have shown that the care actually given may fall far short of that painstakingly prescribed in individualised care plans. Furthermore, nurses soon learn how to document care in a way which favourably influences the audit results (Jelinek *et al*, 1974), and Hegyvary and Haussman (1976) argue that chart audit only serves to improve documentation, not care. Despite all these arguments, auditing nursing records can be useful as part of a quality assurance programme if other measures of care are also recorded.

A broader perspective

A broader definition of medical audit given in 'Working for Patients' is: "The systematic, critical analysis of the quality of medical care, including the procedures for diagnosis and treatment, the use of resources and the resulting outcome and quality of life for the patient".

Within this very broad definition, many operational methods can be developed. An audit can be carried out retrospectively or prospectively. It can include record or chart review, patient and staff interviews, the use of questionnaires, direct observation of activity or any combination of these. Generic (preformulated) measuring instruments can be used. The uses, advantages and disadvantages of some of the most widely available generic nursing audit tools are reviewed by Pearson (1987), Dunne (1987) and Sale (1990). Alternatively, an audit tool can be developed locally to gain insights into a perceived problem. The tool can include items to measure the criteria and level of performance previously agreed in a locally generated standard relating to the problem.

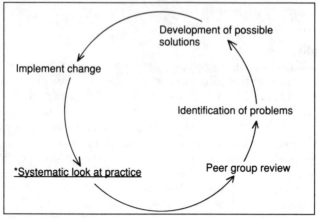

Figure 1. The audit cycle.

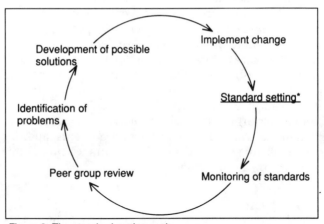

Figure 2. The standard setting cycle.

The principle stages in the audit cycle are summarised in Figure 1; similarities with the standard setting cycle (Figure 2) are immediately apparent. Both have quality assurance as their primary aim and involve:

- peer group review of data;
- problem identification;
- the development of solutions to the problems identified;
- implementing change aimed at overcoming these problems.

There are, however, certain differences. Standard setting involves agreeing ahead the criteria for the process, including an acceptable level of performance and monitoring this, while in a purely audit study there need be no predefined expectations of the process. Audit involves a systematic look at what is actually happening - different practices may be compared but there need be no advanced decision about what constitutes best practice. In reality many standard setting projects have an audit component and in most, if not all, audit studies there are implicit normative standards.

Introducing nursing audit locally

The Strategy for Nursing, Midwifery and Health Visiting in Scotland (SHHD, 1990) highlighted as a key objective the establishment of a system of nursing audit, in tandem with continued development and monitoring of standards of care. We at Stirling saw this as an opportunity to review our priorities in nursing quality assurance initiatives, and out of our deliberations came our model of nursing audit (as depicted on the wallchart) in which we defined audit and explored the audit process and its relationship to standard setting initiatives already well under way.

When developing our strategy we:

- agreed a management statement,

- identified key objectives,

- prepared an action plan and timetable for our short-term goals.

Appropriateness
Meeting the actual needs of individuals, families and communities

Effectiveness
Achieving the intended benefit

Acceptability
Satisfying patients' reasonable expectations

Continuity
Of care and care provider(s)

Accessibility
Availability not unduly restricted by time, distance or finance

Efficiency
Maximising outcomes with the available resources

Table 2. Dimensions of quality of healthcare (based on Shaw, 1986).

We had to agree what we felt nursing audit was, what we were aiming to achieve by it, the nature of the audit process and how to build on the standard setting and quality assurance initiatives already underway. We decided on a definition of nursing audit which would be compatible with that of our medical colleagues, with its emphasis on a critical look at the quality of care and outcomes and quality of life for the patient. We discussed the dimensions of quality as described by Shaw (1986) (Table 2), and using Donabedian's (1969) framework of structure, process and outcome, summarised the key factors to consider when measuring quality of care (Table 3). These aims are what we hope to achieve through nursing audit:

- to improve the quality of patient care;

- to make the most efficient use of resources;

- to foster in nurses a critical questioning approach to their activities and the needs of their patients.

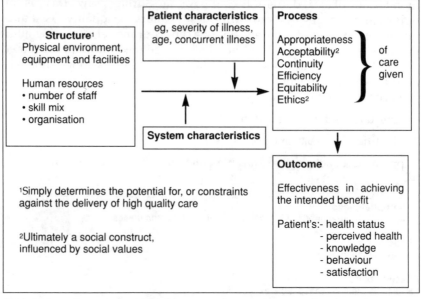

Table 3. Some factors to consider when attempting to measure quality of care (based on Donabedian , 1969; Shaw,1986; Hopkins, 1990).

Creating a climate for audit

A major objective is to create a positive climate for audit, involving the maximum number of practice based nurses in a small way without impinging on their time spent with patients.

It is natural and understandable that people should initially resist being involved in audit. One definition of audit is "a calling to account", which has many negative connotations, and people may feel threatened. Resistance to audit, or to any change, manifests in many ways: rarely as outright aggression, more often as lethargy while paying lip service to the change. Things only get done by the enthusiasts.

It is therefore vital to create a positive climate for enquiry from the outset and to address issues of confidentiality fully and frankly with staff, discussing ways of maintaining patient and staff anonymity. More positively, audit should be regarded as an important component of nurses' continuing professional development, helping them individually to identify their strengths as well as their continuing education and training needs.

Creating a climate for enquiry involves organising an education programme to ensure the nursing staff understand what they are trying to do and how to set about it. Nursing staff themselves should identify and decide the priorities for local audit projects.

Priorities for audit

When deciding our priorities for audit, we felt it was important to ensure we chose topics where the nurse's intervention had most influence on outcome for the patient. We are for instance looking at pressure sore prevention, wound care in the community, nursing care of dying patients and pain control, beyond merely the giving of analgesia. Some topics selected and seen as priorities for audit are summarised in Table 4.

• Pressure sore prevention
• Care of the dying patient
• Bereavement counselling for relatives
• Information giving
• Pain control
• Wound assessment
• Maintaining a safe environment for the confused or aggressive patient
• Source isolation: barrier nursing
• Chemotherapy

Table 4. Some topics seen by staff as priorities for audit.

Integrating nursing audit with standard setting initiatives already underway was identified as a high priority. The essence of the Stirling model is the integration of the two approaches (Figure 3). Quality assurance can start with standard setting or a prospective look at current practice or both concurrently. An example will make this more clear.

We are interested in pressure sore prevention in non-ambulant patients brought to the A&E department, as research has identified these patients to be at high risk. A standard has been written on pressure sore prevention in A&E and a monitoring tool to compare observed practice with the agreed standard is being developed. We have decided to carry out an audit at the same time to help us identify:

- how many high risk patients arrive in A&E over a month and whether there is any pattern to the time of the day the injuries are sustained;

- patients' primary diagnosis;

- how long patients wait in A&E before transfer to the ward;

- the pressure relieving equipment currently available and whether it is in use.

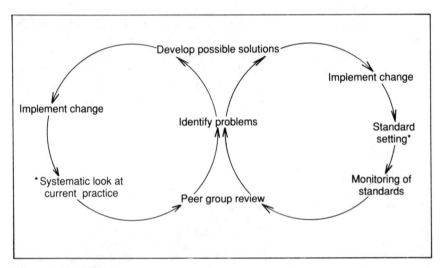

Figure 3. Nursing audit.

It may be helpful to think of our model of nursing audit (Figure 3) as a pair of spectacles which allow nurses to look systematically at their practice and its effectiveness. The audit 'lens' has its ancestry in healthcare research. The standard setting 'lens' represents the existing work on nursing standard setting and quality assurance. Each has a great deal to offer on its own, but together they provide a useful conceptual framework of nursing audit within which a variety of operational methods can be developed. Two lenses give a more three dimensional view of nursing practice than looking at practice through one.

The Stirling model is helping us to understand what we are trying to do, the stages in the audit process, and the relationship between nursing audit and standard setting. It is evolving, as the concept of audit in the NHS is itself evolving, in the light of our experience, but no doubt we have still got a great deal to learn.

References

Department of Health (1989) Working for Patients: Medical Audit (Working Paper No. 6), HMSO, London.

Donabedian, A. (1969) Some issues in evaluating the quality of nursing care. *American Journal of Public Health*, **39,** 10, 1833-36.

Dunne, L.M. (1987) Quality assurance: methods of measurement. *The Professional Nurse* , **2,** 6, 187-90.

Goldstone, L.A., Ball, J.A., Collier, M. (1983) Monitor: an Index of the Quality of Nursing Care for Acute Medical and Surgical Wards. Newcastle-upon-Tyne Polytechnic, Newcastle-upon-Tyne.

Hegyvary, S. and Haussman, R. (1976) Monitoring nursing care quality. *Journal of Nursing Administration.* **6,** 9, 6-9.

Hopkins, A. (1990) Measuring Quality of Medical Care. Royal College of Physicians of London.

Jelinek, D., Haussman, R., Hegyvary, S. (1974) A Methodology for Monitoring Quality of Nursing Care. US Department of Health, Education and Welfare, Bethesda, Maryland.

Mayers, M., Norby, R.B., Watson, A.B. (1977) Quality Assurance for Patient Care - Nursing Perspectives. Appleton-Century-Crofts, New York.

Pearson, A. (Ed.) (1987) Nursing Quality Measurement: Quality Assurance Methods for Peer Review. John Wiley, Chichester.

Phaneuf, M. (1976) the Nursing Audit. Appleton - Century - Crofts, New York.

Redfern, S.J. and Norman I.J. (1990) Measuring the Quality of Nursing Care: A Consideration of Different Approaches. *Journal of Advanced Nursing*, **15,** 1260-71.

Sale, D. (1990) Quality Assurance. Essentials of Nursing Management Series. MacMillan, London.

Scottish Home and Health Department (1990) A Strategy for Nursing, Midwifery and Health Visiting in Scotland. HMSO, Edinburgh.

Shaw, C.D. (1986) Introducing Quality Assurance. Paper No. 64, Kings Fund, London.

Wandelt, M. and Ager, J. (1974) Quality Patient Care Scale. Appleton-Century-Crofts, New York.

Bibliography

Scottish Home and Health Department (1988) Quality Assurance in Nursing: Report of a Working Group of National Nursing and Midwifery Consultative Committee. HMSO, Edinburgh.

Royal College of Nursing (1989) A Framework for Quality. Royal College of Nursing Standards of Care Project. Royal College of Nursing, London.

23

Balancing public concern and patients' rights in HIV testing

Ann Shuttleworth, BA
Editor, Professional Nurse

The issue of HIV testing gained further controversy recently with the news that doctors are being asked to take blood for tests from patients who have not given informed consent. The British Medical Association said insurance companies have been asking doctors to take the blood from people who have applied for life insurance. The doctors are then asked to send the samples to a laboratory who will inform the insurance company of the result. The first indication people have that they are HIV positive could be the refusal of their application for insurance.

The BMA argue that the standard letter issued to applicants, briefly outlining the test with an attached consent form does not constitute informed consent. They insist counselling is essential before a test is given and then after for the result to be followed up correctly. This view is shared by the DHSS (1986).

Implications for nurses

The whole issue of HIV testing has wide implications for nurses, who often take the blood samples. If they do so without the full consent of the patient, they could find themselves defending civil actions for damages or criminal actions on charges of battery. If they knowingly collude with a doctor in taking such a specimen they may face charges of aiding and abetting an assault, while they also risk being struck off their professional register if they mislead patients about the reason for taking blood samples.

In a circular on professional conduct, the UKCC emphasise that nurses must especially heed the first two clauses of their Code of Professional Conduct with respect to people with or suspected of having HIV infection. These state that they must always act in such a way as to promote and safeguard the wellbeing and interests of patients, and ensure that no action or omission on their part or within their sphere of influence is detrimental to the condition or safety of patients.

Sherrard and Gatt (1987), defining informed consent, say that it must be genuine, and not obtained by misrepresentation, fraud, deceit or duress. Surely the prospect of not being allowed life insurance, and therefore a mortgage, could be construed as duress? The law may interpret a test taken in such a situation as being taken without informed consent.

More generally, practitioners taking blood for HIV tests must take account of the patient's 'right of bodily integrity' – the right to determine what is to be done with his or her own body. Sherrard and Gatt say the far reaching implications of a positive result for the patient would probably make implied consent insufficient from a legal point of view. It is not good enough to take a blood sample 'to run a few tests' and assume the patient realises an HIV test will be among them, and consents to this. The patient must explicitly consent to an HIV test. Obviously nurses should beware of taking blood for HIV tests without the explicit consent of the patient. But does anyone benefit from HIV testing anyway – apart from the insurance companies?

Those responsible for planning and allocating services for AIDS sufferers would certainly be grateful for more information on how many people are HIV positive and therefore likely to contract AIDS. Such information is currently in short supply. Nor is there much information on how far HIV infection has spread into the heterosexual community.

The more people who have HIV tests, the more information will be available on the epidemiology of the virus. This would enable services to be more efficiently planned before a situation arises, rather than when it has reached crisis proportions. This is assuming such action would really be taken, which is by no means certain.

Who should be tested?

While mandatory testing of the entire population is logistically impractical and undesirable from the aspect of individual rights, the voluntary testing of certain groups may be beneficial. Pregnant women are one important group, for two reasons. Pregnancy has been shown to make HIV positive women more likely to develop AIDS because the functioning of mother's immune system is lowered so that her body does not reject the foetus (ACHCEW, 1988). This is thought to give the HIV virus more chance to gain ascendancy. Half of HIV positive mothers can also be expected to pass on HIV to their children either during pregnancy or at birth. Testing would give them the option of having an abortion.

Pregnant women could also be epidemiologically extremely valuable. Brain (1988) said that midwives and antenatal women would be unwise to oppose the routine screening of all pregnant women if they are the only group who would give a clue to the spread of the disease into the heterosexual community. She recommended that testing be voluntary and that the women know its full implications. She also expressed concern at reports that a group of antenatal women had been tested without their consent.

The Government is to decide whether or not pregnant women should be tested anonymously – and whether this should be with or without their consent – when it receives a report on surveillance and monitoring for the Expert Advisory Group. However, Britain's Chief Medical Officers recently refused to support a call for such anonymous screening without the women's consent. They were criticised by Black et al (RSM, 1988), who said anonymous testing would be easy to administer, using blood left over from that taken for routine tests, and would provide a sensitive index of the rate at which the disease is entering the heterosexual community. Women could be told their results if they wished, the rest of the samples would be sent to a central laboratory.

The question of who should be tested and under what circumstances is an emotive one which many nurses will feel strongly about. They have their safety and that of patients and colleagues to consider but must also protect their patients' rights, which may be compromised in the quest for information.

Testing certain groups would not only provide epidemiological information and give pregnant women the chance to have an abortion, say Masters, Johnson and Kolodny (1988). Infected people who were unaware of their status could be identified and counselled to modify their behaviour and avoid infecting others.

As well as pregnant women, they recommend testing all people admitted to hospital between the ages of 15 and 60. Again, the epidemiological information would be valuable. The results would also ensure that staff were aware of the hazard of contact with biological fluid from seropositive patients, and that immunocompromised people were not put at unnecessary risk by exposure to contagious illnesses.

How reliable are the tests?

However, there are other factors in the debate about HIV testing. While the tests currently used are highly reliable compared with many other routine medical tests, some errors are made.

The main test used is the enzyme-linked immunosorbent assay (ELISA), which works by mixing serum with protein pieces of HIV in the presence of chemical reagents. These cause a colour reaction if the HIV antibody is present. ELISA is relatively cheap to administer, and under ideal conditions will detect 98-99 per cent of samples correctly. However, high sensitivity means it occasionally registers false positive results, especially in people who have had numerous blood transfusions and women who have had numerous pegnancies.

The effect of a false positive test on a person could be almost as catastrophic as a true positive. They will suffer the same stigmatisation and emotional trauma as if they were infected, and from a practical point of view, are unlikely to be able to get life insurance or a mortgage among other things. While they may not have the same health problems as a seropositive person, the stress of believing themselves to be infected would be likely to have a detrimental effect on their health. ELISA also shows a small percentage of false negative readings.

To guard against a high number of false positive test results, readings are only considered positive if they are consistent with a repeated ELISA and confirmed by a more specific test like the Western blot. This test is carried out only on samples which have given positive readings with ELISA, because it is much more expensive and requires a higher degree of technical skill to administer. This means false negative readings are not retested. The two tests give a high degree of accuracy, but they are not infallible, or free of the possibility of human error.

Compulsory testing

Compulsory testing of either the whole population or certain groups, usually those who are at high risk of infection, is a subject raised from time to time. At present, however, the question is really academic. The purpose of such screening would be to discover all those who are infected with HIV, and presumably to take steps to ensure that they do not spread the infection. The time lapse between infection with HIV and the body producing the antibodies to the virus can be anything from two months to over a year, so even screening the entire population would not give an accurate picture of who was infected. Until a test is devised which isolates the virus itself, rather than the antibodies, the compulsory testing lobby is unlikely to get very far. If such a test does become available, however, nurses may have to defend their patients' right to bodily integrity from more sustained and vociferous campaigns.

The arguments about HIV testing are bound to continue, but common sense on the part of health care professionals can do much to protect both those afraid of infection with HIV and those already infected. For example, nursing care should not change if a person is diagnosed seropositive – body fluids from seronegative patients may contain other biohazards and should be treated as potentially hazardous. This weakens the argument for compulsory testing – why bother if the same precautions are necessary for seronegative and seropositive people?

The case for voluntary testing, either anonymously or otherwise, is probably the strongest. The information such a programme, properly conducted, could yield would be invaluable if it were used to plan services and public education programmes, and full patient confidentiality were retained. If it were simply used to whip up hysteria against minority groups, however, it would be worse than useless. In such a case it would merely deflect attention from the real issue of how to care for people with AIDS effectively and prevent other people from infection. It would discourage people from going for the test, and make the already catastrophic personal situation of being HIV positive much worse. Any testing programme must be carefully conducted.

How nurses can help

By remaining calm and giving effective education to those who need it nurses can help people take reasonable steps to protect themselves from infection and overcome any unreasonable fears they may have. Hopefully they will also be able to ensure that HIV testing is never used in a negative way against those who are infected with the virus.

Nurses have a huge part to play in protecting both their patients' health and their rights. The medical establishment has expressed its voice in the public debate – albeit often in a contradictory fashion. Nurses are often at the 'coal face' in these issues. It is time the nursing profession made itself heard as well.

References
ACHEW (1988) AIDS and HIV Infection (Health News Briefing). Association of Community Health Councils for England and Wales, London.
Brain, M. (1988) President's address to the 1988 RCM annual conference.
DHSS (1983) AIDS. Booklet 3. DHSS, London.
Masters, H., Johnson, V.E., Kolodny, R.C. (1988) Crisis – Heterosexual Behaviour in the Age of AIDS. Grafton, London.
RSM (1988) Anonymous testing for HIV. *The AIDS Letter*, **1**, 5, 7.
Sherrard, M. and Gatt, I. (1987) Human immunodeficiency (HIV) virus antibody testing. *British Medical Journal*, **295**, 911-2.
UKCC (1987) AIDS – testing, treatment and care. Circular PC/87/02. UKCC, London.

24

Counselling: basic principles in nursing

Philip Burnard, PhD, MSc, RGN, RMN, DipN, CertEd, RNT
Director of Postgraduate Nursing Studies, University of Wales College of Medicine, Cardiff

During the past five years the idea that nurses in all specialties should develop appropriate skills in communicating with and helping their patients has received much attention. Often, however, basic counselling skills are taught without supporting theoretical rationale. This chapter sets out some basic principles based on those found in humanistic psychology theory and in the literature on client-centred therapy, with the aim of offering a 'theoretical scaffolding' on which to build good practice. The principles are presented dogmatically for the sake of clarity but, like all principles, they are open to debate, clarification and development. A further reading list is offered to be used as a guide to tracing the ideas back to source.

The terms 'counsellor' and 'client' are used through the chapter. 'Counsellor' means any grade of nurse acting as counsellor. 'Client' means anyone with whom the nurse is interacting in a counselling capacity. Thus a client may be a patient, a colleague or a friend. Table 1 shows the basic principles of counselling.

1. The client knows best what is best for them.
2. Interpretation by the counsellor is likely to be inaccurate and is best avoided.
3. Advice is rarely helpful.
4. The client occupies a different 'personal world' from that of the counsellor and vice versa.
5. Listening is the basis of the counselling relationship.
6. Counselling 'techniques' should not be overused; however:
7. Counselling can be *learned*.

Table 1. Basic principles in counselling.

The client knows what is best for them   We all perceive the world differently having had different personal histories which colour our views. Throughout our lives we develop a variety of coping strategies and problem solving abilities which we use when beset by personal problems. Central to client-centred counselling is the idea that, given the space and time, we are the best arbiters of what is and is not right for us. We can listen to others, and hear their ideas but in the end we as individuals have to decide upon our own course of action.

Belief in the essential ability of all people to make worthwhile decisions for themselves arises from the philosophical tradition of existentialism. Existentialism argues, among other things, that we are born free and that we 'create' ourselves as we go through life. For the existentialist, nothing is predetermined, there is no blueprint for how any given person's life will turn out. Responsibility and choice lie squarely with the individual.

No one is free in all respects. We are born into a particular society, culture, family and body. On the other hand, our *psychological* make up is much more fluid and arguably not predetermined. We are free to think and feel. One of the *aims* of counselling is to enable the client to realise this freedom to think and feel.

Once a person has to some extent, recognised this freedom, he begins to realise that he can change his life. Again, in humanistic or client-centred counselling, this is a central issue: that people can change. They do not have to be weighed down by their past or by their conditioning (as psychoanalytical and behavioural theory would argue): they are more or less free to choose their own future. And no one can choose that future for them. Hence the overriding principle that the client knows what is best for them.

Interpretation by the counsellor is likely to be inaccurate and is best avoided   To interpret, in this sense, is to offer the client an explanation of his thinking, acting or feeling. Interpretations are useful in that they can help to clarify and offer a theoretical framework on which the client may make future decisions. However, they are best left to the client to make.

As we have seen, we all live in different perceptual worlds. Because of this, another person's interpretation of *my* thinking, acting or feeling will be based on that person's experience — not mine. That interpretation is, therefore, more pertinent to the person offering it than it is to me, coloured as it is bound to be by the perceptions of the other person. Such colouring is usually more of a hinderance to me than a help.

It is tempting for others to lace their interpretations of a person's action with 'oughts' or 'shoulds'. Thus an interpretation can quickly degenerate into moralistic advice which may lead to the client feeling guilty or rejecting the advice because it does not fit into his own belief or value system.

Advice is rarely helpful   Any attempt to help to 'put people's lives right' is fraught with pitfalls. Advice is rarely directly asked for and rarely appropriate. If it is taken, the client tends to assume that 'that's the course of action I would have taken anyway' or, he becomes dependent on the counsellor. The counsellor who offers a lot of advice is asking for the client to become dependent. Eventually, of course, some of the advice turns out to be wrong and the spell is broken: the counsellor is seen to be 'only human' and no longer the necessary life-line perceived by the client in the past. Disenchantment quickly follows and the client/counsellor relationship tends to degenerate rapidly. It is better then, not to become an advice-giver in the first place.

There are exceptions to this principle where advice giving is appropriate; about wound care or medication for example. In the sphere of personal problems, however, advice-giving is rarely appropriate.

Different 'personal worlds' of client and counsellor Because of varied experiences, different physiologies and shifting belief and value systems, we perceive the world through different 'frames of reference'. We act according to our particular belief about how the world is. What happens next, however, is dependent upon how the world *really* is. If there is a considerable gap between our 'personal theory of the world' and 'how the world really is' we may be disappointed or shocked by the outcome of our actions.

It is important that the counsellor realises that her own belief system may not be shared by the client and that her picture of the world is not necessarily more accurate.

A useful starting point is for the counsellor to explore her own belief and value system before she starts. She may be surprised at the contradictions and inconsistencies that abound in that 'personal world'! She is then in a better position to appreciate the difference between her belief system and her client's.

The counsellor's task is to attempt to enter and share the personal world of the client. This is often described as developing empathy or the ability to non-judgementally understand the particular view of the world that a person has at a particular time. That view usually changes as counselling progresses, after which the client may no longer feel the need for the counsellor. When this happens, the counsellor must develop her own strategies for coping with the separation that usually follows.

Counselling is a two-way process. While the client's personal world usually changes, so may the counsellor's. It can, then, be an opportunity for growth for the counsellor as well as the client.

Listening is the basis of the counselling relationship To really listen to another person is the most caring act of all, and takes skill and practice. Often, when we claim to be listening we are busy rehearsing our next verbal response, losing attention and failing to hear the other person. Listening involves giving ourselves up completely to the other person in order to fully understand.

We cannot listen properly if we are constantly judging or categorising what we hear. We must learn to set aside our own beliefs and values and to 'suspend judgement'. It is a process of offering free attention; of accepting, totally, the other person's story, accepting that their version of how the world is may be as valid as our own. Listening can be developed through practice and may be enhanced through meditation. Various experiential exercises have been developed to enable people to learn properly. They need to be used carefully with plenty of time allocated for them.

We need to listen to the metaphors, the descriptions, the value judgements and the words that people use, as they are all indicators of their personal world. Noting facial expressions, body movements, eye contact or lack of it, are all aspects of the listening process.

Many of us have been confronted by the neophyte counsellor whose determined eye-contact and stilted questioning make us feel distinctly uncomfortable! The aim is to gradually incorporate techniques into the personal repertoire. It is important that learner nurses do not adopt, wholesale, a collection of techniques that they have been taught in the school of nursing.

Counselling 'techniques' should not be overused   If we arm ourselves with a whole battery of counselling techniques, perhaps learned through workshops and courses, we are likely to run into problems. The counsellor who uses too many techniques may be perceived by the client as artificial, cold and even uncaring. It is possible to pay so much attention to techniques that they impede listening and communicating.

Some techniques, such as the conscious use of questions, reflections, summary, probing and so forth are very valuable. What one must hope for, is that through practice, such techniques become natural to the counsellor. The process takes considerable time and must be rooted in a conscious effort to appear natural and spontaneous to others.

Counselling can be learned   Counselling is not something that comes naturally to some and not to others. We can all develop listening skills and our ability to communicate clearly with other people, which is the basis of counselling. The skills can only be learned through personal experience and lots of practice, which may be gained in experiential learning workshops for development of counselling skills.

The list of principles outlined here is not claimed to be exhaustive. It attempts to identify *some* of the important principles involved and to explain them. The next stage is to develop counselling theory and skill further through reading and counselling skills courses. The bibliography identifies some sources of further ideas regarding the theory of counselling. These are not the *only* books on counselling but they are up-to-date, readable and currently available in bookshops.

Counselling skills courses are run by a variety of university extra-mural departments; by specialist counselling organisations and, increasingly, as part of the continuing education programmes organised with schools of nursing.

Bibliography
Bond, M. (1986) Stress and Self Awareness: A Guide for Nurses. Heinemann, London.
    A practical book which explores methods of coping with emotions and personal problems.
Burnard, P. (1985) Learning Human Skill: A Guide for Nurses. Heinemann, London.
    An introductory text on self-awareness and experiential learning. Contains a series of exercises on counselling skills training.
Burnard, P.(1989) Counselling Skills for Health Professionals. Chapman and Hall, London.
    A guide to many aspects of counselling theory and skills.
Claxton, G. (1984) Live and Learn: An Introduction to the Psychology of Growth and Change in Everyday Life. Harper and Row, London.
    A stimulating and eclectic approach to the question of how people learn and change. A very readable book.
Nelson-Jones, R. (1981) The Theory and Practice of Counselling Psychology. Holt, Rinehart Winston, London.
    A very comprehensive account of most aspects of counselling.
Rogers, C.R. (1980) A Way of Being. Houghton Mifflin, New York.
    A sensitive book by the late Carl Rogers founder of 'client-centred' counselling, which explores the nature of empathy and the therapeutic relationship.

25

Bereavement: the needs of the patient's family

Jenny Penson, MA, SRN, HVCert, Cert Ed, RNT
Senior Lecturer in Nursing Studies, Dorset Insitute of Higher Education

Through this chapter bereaved people are referred to as "family" or "relatives" for ease of comprehension. Terms such as "key people" or "significant others", while rather unwieldy, may more accurately describe the grieving person who is, for example, a life-long friend.

"Bereavement" means "to be robbed of something valued" – this definition seems particularly helpful as it indicates that this someone or something has been wrongly or forcibly taken from you. A key concept to understanding bereavement is that of loss. As Caplan (1964) and others have suggested, the grief experienced after losing someone close to you may be similar to the emotions felt after other types of loss, life transitions such as redundancy, divorce, failing an important exam or losing a much loved pet. As nurses we become aware of the emotions that patients experience after operations such as mastectomy, amputation of a limb or the loss of body image caused by suffering from a disfiguring disease.

When people are bereaved they suffer not only the loss of a person but also a substantial part of themselves, because everything they have shared with that person cannot be repeated with anyone else. The bereavement experience, therefore, is one of strong, violent and sometimes overwhelming reactions. These feelings actually begin from the moment the relative is told that the patient will not recover, referred to by Lindemann (1944) as "anticipatory grief".

The patient

Kubler Ross (1970), states: "We cannot help the terminally ill patient in a really meaningful way if we do not include his family." She determined that family members undergo stages of adjustment similar to the five phases she described for dying patients – denial, anger, bargaining, depression and acceptance as they come to terms with the reality of terminal illness in the family. She advocates that when there is time to do so, the family should be encouraged to express grief as much as possible prior to the death of a loved one which serves to alleviate, to some extent, the pain that is felt afterwards. If members of a family can share these emotions they will gradually face the reality of the impending separation and come to an acceptance of it together.

Unresolved family stress can significantly affect the outcome of the patient's illness, so the care of the family is part of the total care of the patient. It is also about understanding him as a member of the family group, and being aware that he and his family are not separate entities. Each constantly influences the other, thus affecting the health and happiness of both. It is possible that nursing actions may affect the long-term adjustment of the bereaved relatives after the death of the patient.

Molter (1979) studied family needs as they identified them, and looked at whether these were being met, and if so, by whom. The results showed that relatives could identify their needs during an intensive phase of hospitalisation. Their universal and strongest need was for hope. Nurses can go some way towards meeting this need by helping to set short-term goals for the patient. A weekend at home, a visit from a favourite friend, planning something special to enjoy together all helps to relieve that sense of helplessness which is often felt. They also go some way towards providing good memories to look back on. Reassurance that the patient will not be allowed to suffer pain or great distress, that someone will be with them when they die, and that support is available after the death if they need it, are all significant to those for whom no hope of an ultimate recovery can be given.

Hampe (1975) also found that spouses believed that the nurse's primary responsibility was to the patient and therefore they would be too busy to help relatives. One of the principal needs she identified from her study was for the family to be able to visit the dying patient at any time and for as long as they wished. They also wanted prompt help with the physical care and a demonstration of friendliness and concern in their relationship with the nurse.

My own experience indicates that encouraging involvement of the family in the care of the patient may minimise feelings of guilt during bereavement. There is a sense of not having failed when one was needed and the satisfaction of having done something tangible to give comfort and show love.

Hospital or home care?

This must be borne in mind when discussing the pros and cons of hospital versus home care. Where dying at home is possible because both the patient and their relatives want it, and there are enough resources available when needed, the family are likely to feel a sense of achievement, of not having failed the patient. On the other hand, relatives do derive comfort from the security of constant professional expertise and the knowledge that any emergency will be dealt with by a 24-hour service. However, they still need to feel involved and should be encouraged to give to the patient in any way they can. This might range from helping with nursing care to arranging photos and flowers or bringing in special food or drink that the patient may ask for which the hospital cannot supply.

To tell or not to tell

Whether or not to tell the patient of his diagnosis and prognosis is a dilemma which causes much distress to family, patients and nurses. Sometimes relatives are advised by doctors and/or nurses not to be truthful with the patient and this can create a barrier between them, described by Solzhenitsyn (1971) as "a wall of silence" which separates them.

There is an obvious conflict in many relatives' minds between the idea of the patient's right to autonomy to knowing the truth if he wishes it, and the idea of paternalism, having the right to withhold it on the grounds of protecting the patient and giving him hope. Relatives will often say such things as "it will be too much for him", "he will give up", "I know he won't be able to stand it", "he will be frightened". These sort of statements may well be true but they may also reflect the relatives' own fears.

The cue to how much information is given should lie with the patient and the nurse's role with the relatives is often to explain to and sustain them during that gradual realisation that comes to most patients near the end. This may or may not be expressed and shared. However, when a patient and family can openly discuss their situation together, their relationship can be deepened and this can give great comfort to the bereaved person afterwards. It also creates a basis of honesty and trust which facilitates the relationship between patient, family and carers. Ann Oakley (1985) described when her father, Richard Titmuss, was dying: "You said things you never would have said had you not known you were dying – and that is how I knew you were."

That families fail to share their feelings openly with one another when faced with terminal illness may be due to the defence of denial and also a function of experience. Although we, the health workers, have been enlightened about combating this so-called conspiracy of silence which surrounds the topic of death, it is also possible that some families have been over-exposed to that viewpoint. As Bowen, (1978) points out, in spite of whatever attitudinal change that may have taken place the "basic problem is an emotional one and a change in the rules does not automatically change the emotional reactivity."

Support

So, should staff be so involved as to sit and weep with the relatives? Is this what sharing and support is about? Kubler Ross, (1974), suggests that we ask ourselves whether we would judge someone who cared enough to cry for us. "A display of emotions on the part of the therapist is like drugs, the right amount of medicine at the right time can work wonders. Too much is unhealthy – and too little is tragic."

It has been suggested that nurses are in a prime position to meet the family needs through active listening and supporting. They found that relatives wanted support but they tended to feel they should not burden the "too busy" nurses with their problems. It is important, therefore, that a sense of availability is conveyed to families so that they will not feel guilty when sharing fears and worries with the nurse. Families usually appreciate information and explanation about nursing procedures, tests, treatments, medications. This helps them to feel they are part of the life of the patient and increases feelings of control, which can enable them to cope more realistically and effectively with the immediate future.

Relatives who feel that they have not been "told enough" are suffering from a lack of sustained professional interest. Effective nursing care is *planned* care and relatives can and should be involved in this. Short-term objectives for the patient such as an improved night's sleep, can be explained to relatives and are positive indicators that there are always things which can be done to improve the quality of life for the patient.

There is often an accompanying aspiration or, for many people, a desperate need to find that the experience of grieving does have some meaning. This may lead to a turning or returning towards religion, or other philosophies of living. The nurse can often meet this need with tact and sensitivity by introducing the hospital chaplain or family priest at an appropriate moment. Their availability to families as well as patients gives comfort, and helps them to explore their own beliefs and what they mean.

Physical fitness is related to the ability to cope with stress and measures to maintain health may be more acceptable to the family if they are seen in terms of enabling them to support and be with the dying patient. They also serve to reinforce the message that the grieving relative *is* an important individual whose needs are also the nurse's concern. Simple relaxation techniques to promote sleep and encouragement to eat regularly are all part of this care.

Interpersonal skills

It is important, therefore, for nurses to develop interpersonal skills to enable them to meet the needs of the patient's family. The creation of a trusting relationship, the ability to give information in a clear and sympathetic manner, the ability to listen actively to their concerns and to help them to clarify problems and options all involve skills which can be learned and practised.

As Frederick and Frederick (1986) point out, although there is a great deal of controversy surrounding anticipatory grief, it appears that it may be a way of doing some of the work of mourning before the death occurs. In this way, it may soften the impact of the actual death on the bereaved.

The nurse is in a unique position, being in constant contact with the family. Her attention to their needs may have long-term beneficial effects on their adjustment to bereavement and is likely to enhance the quality of their remaining time with the dying patient.

References
Bowen, M. (1978) Family reactions to death. In: Family Therapy and Clinical Practice. Aronson, New York.
Caplan, G. (1964) Principles of Preventive Psychiatry. Basic Books, New York.
Frederick, J.F. and Frederick, N.J. (1985) The hospice experience: possible effects in altering the biochemistry of bereavement. *Hospice Journal*, **1**, 3, 81-89.
Hampe, S. (1975) Needs of the grieving spouse in a hospital setting. *Nursing Research*, **24**, 20.
Kubler-Ross, E. (1970) On Death and Dying. Tavistock, London.
Kubler-Ross, E. (1974) Questions and Answers on Death and Dying. Macmillan, London.
Lindemann, E. (1944) Symptomatology and management of acute grief. *American Journal of Psychiatry*, 101, 141-149.
Molter, N.C. (1979) Needs of critically ill patients: a descriptive study. *Nursing Research*, **8**, 2.
Oakley, A. (1985) Taking it Like a Woman. Penguin, London.
Solzhenitsyn, A. (1971) Cancer Ward. Penguin, London.
Ward, A.W.M. (1976) Mortality of bereavement. *British Medical Journal*, **11**, 700-102.

Bibliography
Penson, J. (1990) Bereavement: A Guide For Nurses, Harper Collins, London.

26

It's OK having asthma . . . young children's beliefs about illness

Christine Eiser, BSc (Hons), PhD
Senior Research Fellow, Department of Psychology, Washington Singer Laboratories, University of Exeter

Children's knowledge of and attitudes towards health and illness change with age. It is important for health professionals to understand these changes if they are to communicate successfully with children about their illness and treatment, and to realise that each child's development is unique and cannot be rigidly categorised.

Why understand children's views?

Health education   All children need to develop positive attitudes to self-care and health behaviour; partly for their own immediate benefit and partly because such habits are likely to promote positive healthcare behaviour in adulthood. For example, attitudes toward smoking develop early, and early tobacco use appears to increase the likelihood that illegal drugs will be used in later adolescence. Positive adult attitudes to dental care can be promoted by health education in the young (Eiser, 1989).

Hospital admission for acute illness   Children seem to suffer less stress associated with short-term hospital admission when they are given information about their treatment and what to expect.

Chronic disease   Children with chronic diseases (eg, epilepsy, diabetes, asthma) are often encouraged to become responsible for many aspects of their treatment. It is therefore necessary to explain what needs to be done; when, how and why.

Given the range of situations in which effective communication about illness is necessary, much research has centred on what illness means to young children. There appear to be age-related changes in beliefs about illness: older children explain illness in more complex terms, refer more frequently to internal body cues, are more focused on specific diseases and can better describe process and cause (Bibace and Walsh, 1981).

More specifically it has been argued that children under seven years of age tend to believe illnesses are a punishment for wrong-doing, occur by some magical process, or towards the end of the age-period, are 'caught' from others. From seven to 11 years, they believe illnesses are contracted through contact with germs, and it is not until approximately 11 years of age that they understand enough about their bodies to realise that illnesses can also result from a failure of some specific body part.

These results have been taken to imply that children go through a series of stages in their beliefs about illness, and that these stages parallel those described by Piaget to account for development in physical concepts, such as space or time. A corollary of this approach is that children need a certain kind of explanation of illness which is 'matched' to their cognitive level, and will be unable to understand more advanced explanations. Thus, the seven-year-old is likely to understand the cause of illness if this is explained in terms of contagion, but will not understand a physiologically based explanation. There is, however, a danger in over-interpreting these findings and being too rigid in giving explanations to children.

There are both methodological and theoretical difficulties in the interpretation of this work. Methodologically, researchers often use prolonged and unnatural questioning with children; there is little comparability across studies in the kinds of questions asked, and work is invariably based only on small samples of healthy children. Theoretically, there has been no adequate explanation of how children shift from one stage to the other, nor of the role of emotions or personal experience in determining children's explanations. It is perhaps this lack of awareness of how experience affects children's understanding that has been especially damning to the stage approach.

Children's knowledge   Given these criticisms, our research in this field (Eiser, Eiser and Lang, 1989) was based on a model that emphasises what the child knows and the role of the experience. According to 'script' theory (Nelson, 1986) children learn through participation in routine everyday events, so the study began by asking 20 children from two age groups (five and eight years) "What happens when you go to the doctor (or dentist, or hospital)?". All the children attended the same small primary school and there were equal numbers of boys and girls in each group. The conversations with the children took place immediately before the whole school embarked on a project about health and illness.

Children of both age groups were able to give well-ordered accounts of the sequence of events involved, ie they organised their descriptions according to the following sequence:

• **Cause** Some children discussed why the visit to the doctor/dentist/hospital was necessary, or why they were unwell or needed an operation. These precursors to the main event were discussed in terms of symptoms ("I had toothache"; "My throat was sore") or accident ("I fell out of a tree").

- **Journey** Children may describe the journey to the surgery ("We take the bus into town"; "They wheel you along the corridor on a trolley").

- **Reception** This refers to the time spent in the waiting-room prior to seeing the doctor or dentist ("We wait outside and Mummy reads me a story"; "We wait till the nurse calls our name").

- **Inspection/diagnosis** This refers to the main diagnostic interview ("You open your mouth and the dentist looks inside with his mirror"; "Mummy tells the doctor what's wrong and he listens to your heart").

- **Treatment/cure** This refers to the treatment offered ("The dentist cleans your teeth"; "They take your tonsils out"; "You stay in bed and have some medicine").

- **End of treatment** This describes the acts that signal the end of the encounter with medical personnel, and occurred most frequently in the 'dentist' script ("The dentist gives you a sticker"; "We make an appointment for next time").

- **Journey home** ("We walk home"; "We go shopping and Mummy buys me a treat").

- **Recovery** ("When I'm better, I go back to school").

Ordering experiences

Children appear to organise their knowledge about hospitals and medical visits in terms of sequences of events, and this may well enable them to predict what will happen in future encounters, but this study was conducted with children of school age, and required them to verbalise their descriptions. In a further study, a picture-sequencing task was used to see if four-year-olds could also order their experiences (Eiser, Eiser and Jones, 1991).

Each child (n=90) was shown five photographs of hospital scenes. The scenes made up from Playmobil toys and showed an ambulance, children eating on a hospital ward, children playing in a hospital ward, a surgery and a more formal scene where children were in hospital beds in rows, with less sign of ordinary games activities. The four-year-olds agreed on the ordering of the photographs: the ambulance was placed first, followed by the surgery, meal-times, formal ward scene and finally the less formal play scene. This implies that even young children without personal experience of hospital admission were aware that people go to hospital by ambulance, and are not allowed to eat until after surgery.

Half the children were then shown the informal play scene and the remainder the formal scene, and asked to look at it carefully for 10 seconds. They were then shown 12 photographs, each depicting one item. Four of these items had appeared in the original photograph (correct), four showed objects that might have been in a hospital scene but weren't on the photograph (plausible) and four showed items that would never be found in a hospital (implausible). The mean number of correct items was high (mean for formal scene = 3.27, informal = 3.11). More importantly, children were more likely to make plausible than implausible errors. Ignoring ties, 17 children chose more plausible than implausible items in the informal scene, and four chose more implausible. In the formal scene, 26 children chose more plausible items and none more implausible items. This suggests children even of this young age have well-developed beliefs about what happens in hospital, and that this allows them to make inferences about what they might see, rather than simply recall what was in the photograph.

Taken together, these data suggest that, from two years of age, children have well-ordered ideas about what hospital is like and what happens there, and that this information must be gained from such sources as television, books or other people's accounts, rather than their own experience. The fact that children have such information is both an advantage and disadvantage. It is an advantage to the extent that it allows them to make some predictions as to what hospital is like and what happens there; but a disadvantage if their experiences clash with these expectations. Children with serious or chronic diseases are especially likely to find that their experiences do not match expectations.

Children with chronic disease

Chronic diseases and their treatments can be particularly difficult for children to understand. Sometimes (as for children with leukaemia), they can feel quite well before a hospital appointment, but much worse afterwards. Treatments often continue for many years, and also require children to become increasingly responsible for their own health. Those with diabetes for example, must monitor their diets, test blood sugar levels and self-inject insulin. It is often difficult for children to understand why these tasks are necessary, and it is understandable, therefore, that some children perceive them as some kind of punishment. Despite careful explanations, some children with diabetes seem to feel that not being allowed to eat sweets is a punishment for eating far too many before their diagnosis. However, this emphasis on punishment is not necessarily the norm. In a study of 47 children with diabetes, 34 felt it was a 'good' thing, arguing that not being allowed to eat sweets meant that they were less likely to get fat or have spotty skin and more likely to have strong teeth compared with their 'healthy' friends (Eiser *et al*, 1988).

It is often difficult for adults to appreciate which aspects of a disease are the most difficult for a child to cope with. Given the range of aggressive and painful treatments experienced by children with leukaemia, for example, it is surprising to find that many feel that the relatively innocuous finger-prick is the worst thing that happens to them.

For the eight-year-old boy quoted left, having asthma means he might make a fool of himself in front of his class. He understands that his father had asthma as a child, but no longer suffers, and his knowledge results in a rather confused understanding that asthma can be shared around, more like a contagious disease than an inherited condition. There are other indications that children can feel shame or embarrassment about their condition. Colland (1988) for example, found that children described their asthma in the following ways: "I make high noises and everyone can hear me"; "I am ill and often wheezy"; "I cannot go to the zoo"; "I cannot have a dog"; "I am afraid to die"; "Other children tease me"; "I have to take stupid medicines every day". Asked how they managed to take medication at school, they replied:-"Quickly, so no-one can see"; "After everyone has left the classroom and gone outside"; "I don't take them"; "In the toilets so no-one can see".

It is one thing to explain a disease and its treatment to a child in terms of physiological processes; it is quite another to address issues of shame, guilt and embarrassment that can be associated with diagnoses.

A range of understanding

Children vary enormously in their abilities to understand illness and treatment, and this understanding is determined as much by their personal experience as any maturational process. Illness experience is in any case, very idiosyncratic. In the process of conducting research we recently asked eight-year-olds and 11-year-olds to tell us the names of all the illnesses they knew, expecting that the eight-year-olds at least would be limited to knowledge of childhood infectious diseases. Although this was true for a small percentage, the range of cited diseases was extremely wide. One child only knew about diseases contracted by horses! Others (who admitted to watching lots of television), knew about Aids, heart attacks and nervous breakdowns. Still others knew more about leprosy than anything else. The moral is that we should never assume a child's knowledge; they can be surprising both in terms of what they know and what they don't know.

Healthcare professionals must be more prepared to use a variety of methods to elicit children's knowledge, rather than rely on verbal questions and answers. Toys that are familiar to young children are specially useful.

We also need to be aware that increasing children's knowledge of illness is not necessarily a good thing, especially if the illness is chronic or life-threatening. Children who had greater awareness of diabetes have been found to be more distressed and anxious than those who were less well-informed (Allen *et al*, 1984). Making children more knowledgeable about their illness must, therefore, go hand-in-hand with a preparedness to tackle the social and emotional consequences of that knowledge. There is increasing evidence that it is emotional development, far more than the cognitive or intellectual, that is attenuated in sick children. Harris (1988) found that children hospitalised briefly for acute illness were less aware that emotional reactions could determine the course of recovery from an illness than age-matched healthy controls.

Children's beliefs about illness will be determined at least in part from those of their family. Among those with diabetes, children from poorly functioning families are likely to experience difficulties in compliance and haemoglobin control (Hauser *et al*, 1986). Children from families that function well are less likely to experience similar difficulties. Communications with children must take into account the beliefs and understanding about illness and treatment held by the child's whole family.

Finally, it is often assumed that from 11 to 12 years of age, children's knowledge and ability to understand information conforms increasingly to medical doctrine. Certainly, adolescents' biological knowledge becomes much more extensive (Carey, 1985), but there continue to be widely held myths and confusions over many issues. While the concern with how to improve communication with young children is welcome, it needs to be seen as part of a much wider issue. There is a continuing need to integrate medical knowledge within an individual's general framework for understanding illness. Within this perspective communicating with patients, whether children or adults, demands the treading of a delicate balance between the need to impart high technology information as quickly as possible with individual beliefs, drawn from a variety of sources over an extended period of time.

References

Allen, D.A., Affleck, G., Tennen, H., McGrade, G.J., Ratzan, S. (1984) Concerns of children with a chronic illness: a cognitive-developmental study of juvenile diabetes. *Child Care, Health and Development*, **10**, 211–18.

Bibace, R. and Walsh, M.E. (1981) Children's Conceptions of Health, Illness and Bodily Functions. Jossey-Bass, San Francisco.

Carey, S. (1985) Conceptual Change in Childhood. MIT Press, Cambridge, Mass.

Colland, B. (1988) Outwikkelings-psychologische aspectin by astma. *Kind en Adolescentie*, **9**, 85–97.

Eiser, C. (1989) Children's Concepts of Illness: Towards an alternative to the stage approach. *Psychology and Health*, **3**, 93–101.

Eiser, C., Eiser, J.R., and Jones, B.A. (1991) Scene schemata and scripts in children's understanding of hospital. *Child Care, Health and Development*, **16**, 303-17.

Eiser, C., Eiser, J.R., and Lang, J. (1989) Scripts in children's reports of medical events. *European Journal of Psychology of Education*, **IV**, 377–84.

Eiser, C., Swindell, A., Eiser, J.R., Penfold, J., Mann, L. (1988) Interviews with Diabetic Children. Flinders University of S. Australia, unpublished report.

Hauser, S. *et al* (1986) Children with recently diagnosed diabetes: Interactions within their families. *Health Psychology*, **5**, 273–96.

Nelson, K. (1986) Event Knowledge: Structure and Function in Development. Lawrence Erlbaum, New Jersey.

Acknowledgements

The author is supported by the ESRC, England.

27

Taking children at their word: pain control in paediatrics

Suzanne Alder, SRN, RSCN, DN Cert
Clinical Nurse Specialist, Great Ormond Street Hospital for Sick Children

Young children have a limited ability to understand what is happening to them and being asked of them when they are ill. Their limited experience of pain and our lack of understanding of the child's developing nervous system can only add to the obvious difficulties in measuring and, therefore, treating pain in children.

Various methods have been devised and studied to assess paediatric pain. These differ in suitability depending on the child's age, the type of pain and whether the assessment is for clinical or research purposes. Pain is subjective, so assessors must be aware of their own biases – for example culture, sex or experience, and try to remain uninfluenced by them.

Methods of assessing children's pain

Questioning Questioning children and their parents remains one of the most common methods of pain assessment, and is useful depending on the child's age and ability to express her- or himself. The usefulness of this method can, however, be questionable.

Visual analogue scale (VAS) Consists of a 10cm line, vertical or horizontal, with 'no pain' written at one end, and 'severe pain' at the other. Children over seven years can show how much pain they are feeling by marking this line.

Faces Faces scales are an attempt to provide a VAS for younger children. The 'Oucher' developed by Beyer (1984) shows six expressive photographs of young children matched with a numerical scale, ranging from 0 (content) to 100 (full-blown crying). The child chooses the face which most closely approximates his or her feelings.

Poker chips In 1979 Hester developed a numerical method in which children were given four white poker chips, and asked to select one chip if in a little pain and up to four if in great pain. This type of tool can be used successfully by children aged between four and seven years.

X marks the spot Helps children demonstrate the site of pain, although it does not quantify it. A drawing of a body outline is shown to children (aged four to 10 years) who put a cross where it hurts. A study by Eland (1977) showed that 168 of 172 children correctly placed a cross on a body outline and told the investigator why that area hurt.

Verbal scales Verbal scales such as the McGill-Melzack scale developed in 1975 are useful for adolescents who can understand adjectives such as 'lacerating' and can therefore match their pain with such a description. Younger children, however, are not able to this this so easily. Eland and Anderson (1977) describe how a six-year-old child with polio complained of his affected leg feeling like a lemon. After careful questioning, his mother established that he experienced a shrivelled-up feeling, similar to that experienced after sucking a lemon drop for a long time! It is vital to talk and listen carefully to children and establish exactly what they mean.

Pain diary These can be helpful especially to record the pattern of chronic pain, avoiding the discrepancy between reports by children and their parents, and to assess the effects of treatment prescribed.

Some people choose to measure children's pain by observing their behaviour. This can be successful, but difficulties arise distinguishing between pain and other forms of distress, defining 'normal' behaviour and observing children accurately and consistently. Formal behaviour charts are sometimes used in research, although for a young baby or child drowsy following general anaesthetic, informal observation may be the only method available of assessing pain.

Crying is the usual way parents or healthcare professionals assess whether a baby or child is in pain. Wolff (1969) described how the pain cry differs from a hunger cry, but in real life this is not always so clear.

Other forms of behaviour associated with pain in babies and children include change of facial expression, body rigidity and movement of the affected part. Even if young children can demonstrate the presence of pain by such behavioural changes, it must be remembered a child suffering from chronic pain may be able to 'mute out' behavioural responses even when still in pain.

Although observing physiological changes in both children and adults has been used widely as a method of pain assessment (blood pressure, pulse, respiration rate, sweating and hormonal changes), this has rarely proved useful in children, as these signs are influenced by too many variables, such as fear, stress or the illness itself. They have, however, proved useful in babies. Williamson and Williamson (1983) showed infants who received a penile block for circumcision had lower heart rates than those who received no anaesthetic block. Anand *et al* (1985) used these techniques to condemn the practice of ligating patent ductus arterioses in babies with inadequate analgesia.

Pain is made up of physiological, psychological, social, ethnic and cultural components. In most situations more than one of these contributes to what the child feels, while staff attitudes to assessment and treatment also affect the child. Fear and anxiety contribute towards pain, and in hospitalised children feared or actual separation from their parents can add to the fear of medical procedures.

Previous pain experience and parental influence are significant factors in the amount of pain felt by children. After the age of six months, for example, a child will remember certain aspects of an injection procedure such as the needle, a white coat, or being restrained, and might act fearfully if required to repeat the experience. Adolescents whose parents are over-protective or over-involved in their child's activities, seem less able to cope with pain than those whose parents are not as intrusive.

Different cultures respond to pain in different ways: Italians, for example, believe it is natural to cry and moan when in pain and therefore are seen as having a low pain tolerance. Children naturally follow their parents' reactions – in our society it is commonly accepted that 'men don't cry', and therefore adolescent boys experiencing pain may try to hide their suffering, as they feel they are expected to be brave. Even young children can be affected by these beliefs. Eland and Anderson (1977) describe how a six-year-old boy who received multiple injuries after being struck by a car denied feeling any pain when asked in the presence of his father. The child was interviewed the following day, this time when his aunt was in the room. When asked about pain he burst into tears – he was able to say in front of his aunt that he was in pain and had been on many occasions since the accident.

Nurses' own fears influence pain management. Many believe that by giving an unwilling child an injection, for example, they will come into disfavour with the child. Some nurses are so worried about being seen as a 'baddie' that their fears actually stop them giving a much needed injection to a child in pain.

Nurses and other healthcare professionals can also make subjective judgements about the pain level a child is experiencing, regarding a child as a 'sissy' or having a low pain threshold if he or she complains. "Children do not experience pain with the intensity that adults do" and "Narcotics always depress respiration in children" are opinions voiced on and off the ward. It is not surprising therefore, that children are sometimes left to suffer from untreated pain.

Acute pain

Peri/postoperative pain A common cause of pain in children, this is now more readily acknowledged (Goldman and Lloyd-Thomas, 1991). However, until recently there has been "traditional reluctance to prescribe analgesic drugs to alleviate postoperative or other pain" in neonates and young children, due to doubts as to whether neonates feel pain and concerns over potentially harmful effects of powerful analgesics, such as respiratory depression or even addiction (Hatch, 1987). Anyone who has witnessed the restraint needed for a newborn undergoing a simple operative procedure such as circumcision without general anaesthetic, will have little doubt of a neonate's ability to feel pain (Eland and Anderson, 1977). Patient controlled analgesia is a method of postoperative pain control used with adults, which is beginning to be explored in paediatrics.

Medical interventions   All children are subjected to pain from medical procedures at some time during their lives, such as heel pricks when tiny babies, or immunisations. There is evidence that children who are subjected to frequent interventions become sensitised to these procedures, and their fears become greater each time they visit the hospital. Doctors and nurses, however, frequently ignore this aspect of pain, with comments like "it will only take a few seconds" or "are we going to be brave today?"

Accidents and injuries   Accidents are the biggest cause of death in children, and accidental injury is one of the biggest causes of childhood pain. Accidents such as car crashes, falls, burns and scalds, cuts and lacerations are extremely common.

Chronic pain

Juvenile chronic arthritis   Passo (1982) found that 4.5 per cent of children have sufficient pain to interfere with their daily activities for more than three months. Juvenile chronic arthritis can seriously debilitate children and cause extended periods of pain and suffering.

Abdominal pain   Caused by a variety of disorders, recurrent abdominal pain can occur with no detectable organic cause. This problem is quite common, affecting 12.3 per cent of girls and 9.5 per cent of boys (Apley and Naish, 1958). If no organic cause is found, it should not simply be assumed that the pain is psychogenic.

Headache   Most of us suffer from headaches at some stage in our lives. Despite the multiple obvious causes of headache, there are some children who suffer ongoing headaches for no apparent reason.

Cancer   Most children suffering from cancer suffer pain at some stage. The psychological effects and implications can often increase this pain dramatically, especially if they are not attended to sympathetically. It can be difficult – sometimes impossible – to untangle the physical pain felt by the child from the psychological pain caused by fear, watching distraught parents and worrying about the outcome of the disease.

Treatment of pain

There are many treatments for children's pain and those chosen will depend on the assessment of the pain and its cause. It is important to remain objective when planning treatment, but the causes of pain and any relevant social and cultural factors must be taken into account.

Numerous analgesics are available and it helps to remember a few important points. The correct strength analgesia should be given to correspond with the amount of pain the child is suffering. The 'analgesic' ladder is important to remember when prescribing drugs for children, as if the chosen drug is too mild it will not have the desired effect and the child may refuse further pain relief. If the drug is too strong, or the dose too high, it will have adverse effects on the child. It is better to know a few drugs well than to have a poor understanding of a wide range.

In chronic pain, always give analgesia regularly so the child is not experiencing peaks and troughs in pain control. Mild analgesics such as paracetamol and aspirin can be effective, especially if given regularly (every four to six hours), and dosage depends on the child's age and weight. It often surprises people that in the control of chronic pain from cancer, mild analgesics will often keep the child pain free for several weeks before a stronger drug is required.

The next rung on the ladder are mild opioids such as Dihydrocodeine and codeine which should be given on a regular basis, with dose depending on the age and weight of the child.

If the mild opioids are no longer effective, the next and final step are strong opioids such as morphine and diamorphine. Again, these must be given regularly to ensure adequate pain relief. Morphine sulphate slow release tablets (MST), have a long half life and therefore only need to be given every 12 hours. This can obviously be helpful to parents, who may have previously been battling with their child every four hours to encourage him or her to take medication. The starting dose for MST is 1mg/kg twice daily. Pain caused by nerve compression can be difficult to manage, and is not usually responsive to opioid drugs. Tricyclic antidepressant drugs such as amitriptyline may be helpful. Also anti-epileptic drugs such as carbomazepine may be helpful for neuropathic pain.

Routes of administration

Once an analgesic has been selected, an appropriate route of administration must be chosen. The oral route is first choice, but unfortunately is not always as easy as it sounds – we've all tried administering medicine to a toddler, ending up with most of it in our laps! Even though many modern medicines are pleasant tasting, trying to persuade children to take them can be extremely difficult. Parental involvement, the use of play including dolls and teddies being given medicine first, disguising tablets with sugar and jam, and nurses' patience and attitudes are all important.

When a child cannot take oral medication, another route must be chosen. Intramuscular codeine phosphate is often the drug of choice for babies postoperatively, especially when they are breathing spontaneously and strong opioids are being avoided, whereas intramuscular omnopon is often prescribed for bigger children.

Infusion if a more effective way of administering postoperative analgesia, however, giving the child constant pain relief rather than peaks and troughs, and alleviating the need for constant injections. Diamorphine is sometimes given at doses of 0.5mg/kg over one to two days. Postoperative epidural analgesia is extremely effective but depends on nurses being trained to look after the infusion and is not always practical in a busy surgical environment. Patient controlled analgesia is a means of postoperative analgesia also used in some units for children over eight years old (Llewellyn, 1991).

In terminally ill children who can no longer tolerate oral medication, subcutaneous diamorphine is effective. This is given via a syringe pump, which is easy to use and fairly inexpensive, so parents, or even the children, can often learn to operate it. The small size of the machine allows children to remain active for as long as their condition allows.

Intravenous diamorphine can also be given continuously via a syringe driver, but there is no advantage over the subcutaneous route. However, if a long line such as a Hickman line is *in situ*, this will avoid inflicting more needles upon the child. Rectal morphine is also available for children for whom other routes are not appropriate, but steady pain control can be difficult to achieve, probably due to absorption problems.

Problems with morphine and diamorphine

Although opioids are extremely effective in relieving pain in children, their use will always incur some anxiety. Parents sometimes become worried at the thought of their child using opioids, fearing he or she might become hooked on drugs. It is, therefore, important to prepare parents who may also worry about physical changes and respiratory problems – showing them pictures of other children on similar drugs, and who still look the same and are continuing with their normal lives will help.

Unfortunately, many professionals still believe some of the myths about morphine and diamorphine, denying analgesia to children in intense pain (Eland and Anderson, 1977). A study of adults and children with identical diagnoses matched only 18 of the 25 children by diagnosis. The 18 adults received 372 narcotic analgesics and 299 non-narcotics – a total of 671 doses, while the 25 children received a total of 24 doses of analgesics. Although incidences of respiratory depression have occurred in neonates, probably because of altered pharmacokinetics and increased sensitivity to opioids related to the blood brain barrier, safe use of opioids in children is possible providing the correct dose is given. If respiratory depression does occur, it can be reversed by giving Naloxone.

Reluctance to use these drugs must be weighed up against the often troublesome side effects of reduced movement and the humane aspect of human suffering. Fears of addiction also prevent some doctors from prescribing opioids to children, but if the correct dose is given and this is titrated as the child recovers, dependence is easily controlled. There are few side effects, but they affect most children to a greater or lesser degree (Table 1). However, the benefits usually outweigh the side effects in most parents' minds.

Drowsiness Quite a common effect in the first few days, but almost always wears off once the child is accustomed to the drug.
Constipation Common with all forms of opioid analgesia, if constipation is recognised early, or better still, prevented by giving a laxative regularly, it can be controlled.
Nausea and vomiting These are uncommon in children, and can usually be controlled with the use of appropriate anti-emetics and careful diet. May be due to an incorrect dosage.
Hallucinations and nightmares These problems occur occasionally when a child is commenced on opioids, and usually wear off within 48 hours.
Itching This can be quite a problem to some children. It usually wears off when the child is accustomed to the drug, but may be eased by topical or systemic antihistamines or calamine lotion.

Table 1. Side effects of opioid drugs.

Psychological methods of pain relief

Fear can add to the painful experience of being ill and is a problem which should be tackled actively and sympathetically. Many hospitals now produce pamphlets and books for young children to see before a planned hospital admission, and parents are encouraged to stay with their children in hospital, participating as much as possible in their care. Brothers and sisters are also encouraged to visit, and in Nottingham, even pets are encouraged on to the children's unit (Ainsworth, 1989).

Allowing a terminally ill child and his or her family the choice to go home, providing adequate support is available, is of the utmost importance. Most families, given this choice, will wish to take their child home, and a dying child can then spend the last days away from the stresses of hospital life, in the comfort and security of home.

Full explanations and constant reassurance are vital to keep children as relaxed as possible and maintain their trust. Children often believe pain is a punishment for having done wrong, and all sorts of ideas and fantasies may fill their minds if they are not kept informed of what is happening to them and why.

Hypnosis has been found to be successful in dealing with children's pain in many cases. Particular problems such as needle phobia and pain during medical procedures can be helped using this method.

Distraction techniques and the use of imagery and relaxation methods are similarly helpful, especially if parents join in too. These require relatively little time to learn, are cheap and unobtrusive and allow older children to gain some control over their fears. These techniques are demonstrated in a Canadian video 'No Fears, No Tears'.

Local methods of pain control

There are various other methods to reduce pain, which can be valuable alongside other forms of analgesia:

EMLA (enteric mixture of local anaesthetics) is a local anaesthetic cream which prevents pain during venepuncture. It should be applied to the chosen area one hour before the procedure and covered with an occlusive dressing. This cream helps many children overcome their fear of needles.

Skin coolant sprays can also be used before childhood immunisations, while topical heat, in the form of heat pads, and cold such as ice packs, are useful for complaints such as abdominal pain or bruising.

The use of transcutaneous electrical nerve stimulation (TENS) can be helpful for phantom limb pain, postoperative pain, and even pain from more serious conditions such as deaferentation pain from cancer.

Radiotherapy is a painless procedure which can be used particularly for children with localised pain from cancer, and is very useful for dying children, whose quality of life can often be improved for days or even weeks, by a short course of radiotherapy to a problem area. Entonox (nitrous oxide and oxygen) has proved effective and safe in children of four years and over. It is self-administered via a mask or mouthpiece, and can be used during short procedures such as suturing, plastering, removing sutures and changing dressings.

Homoeopathic remedies and acupuncture are chosen by some parents for their children – indeed may be the first choice of treatment in some instances. We must remember that freedom of choice is everyone's perogative, and even if our beliefs differ we are not necessarily right.

Pain suffered by young children can be reduced by a wide variety of remedies. Each child will feel pain of differing levels and degrees, and react to, and cope with this in their own way. As healthcare professionals, we have an obligation to children suffering from pain – the choice of pain relief methods and the tools available to measure and assess pain mean there is little excuse or reason for any child to suffer. The lack of research, at least until recently, into paediatric pain, means more exploration and assessment are required to help us tackle the problem effectively. We have a duty to dispel some of the old myths about paediatric pain.

References

Ainsworth, H. (1989) And the guinea pig came too. *Nursing Times*, **85**, 39, 55–56.

Anand, K.J.S. and Aynsley-Green, A. (1985) Metabolic and endocrine effects of surgical ligation of patent ductus arteriosus in the human preterm neonate: Are there implications for further improvement of postoperative outcome? Mod. Pr *Paediatrics*, 23, 143–157.

Apley, J. and Naish, N. (1958). Children with recurrent abdominal pains; a field survey of 1,000 School Children. *Archives of Disease in Childhood*, **33**, 165–170.

Beyer, J.E. (1984) *The Oucher: a user's manual and technical report.* The Hospital Play Equipment Co., Evanston, Il.

Eland, J.M. (1977). *Children's Experience of Pain: A Descriptive Study.* Unpublished data.

Eland, J.M. and Anderson, J.E. (1977) *Pain*. Little Brown & Co, Boston.

Goldman, A. and Lloyd-Thomas, A.R. (1991) Management of pain in children and neonates. British Medical Bulletin, **47**, (3) 676-89.

Hatch, D.J. (1987) Analgesia in the neonate. *BMJ*, **294**, 6577, 920.

Llewellyn, N. (1991) A headache all over my body. *Paediatric Nursing*, **3**, 7, 14-16.

McGrath, P.J. and Unruh, A.M. (1989) *Pain in Children and Adolescents*. Elsener, pp 73-104.

Melzack, R. (1975) The McGill-Melzack Pain Questionnaire: major properties and scoring methods. *Pain*, **1**, 277-99.

Passo, M.H. (1982). Aches and limb pain. *Paediatr. Clin. North Am*, **29**, 209-19.

Williamson, P.S. and William son, M.L. (1983). Physiologic stress reduction by a local anaesthetic during newborn circumcision. *Paediatrics*, **71**, 36-40.

Wolff, P.H. (1969) The natural history of crying and other vocalisations in early infancy. In: B.M. Foss (Ed). *Determinants of Infant Behaviour*, Vol 4, Methuen, London.

28

Tablets to take away: why some elderly people fail to comply with their medication

Sally Quilligan, RGN, DipN
Currently studying BEd (Hons) at South Bank Polytechnic

In 1981, Bliss revealed that drug related problems accounted for 10 per cent of all hospital admissions in elderly people. While some of these could be explained by the age-related changes in physiological and metabolic processes and by polypharmacy, some were also a consequence of patients failing to take their medications correctly (Bliss, 1981). My own experiences as a medical ward sister appeared to support this finding and stimulated me to investigate the problem at a local level. In doing so I was surprised to see that, although nursing studies about discharge planning and self-medication briefly mention the problem of non-compliance with medication, there have to date been few detailed nursing papers (Entwistle, 1989).

Increased life expectancy

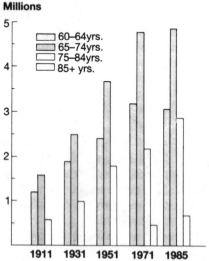

Figure 1. Population trends above 60 years, adapted from Social Trends (1987).

In 1980, Williamson reported that one quarter of all elderly patients admitted to hospital suffer from four or more chronic conditions, and that 80 per cent of all elderly patients take some prescribed medication. Statistics (Figure 1) clearly demonstrate that elderly people have an increase in life expectancy, and although this demographic trend may be attributed to many causes, a major factor is medication.

There is, however, strong evidence to suggest that elderly people frequently fail to comply with their medication regime – the Royal College of Physicians (1984) emphasised this in their report demonstrating that 75 per cent make errors in their compliance to prescriptions, of which 25 per cent are potentially serious. An extensive literature search seems to demonstrate that compliance with long-term medication is about 50 per cent. Non-compliance with a drug regime may disrupt or reverse the possible benefit of the preventive, curative or palliative effect the drug provides. It may involve the patient in further investigative procedures, cause discomfort and physical suffering. Illness

1. The medication to take home is checked by a trained nurse, but invariably given to the patient by a student nurse.

2. The medication is handed to the patient at their bedside less than an hour before discharge.

3. Little attempt is made to check the patient's knowledge about the medication.

4. With the occasional exception of patients on Warfarin and steroids, no explanation of likely side-effects is given.

5. Patients' ability to open containers, dispense their medication, or read the labels is not checked.

6. No mention is made about the danger of hoarding previously prescribed medication.

7. Occasionally, family members are told when to administer the drug, but there are no planned teaching sessions.

8. No explanation is given of how to obtain a new prescription unless the patient asks.

9. No reference is made in the care plan to this aspect of discharge preparation.

Table 1. Outcome of observations.

and possible readmission to hospital may upset daily routines, disrupt social relationships with family and friends and possibly induce deep anxiety for the elderly person. With dwindling resources and the current NHS crisis, the additional cost generated must also be considered.

This appears to suggest that failure of elderly people to take their medicines correctly after discharge from hospital does have far-reaching consequences. It is surely in the healthcare professional's and society's interest to ensure elderly people are able to administer their drugs safely and correctly.

Fully aware of the importance of correct medication administration among elderly people after discharge from hospital, I decided to review current practice within my own clinical area, a four ward medical unit. This proved a salutary experience as shown by the outcome (Table 1), and I would suggest that the results might be mirrored on hundreds of other wards up and down the country.

Factors affecting non-compliance

"Reasons for error and non-compliance are varied and . . . external factors such as poor record keeping by healthcare professionals . . . inadequate labelling, packaging and presentation may all contribute to the problem, as may the patients' knowledge of their medication and the availability or lack of adequate instructions in their safe and appropriate use" (Parish, 1983).

Size, shape and colour of pills   "The white one is my water pill." Past experience has shown me that some patients relate the action of their drug to its colour. The World Health Organisation (1981) recognises this and suggests that where several drugs are prescribed they should be of different shapes and colours. This may however be failing to treat the patient as an individual, assessment might reveal many elderly people who would know exactly which tablets and what dose to take. The shape of the tablet also needs to be easy to handle. Limited movement and painful joints are a feature of the lives of many old people and they may find it difficult to pick up small, round tablets. Even if a suitable form of medication is prescribed, a repeat prescription may, as Warren (1985) notes, be a different brand or generic product, and this variation in the tablets' appearance may be a contributing factor to drug non-compliance.

Containers   "We have established beyond reasonable doubt that it is difficult, if not impossible, for some elderly patients to open childproof containers and remove tablets from bubble packs without shooting them across the floor" (MacGuire, 1987). In 1983 Parish clearly stated that healthcare professionals should be alert to the fact that child resistant containers are a potential source of medication error. This is reinforced by Halworth's (1984) outpatient study of 92 elderly people, in which he found that a quarter of them admitted to having transferred their tablets to an alternative container. Clearly, blister packaging, foil packaging and childproof containers present difficulties, indeed childproof would appear to generally be synonymous with elderly proof.

Davidson (1973) demonstrated that a glass container with a screw top lid was the most convenient for elderly people to use. However, this requires a firm handgrip, and handgrip becomes progressively weaker with age, which may explain Bellamy's (1981) more recent finding that many elderly people could not completely close screw-capped containers. The ability to open a container depends on eyesight as well as manual dexterity, and Coote (1984) proposes that people with poor eyesight should place each prescription in a different shaped bottle. In my experience I have found patients prefer a clear glass palm-sized bottle with screw cap or push-on lid. There are, however, those with particular needs who will find even these difficult. Coote (1984) suggests that for people with severe hand tremors, the use of Dines high impact polystyrene tubs with pull-off lids may be beneficial.

Labelling   "Pharmacists should provide typewritten labels with clear and complete instructions and ensure that the patient can read and understand the label" (*Drug and Therapeutics Bulletin*, 1980).

It is common knowledge that part of the ageing process results in a loss of visual acuity and may result in a loss of ability to read effectively. Although labels are now computer printed, they are often too small and difficult for elderly people with poor eyesight to read. It is, then, somewhat alarming to consider that in Halworth's (1984) outpatient study, 34 per cent stated that if the instructions were not on the label they would not remember how to take their drugs correctly. It is also disturbing to note that Bliss (1981) revealed that 50 per cent of GPs' repeat prescriptions have no instructions other than take as directed.

Instructions themselves can cause problems if ambiguous. 'One tablet three times daily', or 'one tablet at breakfast, lunch or dinner' may, as MacGuire (1987) notes, cause problems – when is dinner, what is lunch? It may then be better to state take one tablet at 08.00 hrs, 12 noon, 18.00 hrs. What is certain is that research has demonstrated associating specific times of day with medication may improve compliance (*Drug and Therapeutics Bulletin*, 1980).

Written instructions   "Written information about the medication each patient is taking, which they could take home, may help to increase their knowledge level and indirectly compliance" (Waters, 1987). In 1970, Skeet argued that written instructions for patients to take home would increase understanding and memory. Although not all elderly patients need additional instructions, those with memory or hearing impairment may find some useful.

The progressive hearing loss associated with ageing results in a progressive loss of ability to hear high frequencies and may significantly affect ability to understand speech. In a community survey of over-70 year-olds, Gilhome (1981) found 60 per cent had some hearing impairment and, of more concern, 25 per cent of these refused to accept any suggestion that they might have a hearing impairment. This must alert nurses to the fact that elderly people may try to hide their hearing loss and that verbal instructions may often need to be written down.

Memory aids   "Intellectual decline is not a universal and inevitable part of growing old" (Redfern, 1985), but 25 per cent of the population over 80 are moderately severely demented (Cormack, 1985) and many others who are not demented experience short-term memory loss. People with memory or orientation problems may experience difficulty and fail to take their medication as directed, and will require to be given extra time when preparing for their discharge. Even after this, some may have such severe problems that they are unable to manage, but others may benefit from learning to use a memory aid.

Memory aids range from the simple device made by the family, such as setting out doses for a day or week in egg cartons, to the more complex commercial product such as the Dosett Box. I could find no recent research to support the type of simple device already discussed, but it may act to encourage the family and or friends to become involved in reminding the patient about adhering to the drug regimen. The use of commercial aids to improve compliance is somewhat debatable. A ward using the Dosett Box system within my clinical area found it complicated, and the *Drug and Therapeutics Bulletin* (1980) notes that they may be difficult to use and awkward to refill.

Patient teaching   "We believe that teaching patients to take their medication correctly should form part of the rehabilitation programme for patients leaving hospital" (Crome *et al*, 1980). The review of current practice indicated that the information given to patients about their medication was hopelessly inadequate, and Wilson Barnett (1985) suggests that the implication of discharging patients home unprepared and without adequate knowledge is that they will fail to cope.

The benefits of using teaching plans as a means of improving knowledge and compliance have been clearly demonstrated (MacDonald, 1987). However, the author found little evidence that nurses recognise their role in relation to teaching about medication, and no reference to formal teaching on medication on any of the care plans.

The literature does appear to identify that there is no framework for patient education. Instruction is sometimes given in the form of informal chats in response to questioning, or as Price (1984) notes, as a menu or list of facts to be taught after a specific operation or procedure. This type of patient education is self-limiting and a framework is required which all nurses, including students, can use with ease. The familiar format of the nursing process as utilised by Wilson Barnett (1985) provides a basis for such patient teaching.

The way forward
This review of the literature has shown that many of the factors that influence medication compliance have been recognised for as long as a decade. It is suggested that in many clinical areas the importance of this information is being ignored and that nurses need now to consider the significance of their role in this important aspect of care.

References
Bellamy, K. *et al* (1981) Letter: Granny-proof bottles. *Journal of the Royal College of General Practitioners*, **31**, 2, 124.
Bliss, M.R. (1981) Prescribing for the elderly. *British Medical Journal*, **283**, 203–06.
Coote, J. (1984) Helping the elderly with their medicines. *The Pharmaceutical Journal*, November 17, 608–09.
Cormack, D. (Ed) (1985) Geriatric Nursing – A Conceptual Approach. Blackwell Scientific Publications, Oxford.
Crome, P. *et al* (1980) Drug compliance in elderly hospital in-patients. *The Practitioner*, **224**, 782.
Davidson, J. (1973) Presentation and packaging of drugs for the elderly. *Journal of Hospital Pharmacy*, 31, 180–84.
Drug and Therapeutics Bulletin (1980) Helping elderly patients to manage their medicines. *DTB*, **18**, 23, 89–91.
Entwistle, B. (1989) A problem of compliance. *Nursing Standard*, **20**, 3, 33–35.
Gilhome-Herbst, K.R. and Humprey, C.M. (1981) Prevalence of hearing impairment in the elderly living at home. *Journal of the Royal College of Practitioners*, **31**, 155–60.
Halworth, B.R. and Goldberg, L.A. (1984) Geriatric patients' understanding of labelling of medicines. *British Journal of Pharmaceutical Practice*, **6**, 6–14.
MacDonald, E.T. *et al* (1977) Improving drug compliance after hospital discharge. *British Medical Journal*, **2**, 618–21.
MacGuire, J. *et al* (1987) Two pink and one blue. *Nursing Times*, **83**, 2, 32-33.
Parish, P. *et al* (1983) The elderly and their use of medicine. Kings Fund Project Paper, No. 40, Kings Fund, London.
Price, B. (1984) From hospital to home. A framework for patient education. *Nursing Times*, **80**, 8 Aug, 28–30.
The Royal College of Physicians (1984) Medications for the Elderly. Report of the Royal College of Physicians. *Journal of the Royal College of Physicians*, **18**, 7–17.
Skeet, M. (1970) Home from Hospital. Macmillan, London.
Waters, K. (1987) Discharge planning: an exploratory study of the process of discharge planning on geriatric wards. *Journal of Advanced Nursing*, **12**, 71–83.
Williamson, J. (1978) Principles of drug action and usage. In: Isaacs, B. (Ed) Recent Advances in Geriatric Medicine. Churchill Livingstone, Edinburgh.
Wilson-Barnett, J. (1985) Principles of patient teaching. *Nursing Times*, **81**, 13, 28–29.
World Health Organisation (1981) Health Care in the Elderly. Report of the Technical Group on use of medicaments by the Elderly. *Drugs*, **22**, 279–94.

29

When should you take your tablets? Teaching elderly people about their medication

Sally Quilligan, RGN, DipN
Currently studying BEd (Hons) at South Bank Polytechnic

If 10 per cent of hospital admissions of elderly people can be linked to drug-related problems (Bliss, 1981), this must in part reflect that the present level of patient teaching about medication is inadequate. As Wilson Barnett (1985) has suggested, the implication of discharging a patient home without adequate knowledge is that they will fail to cope.

In 1977 MacDonald found that a predischarge counselling session of 15 minutes improved compliance by as much as 50 per cent, and there is much recent evidence to demonstrate that teaching is beneficial and may improve knowledge and compliance (Johnston, 1986). There is, however, little documented data to show that nurses recognise their role, in relation to teaching about medication. Within my own clinical area, while patient teaching was viewed as important, it was often omitted when the ward was busy. In addition, there was no reference to formal teaching about medication on any of the care plans. This accords with Water's (1987) experience in the North of England.

Lack of framework

What the literature does appear to identify is that there is no framework for patient education. Instruction is sometimes given in the form of informal chats in response to questioning, or as Price (1984) notes, as a menu or list of facts to be taught after a specific operation or procedure. This type of patient education is self-limiting – we need a framework which all nurses, including students, can use easily. The familiar format of the nursing process (Wilson Barnett, 1985) provides such a basis.

Who should perform the teaching? This appears to be another point for debate. Many writers suggest pharmacists should counsel patients (Sweeney, 1989; Johnston, 1986), whereas others suggest that because nurses spend most time with patients, it should be primarily their role (Royal College of Physicians, 1984). I would argue that it is the teaching *per se*, rather than who does the teaching, that matters.

Teaching patients to take their medication correctly should, as Crome (1980) suggests, form part of the rehabilitation programme, and should begin with the first nursing assessment following admission. The nurse must assess what precipitated this admission and ask the next of kin to bring in all the tablets patients have at home. It may also be necessary to ascertain how willing the family are to become involved in a teaching plan. As patients' conditions improve, the drug round can be used to assess their knowledge about both their disease and why they have to take their medication. Drug rounds thus become part of the learning process, and where appropriate, this could eventually be in the form of carefully supervised self-medication. Patients would then have a chance to familiarise themselves with their medication and discuss any needs or worries, while the nurses would have the opportunity to assess patients' knowledge, evaluate previous teaching and also identify those patients who may fail to take their medication due to physical or mental impairment and thus alert the community services. Following the drug rounds, nurses and patients could establish new goals – further individualised teaching sessions, involving patients' families wherever possible, can then be planned around patients' needs.

The drug round could thus provide continuous assessment and evaluation, and nurses would, as Redfern (1985) suggests, prepare patients for discharge throughout their hospital stay. Progress and teaching sessions given could then be formally documented within patients' care plans.

Suggested framework

The following framework is one way of ensuring elderly patients are given enough support in learning about their medication. It takes the steps of the nursing process as its structure.

Patient assessment

1. Does the patient understand his or her disease, and why their tablets must be taken?
2. Does the patient want to learn? Is he or she able to learn?
3. Can family be involved in the process?

Planning teaching   Use realistic, clear, *joint* goals on agreed topics and if possible arrange discussions when family can be present. Set dates and times for the sessions to ensure they are not missed.

Implement   Limit teaching to three topics in each session. Discuss the patient's worries and check previous knowledge. Remind the patient of the topic and goal, and limit the session to 15 minutes maximum.

Evaluate   On-going assessment of medication and the teaching programme is required (see Table 1).

By using this simple framework the patient's individual needs may be accounted for. Below is a checklist of areas that, ideally, most patients

1. Patient must be able to explain to the nurse at the end of session what has been discussed.
2. The patient's knowledge, needs and worries should be reassessed when he or she receives drugs on drug round, thus demonstrating change in knowledge.
3. A follow-up questionnaire should be conducted on discharge, to gain feedback on whether the teaching helped.
4. The nurse should assess the experience and recognise any lack of knowledge.

Table 1. Evaluation.

should be aware of.

Many intrapersonal factors such as motivation may influence compliance with medication following discharge and over this the nurse has no control. With a little planning the nurse can provide the elderly person with a real choice. With a sound knowledge base and user friendly medication they can now decide whether or not to comply rather than being in many cases simply unable to comply.

References

American Society of Hospital Pharmacists (1984) Guidelines on pharmacist conducted patient counselling. *American Journal of Hospital Pharmacy*, **41**, 331.

Bliss, M.R. (1981) Prescribing for the elderly. *British Medical Journal*, **283**, 203–06.

Crome, P. *et al* (1980) Drug compliance in elderly hospital in-patients. *The Practitioner*, **224**, 782.

Gooch, J. (1985) Medication to take home. *Professional Nurse*, **1**, 1, 15–16.

Johnston, M. *et al* (1986) Facilitating comprehension of discharge medication in elderly patients. *Age and Ageing*, **15**, 304–06.

MacDonald, E.T. *et al* (1977) Improving drug compliance after hospital discharge. *British Medical Journal*, **2**, 618–21.

Price, B. (1984) From hospital to home: a framework for patient education. *Nursing Times*, **80**, 32, 28–30.

Redfern, S. (1985) Nursing Elderly People. Churchill Livingstone, Edinburgh.

The Royal College of Physicians (1984) Medications for the Elderly. Report of the Royal College of Physicians. *Journal of the Royal College of Physicians*, **18**, 1, 7–17.

Sweeney, S. *et al* (1989) the impact of the clinical pharmacist on compliance in a geriatric population. *The Pharmaceutical Journal*, Feb 18, R4–R6.

Warren, J. *et al* (1985) Drug compliance in the elderly after discharge from hospital. *The Pharmaceutical Journal*, April 13, 472–73.

Waters, K. (1987) Discharge planning: an exploratory study of the process of discahrge planning on geriatric wards. *Journal of Advanced Nursing*, **12**, 1, 71–83.

Wilson-Barnett, J. (1985) Principles of patient teaching. *Nursing Times*, **81**, 8, 28–29.

Issues in Clinical Management

30

Time to dispense with the rituals: changing infection control practice

Diane Thomlinson, BSc, RGN, ONC
Senior Nurse, Infection Control, Worcester Royal Infirmary

Ritualistic practices have long stood in the way of effective infection control. However, they may well meet their match in the 1990s if, as many predict, cost-effectiveness, clinical efficiency and environmental concerns come to dominate infection control programmes (Daschner, 1989; Kunin, 1989).

Programmes which give due weight to these criteria will be forced to confront existing practices in disinfection, aseptic techniques and isolation nursing – all areas steeped in ritual (Horton, 1985; Merchant, 1988; Bowell, 1989). To be effective, however, such programmes will need to change more than these practices – they will have to change the way nurses think about infection control.

Ritualistic practices

There is a mistaken belief that rituals provide a general level of safety for patients. This is not necessarily true – their use often distracts from more important infection control measures. For example, handwashing is the most important factor in the prevention of hospital infection, but it is often displaced, probably because other infection control practices, even unnecessary ones, are seen as more exciting. Crow (1982) found that although theatres may have numerous infection control rituals, 66.7 per cent of anaesthetists failed to wash their hands before a case.

Rituals are, by definition, practices carried out according to custom, often without thinking about reasons for them (Jackson, 1984). Rather than providing a safe environment for patients this approach can have disastrous consequences, as is well illustrated in the following description of an outbreak: "Originally our thermometers were stored in chlorhexidine and spirit (pink) – however this gradually altered to pharmacy prepared mouthwash (also pink) and in turn to ward prepared mouthwash (also pink) placed in each thermometer holder on a 'top up' basis. The result – several cases of *pseudomonas* colonisation." (Newsom, 1984).

Disinfection

It is ironic that in Newsom's description, the principle behind the original procedure was the action of alcohol (spirit); chlorhexidine has no value for disinfection of instruments, but would have coloured the preparation pink, as a pink stain had been used in its preparation. Due to a series of 'slips' over a 10-year period, however, only the 'pink' from the original procedure remained.

What helps sustain rituals in disinfection? Misconceptions are held by many nurses about chemical disinfectants (identified by Ayliffe and Collins in 1982), and these are similar to those held by the general public and stringently reinforced by some advertisers. The researchers found many nurses thought all bacteria were more or less equally infective and undesirable and all spread by air. They thought disinfection of floors and ceilings would reduce the spread of infection and that bacteria remain viable until killed by disinfectant – which they saw as being equally effective regardless of the concentrations. Finally, they thought disinfectant will continue to kill bacteria after it was dried.

The BMA guide to infection control (1989) illustrates how these common misconceptions are reinforced: "Pouring disinfectant into a toilet bowl will not prevent little Jimmy spreading sonnei dysentery to his friends at nursery school; washing round the toilet seat might, but it is not the sort of glamorous activity easy to depict on a television screen."

Information staff are given in hospital may well contradict that which they receive from advertisers and other influences outside work, and those involved in infection control educational programmes should be aware of this. Several years ago I was involved in the implementation of research-based disinfection policy. Domestic staff were so horrified that disinfectants were no longer to be used to routinely clean floors that they brought in their own from home. An educational programme went some way to alleviating the situation, but complete compliance only occurred after a lemon-scented detergent was introduced. Perhaps this touched on further misconceptions:

Misconception: Disinfectants smell antiseptic, therefore they work.

Misconception: If it smells of antiseptic or pine, it must be a good disinfectant.

As a result of the Control of Substances Hazardous to Health (COSHH) regulations, all hospitals in the UK will be examining their disinfection practices in 1990. This is an ideal opportunity to promote cost-effective, environmentally-conscious, research-based practice. Where possible, chemical disinfection and sterilisation should be replaced by heat, which is rapid, cheap, reliable and non-toxic. A number of manufacturers are experimenting in either producing medical equipment able to withstand high temperatures or in providing compact heat disinfection or sterilisation units for areas such as outpatient departments, where a rapid turnover of equipment prohibits the return of instruments to hospital sterilisation units. Both approaches will clearly lessen the necessity for chemical disinfection.

Environmental concerns will also require us to review our use of disposable equipment. While the introduction of some items such as needles and syringes has been of enormous benefit to infection control, others are an unnecessary environmental hazard. This may well mean a return to using reusable equipment, which will require nurses to have a deeper and more extensive understanding of disinfection and sterilisation practices.

Unfortunately, unless nurses take this opportunity to examine more traditional practices, some useful ones may well be lost in the cost-effectiveness drive. An example of this is the withdrawal of lavender water (popular in many elderly care units) on the grounds that it has no disinfectant properties. More recent work in aromatherapy has shown that its use may well be beneficial to patients and an important part of nursing care, so infection control may not be the only consideration.

Aseptic techniques

Merchant (1988) made an interesting examination of rituals in the aseptic wound dressing technique, and noted that many of the dressing packs and procedures in use had their origins in the 1940s and had changed little since. Dressing packs designed with six pairs of forceps may have been useful in the 1940s, to remove materials from sterilisation drums, but it is difficult to justify their use today. Equally, dressing towels are often habitually provided, although they have not been recommended for routine use since the 1960s, while cotton wool balls are another item often included but rarely used in modern aseptic techniques.

Advances in wound care products should encourage nurses to examine this area of their work. A number of hospitals have redesigned the content of their dressing packs to avoid wastage of materials. Changes in rigid aseptic procedures will require nurses to increase their understanding of the principles of asepsis.

Isolation

Most nurses would recognise that many of the isolation measures still practised are ritualistic, and this is not a safe approach. It doesn't automatically follow that if overzealous precautions are implemented by staff when caring for a hepatitis B carrier, adequate measures will be taken to isolate a patient admitted to an orthopaedic ward with a discharging abscess. When a patient is diagnosed as having an infection or where there is a strong suspicion of this, a nursing assessment should be made to calculate the risk the patient may pose to others – ie, is there a communicable or contagious aspect to the infection? To plan appropriate and individualised care, Bowell (1989) recommends four aspects should be considered:

1. The site of infection.

2. The organism involved.

3. Additional risks related to symptoms, treatments and the mental ability of the patient.

4. The type of unit or clinical area in which the patient is being nursed.

It is also essential to assess the potential routes by which the infection can be spread by asking:

What is infected?

How does it spread?

What could be contaminated?

How can we prevent contamination?

This information, together with an isolation policy, can then be used to plan the specific precautions necessary to prevent cross-infection. This approach will provide a safe system of care without wasting resources.

Implementing change

Staff education is clearly the key to implementing change, but exactly how it should be conducted is not so clear. An interesting study was recently carried out by an infection control team in Hong Kong (Seto *et al*, 1989). The team monitored different methods of introducing a policy to discontinue the recapping of needles (to avoid the risk of needle-stick injuries). Nurses in the study were placed in one of two groups, 'agreeables' and 'non-agreeables', depending on their willingness to comply with the new procedure. Passive methods (posters/memos) were effective for the 'agreeables', while the inclusion of an active method (lectures/discussion sessions) was needed for the 'non-agreeables'. There are always those who will never change unless compelled, and it was interesting to note that a small number of the 'non-agreeables' didn't alter their practice even after the educational programme. Conversely, nurses working in areas like intensive care, where keeping up-to-date and implementing changes are an integral part of the job, were far more likely to be in the 'agreeables' group and may not have even required an educational programme.

Some infection control measures are not fully realised, due to a lack of motivation, rather than a lack of education. Williams and Buckles (1988) measured the frequency of staff handwashing before introducing a gentle liquid soap and an intensive educational programme aimed at increasing the practice. Although an initial improvement was observed the frequency of staff handwashing returned to baseline levels within six months.

The way forward in the 1990s may be to use a link nurse system described by Horton (1988). Each ward sister and charge nurse identifies a senior member of the trained staff to act as a 'key' person in infection control. These key people are given specialised training in the principles as they apply to patient care practices. They are then responsible for monitoring standards and for educating other staff in their area, elucidating help from the infection control nurse as required. Regular study sessions should be held to update key staff and discuss the implication of new policies.

Another method becoming increasingly popular is infection control audit, where the infection control nurses assesses practices and recommends changes to individual wards and departments. Both these approaches clearly require a strong commitment from managers but could be rewarded by the continuing motivation of staff in their clinical areas to make permanent changes for the better – that are at least cost-effective and possibly cost saving.

References

Ayliffe, G.A.J., Collins, B.J. (1982) Problems of disinfection in hospitals. In: Principles and Practice of Disinfection, Preservation and Sterilisation. Russell, A.D., Hugo W.B., Ayliffe, G.A.J., (eds). Blackwell Scientific Publications, Oxford.

Bowell, B. (1989) Nursing Intervention. In: Applied Microbiology. Caddow, P. (ed). Scutari Press, Oxford.

Crow, S. and Greene, V.W. (1982) Aseptic transgression among surgeons and anaesthesiologists: a quantitative study. *Archives of Surgery*, **117:** 1012–16.

Daschner, F. (1989) Cost-effectiveness in hospital infection control lessons for the 1990s. *Journal of Hospital Infection*, **13,** 325–36.

Horton,, R. (1985) Disinfection through the ages. *Nursing Times*, **81,** 36 Journal of Infection Control Nursing Supplement, 17–19.

Horton, R. (1988) Linking the chain. *Nursing times*, **84,** 36, 44–46.

Jackson, M.M. (1984) From ritual to reason – with a rational approach for the future: an epidemiologic perspective. *American Journal of Infection Control*, **12,** 4, 213–20.

Kunin, C.M. (1989) The future of hospital epidemiology. *Infection Control and Hospital Epidemiology*, **10,** 6, 276–79.

Newsom, W.S.B. (1982) Aspects of Infection Control: Infection Control in Cardiac Surgery. ICI Chemical Industries, Cheshire.

Seto, W.H., Ching, P.T.Y., Fung, J.P.M., Fielding, R. (1989) The role of communication in the alteration of patient care practices in hospital – a prospective study. *Journal of Hospital Infection*, **14,** 29–37.

Williams, E. and Buckles, A. (1988). A lack of motivation. *Nursing Times*. **84,** 22. Journal of Infection Control Nursing Supplement 63–64.

31

Why do we forget to remember handwashing?

Annette McFarlane, RGN, CertCN
Senior Nurse, Infection Control, Royal Shrewsbury Hospital

Handwashing is recognised as the single most important procedure in preventing cross infection in hospital. Hands are bacteriologically contaminated with 103-106 colony forming units (CFU) during various care procedures, and with 102-103 CFU by minor social contact (Zimakoff, 1988). Like the rest of the skin, they have two different microbial flora:

- those that are permanently resident and can only be removed for a few hours;

- transient micro-organisms (often pathogenic) picked up and shed on skin scales during normal activities. These can be effectively removed – or at least reduced to a low level – by adequate handwashing (Gould, 1987).

The practice of handwashing

Many healthcare professionals know about the importance of handwashing in infection control procedures, yet fail to practise it. A study in America (Albert and Condiuf, 1981) showed that less than 50 per cent of direct patient contacts were followed by handwashing, and this statistic was confirmed by a multi-centre study in Denmark and Norway (Zimakoff, 1988).

Reinforcement of the handwashing message also appears to have a limited effect. An extensive campaign was conducted in Liverpool, involving staff education and electronic monitoring of handwashing. A study of handwashing practices six months after the campaign revealed that it was back at the precampaign baseline level (Williams, 1988).

Even when staff do wash their hands, they are often not thorough enough. Taylor (1978) found 89 per cent of staff missed some part of the hand surface; 56 per cent missed part of the thumbs; 28 per cent missed the back of the fingers; 24 per cent missed the back of the hands; 16 per cent missed the area between the fingers and 16 per cent missed an area of the palm.

A handwashing technique

A seven step handwashing routine was devised by Ayliffe (1978). Using running water and soap or antiseptic wash, each step consists of five strokes forward and five backward.

1. Palm to palm.
2. Right palm over left dorsum and left palm over right dorsum.
3. Palm to palm with fingers interlaced.
4. Backs of fingers to opposing palms with fingers interlaced.
5. Rotational rubbing of right thumb clasped over left palm and left thumb over right palm.
6. Rotational rubbing backwards and forwards with clasped fingers of right hand in palm of left hand and vice versa.
7. Hands and wrists rubbed for 30 seconds.

The aims of handwashing

The aim of handwashing is to remove all transient organisms – or to reduce their numbers below the level of an infecting dose – before they are transferred to a susceptible patient or to a piece of equipment. A good washing technique using soap, water and paper towels is all that is needed. Three levels of hand hygiene are recognised in infection control practice (Taylor, 1978).

Social handwashing Washing with soap and water is practised when the hands are soiled, before starting work, visiting another department, handling food or leaving for home, and after visiting the toilet, handling patients' bedding or cleaning sessions.

Hygienic handwashing Washing with an antiseptic handwashing preparation (or handwashing followed by an alcohol-based antiseptic handrub) is practised before any procedure involving high-risk patients or an invasive procedure and after contact with infected patients or contaminated material or equipment.

Surgical handwashing Practised before all major surgical procedures, this technique is taught in the operating theatre. It is usually a three minute handwash using an antiseptic preparation.

If correctly applied to all areas of the hands, alcohol handrubs (70 per cent) are an effective hand disinfectant and can be a substitute for soap and water and antiseptic preparations, particularly in high-risk areas such as special care baby units or if soap and water are not readily available, such as in some community situations.

Why is handwashing neglected?

Research into handwashing has increased our knowledge so that we now know:

How to handwash.

When to handwash.

What to use to handwash.

Why we need to handwash.

Handwashing is a prime example of a cheap and effective infection control method. Research has demonstrated that increased knowledge does not necessarily increase compliance, and this has implications for all hospital infection control procedures. A study of handwashing practice by Williams and Buckles found it to be well below that recommended by the Centre for Disease Control guidelines. Conversely, self-reports from staff of their handwashing habits was three times that actually observed. This suggests staff do realise the importance of frequent handwashing but do not carry it out. Taylor (1978) found nurses to believe that if their hands are not physically soiled – if they cannot see dirt or have not been in contact with a soiled object such as a dirty bedpan – no spread of infection can occur.

These facts suggest that knowledge is not enough to change people's behaviour – motivation is also necessary; but what demotivates nurses from washing their hands often enough? A major cause is probably the side-effect of frequent handwashing – sore hands, particularly in winter. Apart from being unpleasant for the nurse to endure, dry, flaky, cracked skin is in itself an infection risk and can easily become colonised with pathogenic strains of bacteria such as *methicillin resistant Staph. aureaus*. It is essential, therefore, that when handwashing products such as soaps, antiseptic solutions and paper towels are being recommended, their effect on nurses' skin has the highest priority. We cannot preach patient safety and comfort if we ignore those of the nurse.

Nurses can save their hands from becoming sore by using cheap composite plastic gloves for many tasks. These gloves can be washed on the hands and successfully decontaminated in exactly the same way as hands are washed, so this need not be an expensive alternative.

Making a lasting change

While it is essential that nurses are taught microbiology, infection control and the role of handwashing in preventing the spread of infection, research has demonstrated that knowledge is not enough. We have to find products for hand hygiene that can be used frequently without having adverse effects on nurses' hands – or better still ones that are actually beneficial. When such a product exists, we will be able to motivate nurses to practise handwashing as often as necessary.

References

Albert, R. and Condiuf, J. (19981) Handwashing patterns in medical intensive care units. *New England Journal of Medicine*, **304**, 1, 465–66.

Aycliffe, G.A.J, et al (1978) Handwashing techniques. *Journal of Clinical Pathology*, **31**, 923.

Gould, D. (1987) Infection and Patient Care. Heinemann, London.

McFarlane, A. (1989) Reducing the risks to medical patients. The Professional Nurse, **4**, 7, 344–48.

Taylor L.J. (1978) An education of handwashing techniques 1 & 2. *Nursing Times,* **74,** 2, 54 and **74,** 3,108.

Williams, E. and Buckles, A. (1988) A lack of motivation. *Nursing Times,* **84,** 22, 60–64.

Zimakov, J. et al (1988) A multicentre investigation of attitudes to hand hygiene assessed by staff in 12 hospitals in Denmark and three in Norway. Proceedings of the 2nd International Conference on Infection Control.

32

The risks of IV therapy

Susan M. Goodinson-McLaren, BSc, RGN
Lecturer in Nursing Studies, University of Surrey, Guildford

In the 40 years since its inception, intravenous (IV) cannulation has made possible effective, life-saving fluid and electrolyte replacement therapy, parenteral nutrition, drug administration and central venous pressure monitoring in acutely ill patients. Today's IV devices range from single lumen peripheral cannulae with or without attached infusions to the more complex central venous catheters, double or triple lumens, entry ports, multiple infusion fluids and pressure monitoring and cardiac pacing equipment. This chapter deals with preventing thrombophlebitis and infection in IV therapy, looking at what these conditions are and their incidence.

A common practice

IV therapy is extremely common – one European study found an average of 63 per cent of surgical patients have an IV device inserted while in hospital (Nystrom et al, 1983). The major hazards are thrombophlebitis, bacteraemia and septicaemia, which can occur independently or together, and indeed thrombophlebitis increases the incidence of sepsis 18-fold (Maki, 1982).

The reported variation in incidence of thrombophlebitis and infection varies widely. This is probably due to research studies having different methods of confirmation and of defining the features of thrombophlebitis, but the reported incidence ranges from 7.8-28.4 per cent (Nystrom, 1983) and the range for septicaemia is 1.0-8.0 per cent (Maki et al, 1973). Nystrom's study also looked at surgical patients who were not given IV therapy. Among these, 1.5 per 1,000 had a bacteraemia and in 0.5 per 1,000 cases this was identified as being hospital acquired. The corresponding figures for patients with a peripheral IV device were 6.9 and 3.7, and a sobering 59.0 and 44.8 for those with a central venous line. Although the study found a strong correlation between certain types of illness and the incidence of bacteraemia, it also found a strong independent correlation between bacteraemia and the presence of either a central or peripheral venous line.

Nosocomial bacteraemia is the second most expensive infection in terms of extended inpatient stay; it also considerably increases the risk of mortality, irrespective of the underlying disease, and when associated with IV therapy, it increases both morbidity and mortality. Of 97 epidemics of nosocomial bacteraemia reported between 1965-78, about one third were due to IV therapy (Maki, 1982). The significant increase in the number of hospital acquired bacteraemias in recent years has been attributed to the more frequent use of central venous lines.

Preventive action
It seems clear that IV cannulation carries an appreciable risk of iatrogenic disease, and in recognising this problem, it becomes our responsibility to take preventive action. There is abundant evidence that the risk associated with IV therapy can be reduced by a number of measures: limiting the duration of cannulation; using coagulants; using catheters with low thrombogenic properties, and rigorous asepsis during insertion and maintenance of the infusion site. Unfortunately, it seems that these preventive measures are not routinely implemented. A preliminary survey by Doig and Slater (1988) suggests that peripheral IV cannulae are over-used and inadequately managed on some hospital wards. Examples found in a significant number of patients include unnecessarily prolonged cannulation and lack of routine heparinisation. Other studies confirm these findings and ignorance of IV infection control among medical staff.

On a more positive note, specially trained IV therapy teams have been shown to reduce the incidence of IV-related infection dramatically, cutting the incidence of IV-related thrombophlebitis in half and decreasing the incidence of cellulitis and suppurative phlebitis tenfold (Tomford et al, 1984). Nurses on a coronary care unit have also eliminated episodes of systemic sepsis associated with peripheral IV cannulae by introducing a strictly maintained treatment protocol (Collignon et al, 1985). The protocol included early removal or replacement of cannulae, strict asepsis with daily inspection and use of sterile 'op-site' dressings. Infection rates in patients having IV therapy could be reduced by maintaining infection control protocols, but should we rely on IV therapy teams, or work on improving the awareness, skills and compliance of all staff?

The conditions
Thrombophlebitis is the inflammation of a vein associated with thrombus formation, and is characterised by varying degrees of histopathological change, including infiltration, oedema and, in extreme cases, haemorrhage and necrosis of the vein wall. Local redness, pain, warmth, stiffness and a palpable cord are usually present, and Dinley (1976) proposed a grading of severity (Table 1).

If there is no other primary focus for infection, cannula-related sepsis is defined as bacteraemia or fungaemia associated with clinical, microbiological or histological evidence of infection of the intravascular cannula. The pathogens most commonly associated with IV sepsis include *Staph. aureus*, *serratia* and *enterococcus*. Diagnostic features can include fever, tachycardia, leucocytosis, lymphadenopathy, and positive cultures obtained from the blood, suspect cannulae and swabs of the insertion site. Bacteraemia can be difficult to diagnose, since it is most commonly caused by the coagulase negative *staphylococcus*. This is a common blood culture contaminant, and in acutely ill patients, there may be other causes for fever. Weightman et al (1988) suggest this problem can be resolved by comparing blood cultures from one (or more) peripheral vein(s) with that from the catheter itself. A recent comparative investigation of three comparative culture methods found cultures from inside intravascular catheters are the best predictors of infection, as they do not get contaminated when pulled through the skin.

0	No reaction.
1	Tender to touch over the intravascular portion of the cannula.
2	Continuous pain ± redness.
3	Continuous pain, palpable thrombosis.
4	Continuous pain, palpable thrombosis beyond cannula ± swelling.
5	As for 4, with overt infection.

Table 1. Severity of thrombophlebitis.

Suppurative thrombophlebitis is a serious, often lethal infection of a vein segment, denoted by purulent drainage at the cannulation site, although in many cases there may be no local signs of suppuration or inflammation. Bacteraemia occurs at six days, but signs at the IV site may either occur before this or follow its outset by 11 days, so lack of purulent drainage, inflammation or cellulitis does not rule out an IV site as the cause of bacteraemia or sepsis.

Suppurative thrombophlebitis occurs most commonly in plastic catheters left *in situ* for longer than 48-72 hours. Patients with burns, complications of drug abuse, depressed immunocompetence or any serious underlying illness (particularly of vascular origin) are at particular risk. Messner and Gorse (1987) suggest that if all peripheral venous catheters were routinely replaced after a maximum of 72 hours, or ideally 48 hours, the incidence of infection with nosocomial bacteria from peripheral IV lines would be virtually eliminated. The pathogens most commonly associated with suppuration are *Staph. aureus, escheria coli, Staph. epidermis, Staph. hominis, enterococcus* and *klebsiella*, and treatment comprises rapid removal of the cannula, wide, thorough excision of the infected vein segment and its collaterals, and parenteral antibiotic therapy specific to the infecting organism. It is essential that treatment is started promptly to prevent metastatic infection, septic pulmonary embolism and the high mortality rate associated with shock.

Causes

Opinion is divided about the most important causative factors for IV thrombophlebitis and sepsis – theories range from chemical factors such as pH and osmolality of infusate to physical factors such as cannula composition. Properties of specific types of dressing, disinfectant, sources of intrinsic and extrinsic contamination and the need for asepsis in site preparation and maintenance have also been cited as risk factors.

Thrombophlebitis may well begin as a localised response to chemical and physical irritation, but be rapidly converted to bacteraemia or suppuration. The foreign material of the cannula activates the clotting cascade, causing a fibrin sleeve to form on the external intravascular surface of polyethylene and siliconised catheters within 24 hours of their insertion. Thrombi may also be localised to the catheter tip, inside the catheter and associated with the vein wall. Once they form they can become a nidus for bacterial proliferation which can fragment and lead to distant metastatic seeding. The skin flora of either patients or healthcare professionals, and contaminated equipment and infusate can be sources of micro-organisms, which can migrate inwards from the puncture site (most commonly *Staph. aureus* and *Staph. epidermis*). It is not unknown for micro-organisms from distant foci of infection, such as from tracheostomy sites, wounds or the bladder to colonise an IV cannula, probably due to blood borne seeding and/or cross infection from staff. Once established, micro-organisms can penetrate the thrombus, which partially protects them from host defence (Maki, 1973).

Catheter properties

There are a number of ways in which an intravascular catheter can contribute to thrombogenesis and phlebitis. Many plastics are thrombogenic either due to their chemical composition or their biophysical surface properties. Surface etching and irregularities such as grooving or lacunae can cause turbulent blood flow, which can in turn trigger clotting. Williams et al (1982) found that short steel needles caused less thrombophlebitis (8 per cent) than teflon (19 per cent) or silicone (27 per cent). Unfortunately, steel needles were associated with greater risks of extravasation and infiltration, although they were cheap and easy to insert. The authors concluded that teflon, which is associated with a lower incidence of thrombophlebitis than many other materials may be more acceptable. However, Fassolt (1985) compared the phlebito-genic properties of four different catheter materials (polyurethane, teflon, PVC and vialon – a polyurethane-like resin polymer) and found the PVC and vialon cannulae halved the incidence of thrombophlebitis.

Bacterial adherence to cannulae has been found to be lowest in siliconised steel needles and highest in those made of polyethylene (Ashkenazi, 1986). Initial adherence was both to surface irregularities and smooth areas, and was augmented by bacterial slime production.

After a short time, peripheral haloes appeared to surround the bacteria, possibly due to their breakdown of catheter components. Development of a material which decreases the ability of bacteria to adhere to catheters, and particularly decreases the production of slime and cell wall proteins may be the way forward, as may bonding antibiotics to cannulae.

The length and diameter of cannulae have also been implicated in thrombophlebitis; any size can cause mechanical irritation, endothelial shearing and venospasm, all of which contribute to the problem, but the longer and larger the cannula, the greater the trauma. It is vital, therefore, to use the shortest cannula with the smallest bore possible for the size of the vein. Hessov (1985) also recommends using the thinnest possible needle and inserting it into the accessible vein in the arm or hand with the largest diameter and greatest blood flow.

Heparin can be used in a number of ways; bonded to the catheter, added to the infusate, administered systemically or used as a 'flush and lock'. Its anticoagulant action has been reported to act as a significant prophylactic against thrombophlebitis in some research, and while other studies have failed to find conclusive benefits, the weight of evidence suggests its use is beneficial in peripheral intravenous cannulation.

References

Dinley, R.J. (1976) Venous reactions to indwelling plastic cannulae: a prospective clinicial trial. *Current Medical Research Opinion*, **3**, 607.

Doig, J.C. and Slater, S.D. (1988) The misuse of intravenous cannulae. *Scottish Medical Journal*, **33**, 325.

Fassolt, A. (1985) 2ur Phlebitogenitat von Venenkathetern ans vialon. *Infusion Therapie*, **12**, 286.

Hessov, L.F. (1985) Prevention of infusion phlebitis. *Anaesthesiologica Scandinavica*, **29**,33.

Maki, D.G.et al (1973) Infection control in intravenous therapy. *Annals of Internal Medicine*, **79**, 867.

Maki, D.G. (1977) Preventing infection in intravenous therapy. *Current Research*, **56**, 1, 141.

Nystrom, B. et al (1983) Bacteraemia in surgical patients with intravenous devices: a European multicentre incidence study. *Journal of Hospital Infection*, **4**, 338.

Tomford, J.W. and Hershey, C.O. (1984) Intravenous therapy and peripheral venous catheta: associated complications. *Archives of Internal Medicine*, **144**, 1, 191.

Weightman, C. et al (1988) Bacteraemia related to indwelling central venouse cathetas: prevention, diagnosis and treatment. *European Journal of Clinical Microbiology*, **7**, 125.

Williams, D.N. et al (1982) Infusion phlebitis and infiltration associated with intravascular cannulae: a controlled study comparing three different cannula types. *National Intravenous Therapy Association*, **5**, 379.

33

Keeping the flora out: reducing risk of infection in IV therapy

Susan M. Goodinson-McLaren, BSc, RGN
Lecturer in Nursing Studies, University of Surrey, Guildford

In this second chapter reviewing the risk factors associated with intravenous (IV) therapy related thrombophlebitis and sepsis, emphasis is placed on insertion techniques and infusion site preparation and maintenance. Important and controversial issues include where peripheral catheters should be sited, and how the infection site should be prepared and subsequently maintained.

Anatomical location of catheter insertion is important, since both Consentino (1977) Eremin and Marshall (1977) have suggested that placement directly over mobile joint areas such as wrist or elbow *without* immobilisation in a splint, on the back of the hand, or in lower extremities, all increase the chances not only of phlebitis, but also extravasation. The relatively sluggish blood flow in lower extremity veins may also explain the greater risks of infection in catheters sited there.

Sepsis is a major potential hazard for the patient with an indwelling venous catheter. Studies by Cleri (1980) and Maki (1973) have implicated the patient's skin flora as an important source of micro-organisms found on catheter tips. These micro-organisms may gain access from the skin by tracking along the area between the catheter and vein wall, or be introduced by accidental contamination during insertion or subsequent catheter manipulation. Other possible sources of catheter colonisation include blood-borne bacterial seeding from distant loci of infection ie, tracheostomy sites, wounds and urinary tract, although the possibility of cross infection from clinical personnel cannot be excluded. Sources of extrinsic contamination of the IV system may also lead to catheter colonisation.

Minor surgical procedure
Most published guidelines strongly advocate that insertion of a venous catheter should be regarded as a minor surgical procedure, requiring scrupulous aseptic technique in handwashing, site preparation and maintenance. Asepsis is also required in the assembly of equipment and addition of additives (Kaye, 1982; Stratton, 1982; Maki *et al*, 1980;

Messner and Gorse, 1987). Where catheters are inserted in an emergency without adequate preparation, it is recommended that these should be removed and resited as soon as possible.

Microbial flora on the skin of hospital personnel can pose a hazard if such rigorous principles of asepsis are not adhered to. Since approximately 40 per cent of hospital staff may carry Gram negative organisms on their hands and 10 per cent may carry *staph. aureus*, rigorous handwashing is necessary. Sterile gloves should be worn for cut-down procedures and when performing cannulation in immunocompromised patients (Maki *et al*, 1980; Knittle, 1978; Messner and Gorse, 1987).

Selecting and preparing the site

The insertion site should be selected taking account of the anatomical constraints described earlier, using the smallest gauge catheter in the largest vein, and avoiding areas of skin which are painful, bruised, infected or affected by dermatitis. Hecker (1988) suggested the application of small quantities of topical vasodilator drugs (eg, glyceryltrinitrate cream) to the hand may prevent venospasm, improve local blood flow, aid venepuncture and help to prevent chemically induced phlebitis. Wright and Hecker (1985) reported in an earlier study that such measures produced a significant reduction in failure of IV infusions due to phlebitis or extravasation. Readers are advised to consult the research literature for further details on dosage and application (special IV skin patches are also now available). The pain and discomfort associated with venepuncture can be reduced using local anaesthetic creams, which have proved effective in a double-blind trial carried out in children (Maunuksela *et al*, 1986).

Peripheral cannulae are usually inserted into areas of skin which are not abundantly hairy, but the question of whether to shave forearm hair sometimes arises to ensure secure adhesion of dressing tape and the cannula. Maki (1980) commented that methods used to disinfect skin also disinfect hair, so there is no absolute necessity to shave, a point reinforced by the fact that shaving of wound sites in general can cause micro-abrasions which adversely affect the skin microflora. Although the use of depilatory creams has proved a useful alternative to the shaving of wound sites, no carefully controlled, systematic evaluation appears to have been performed on its safe use at IV sites (Seropian, 1971).

For the purposes of skin disinfection, rapidly acting iodine preparations which are bactericidal, fungicidal and sporicidal are recommended. Messner and Gorse (1987) suggest using 1-2 per cent preparations of iodine in 70 per cent alcohol, applied with a swab using a circular motion from the centre to the outer diameter of the insertion site for up to 10cm. Most guidelines suggest the iodine solution should be allowed to dry for 30-60 seconds after skin contact, following which it should be washed off using 70 per cent alcohol, which in turn should be allowed to dry for 30-60 seconds. In patients who are sensitive to iodine, a one minute scrub with iodophors may be preferred, but these should not be washed off, to facilitate the release of free iodine which enhances their bactericidal action. An acceptable alternative to either of these solutions is 70 per cent alcohol used as a one minute scrub after preliminary washing (Maki, 1977).

Turnidge (1984) identified the insertion technique as one of the principal risk factors for cannula-related sepsis. An atraumatic, aseptic, no-touch technique is mandatory. Mechanical difficulty encountered during insertion results in higher infection rate (Bolansky, 1970), hence the skill and experience of the individual performing the insertion is critical. A few studies have highlighted the inexperience of junior medical staff, together with lack of motivation and failure to follow guidelines as contributing to problems (Consentino, 1977; Bentley and Lepper, 1968; Maki, 1973). Atraumatic, aseptic venepuncture is a skilled technique, and this may be one reason why IV therapy teams, who are skilled at catheter insertion and follow rigorous infection control protocols, have been able to exert a significant impact in reducing IV related sepsis (Collingnon, 1985; Tomford, 1984).

After insertion, the cannula should be secured firmly using sterile tape, to prevent any lateral movement which may aid the entry of micro-organisms. The tape should not touch the puncture site, and should be anchored at least 5mm from it. After insertion and before connection to the IV infusate system, flushing the cannula with heparinised saline is sometimes advised to ensure immediate patency.

Dressings
Following insertion, application of a sterile dressing is necessary to facilitate stability of the cannula and easy inspection. Ideally, a dressing should be selected under which bacterial growth is low, in the hope of diminishing catheter colonisation and sepsis.

In 1979 a survey by Bauer and Denson emphasised the importance of using sterile dressing products, after finding high IV infection rates associated with the application of general ward use, non-sterile elastoplast to venepuncture sites. The need for rigorous skin disinfection and use of sterile gauze/tape was also supported by Smallman's study in 1980. Here, the incidence of thrombophlebitis at three days post-cannulation was 34 per cent in a group of patients whose IV sites were disinfected with an alcohol preparation, and secured with a sterile dressing, which was changed daily. In comparison, the incidence of thrombophlebitis was 100 per cent in the group who did not receive skin disinfection and whose IV sites were secured with zinc oxide tape.

The comparative merits of using gauze (sterile) dressings plus tape versus the semi-occlusive, polyurethane transparent films on peripheral IV cannulation sites is not clear. Gantz, Presswood and Goldberg (1984) compared incidence rates of phlebitis, malfunction, cellulitis and septicaemia for short-term indwelling Teflon catheters in 807 patients in the groups described below:

Group I IV sites dressed with sterile gauze, secured with tape; dressing changed at 24 hour intervals.

Group II IV sites dressed as above; dressing changed at 48 hour intervals; IV site inspected 24-hourly.

Group III IV sites dressed with polyurethane film (OpSite); protocol as for Group II.

Results suggested the risk of phlebitis 48 hours following insertion was greater in Group I compared to the other two groups. After 72 hours there was significantly less phlebitis in Group II. Risks of malfunction (leaking, infiltration, extravasation) were greater at 24 hours in Group III than in the other two groups, and loosening of the dressing appeared to be a problem. Recommendations arising from this study were that 'standard gauze' dressings were an acceptable, cost-effective choice for dressing peripheral IV sites; 48 hour dressing changes were advocated, as changing at 24 hour intervals appeared to increase the risk of phlebitis, possibly due to manipulation of the cannula during the dressing procedure.

How do the different types of polyurethane film dressings compare in relation to their special properties in producing inhibition of bacterial growth on forearm skin? One study by Wille and Ablas (1989) investigated this in non-cannulated volunteers. Comparisons were made between Tegaderm, OpSite, Tegaderm Plus (impregnated with povidone iodine) and OpSite CH (impregnated with chlorexidine) as to their effectiveness in reducing bacterial skin colonisation after seven days' application. The numbers of colony-forming units present on skin covered with 'OpSite CH' were significantly lower than those obtained with the other three dressings tested. This interesting comparative study should be repeated on IV infusion sites, in randomised groups of hospitalised patients, to obtain a clearer evaluation on reduction of catheter associated complications.

Whatever dressing is selected, adjunctive use of a splint will give additional support, comfort and help to prevent catheter displacement. If crepe or cotton bandages are applied, the sterile dressing over the site should be left uncovered to enable easy access for inspection. If the semi-occlusive, polyurethane film type of dressing is applied, this should not be covered to facilitate its properties in reducing skin colonisation.

Other aspects of site maintenance

Following insertion, site maintenance is largely the nurse's responsibility. A number of other important points for action have been stressed by the

CDC (1982), Messner and Gorse (1987) and Collignon *et al* (1985), and include the following (as consultation with medical colleagues and hospital policies dictate):

- Check the infusion site at least 24-hourly for signs of thrombophlebitis and infection; ask the patient to report pain and/or discomfort.
- Evaluate vital signs and leucocyte count for fever; removal of the dressing is advocated if an unexplained fever occurs, and removal of the cannula at the earliest signs of inflammation.
- Maintain asepsis at the infusion site using effective disinfectants, sterile dressings and a 48 hour dressing change.
- Initiate investigations regarding the source of fever, which may include cultures from the cannula, its tip, skin insertion site and blood.
- Maintain accurate records in the nursing kardex and care plans of all details of IV therapy. This will provide a basis for decisions on cannula and dressing change.

References
Bauer, E and Denson, P. (1979) Infection from contaminated Elastoplast. *New England Journal of Medicine*, **300**, 7,370.

Bentley, D.W. and Lepper, M.H. (1968) Septicaemia related to indwelling catheters. *Journal of the American Medical Association*, **206**, 1749–52.

Bolansky, B.L. (1970) The hazards of intravenous polyethylene catheters in surgical patients. *Surgery, Gynaecology and Obstetrics*, **130**, 342–46.

CDC: Centres for Disease Control Working Group (1982) Guidelines for the prevention of intravascular infections. In: 'Guidelines for the Prevention and Control of Nosocomial Infections'. DHAA-PS, Bethesda, USA.

Cleri, D.J. (1980) Quantitative culture of intravascular catheters and other intravascular inserts. *Journal of Infectious Diseases* **141**, 781–86.

Collignon, P.J. (1985) Prevention of sepsis associated with the insertion of intravenous cannulae. *The Medical Journal of Australia*, **142**, 346–49.

Consentino, F. (1977) Personnel-induced infusion phlebitis. *Bulletin of the Parenteral Drug Association*, **31**, 288–93.

Eremin, O. and Marshall, V. (1977) Complications of intravenous therapy. *Medical Journal of Australia*, **2**, 16, 528–31.

Gantz, N., Presswood, B., Goldburg, R. (1984) Effects of Dressing type and change interval on IV therapy complication rates. *Diagnosis of Microbiology of Infectious Diseases*, **2**, 325–32.

Hecker, J. (1988) Improved techniques in IV therapy. *Nursing Times*, **84**, 34, 28–33.

Kaye, W. (1982) Catheter and infusion related sepsis. *Heart and Lung*, **11**, 3, 221–28.

Knittle, M.A., (1978) role of hand contamination of personnel in the epidemiology of Gram negative nosocomial infections. *Journal of Pediatrics*, **86**, 433–37.

Maki, D.G. (1973) Infection control in intravenous therapy. *Annals of Internal Medicine*, **79**, 867.

Maki, D.G. (1977) Preventing infection in intravenous therapy: current research. *Anaesthesia and Analgesia*, **56**, 1, 141–53.

Maki, D.G. (1982) Infections associated with intravascular lines. In: Remington, J. and Swartz, M. (Eds) Current Topics in Infectious Diseases. McGraw-Hill, New York.

Maunuksela, E.L. and Kopela, R. (1986) Double blind trial in evaluation of lignocaine-pilocaine cream (EMLA) in children. *British Journal of Anaesthesia*, **58**, 1242–45.

Messner, R.L. and Gorse, G.J. (9187) Nursing management of periperal IV sites *Focus on Critical Care*, **14**, 2,25–33.

Seropian, R. (1971) Wound infection after preoperative depilatory versus razor preparation. *American Journal of Surgery*, **121**, 251–54.

Smallman, L. *et al* (1980) The effect of skin preparation and care on the incidence of superficial thrombophlebitis. *British Journal of Surgery*, **67**, 861–62.

Stratton, C.W. (1982) Infection related to intravenous infusions. *Heart and Lung,* **11,** 2, 123–37.

Tomford, J.W. *et al* (1984) Intravenous therapy team and peripheral venous catheter-associated complications. *Archives of Internal Medicine,* **144,** 6, 1191–94.

Turnidge, J. (1984) Hazards of peripheral intravenous lines. *Medical Journal of Australia,* **141,** 1, 37–40.

Wille, J.C. and Albas, A.B. (1989) A comparison of four film-type dressings by their antimicrobial effect on flora of the skin. *Journal of Hospital Infection,* **14,** 153–58.

Wright, A.and Hecker, J. (1985) Use of transdermal GTN to reduce failure of intravenous infusions due to phlebitis and extravasion. *Lancet,* **10,** 1149–50.

34

Urinary incontinence: a many faceted problem

Patricia A. Black, BA(Hons), RGN, PG Dip HV
Health Visitor, Croydon Community Health Trust

Urinary incontinence affects approximately two million people in Britain, mainly women. With the associated emotional and monetary costs, it clearly poses a challenge to healthcare professionals (HCP) to find the best way to help sufferers cope (Townsend, 1988). Since more women than men suffer from urinary incontinence the feminine pronoun will be used throughout this chapter and the anatomy will also refer to the female.

The sufferer should be seen as an active participant in the healthcare process, becoming involved in decisions which affect the management of her condition. If she is not consulted and kept informed as to the reasons for actions taken, compliance is likely to be minimised. This may show as failure to attend for check-ups at the appropriate time or failure in the management of hygiene (Bewley, 1988).

Patient information

People vary in their basic knowledge of biological function and abilities to understand and communicate, so it is up to the HCP to devise an

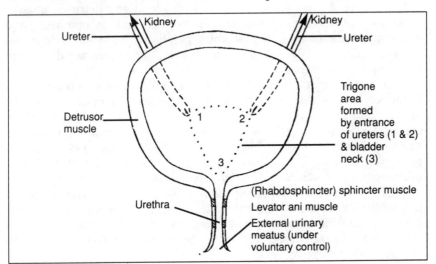

Figure 1. Schematic diagram of the bladder and urethra.

effective method of 'getting the message across'. One way is to begin with a straightforward explanation of urinary tract function accompanied by a schematic diagram of the bladder and urethra (Figure 1). Since anxiety inhibits people's ability to retain information, it is helpful if the diagram and explanation is photocopied and made available to be taken home, so it can be used as a source of reference when the patient is more relaxed (Wilson-Barnett, 1978). If possible, this information should be translated into several languages.

Although the information given to the patient may be fundamental, HCPs should have more detailed knowledge if they are to offer help in a way that is best tailored to the individual's requirements.

Anatomy

The lower urinary tract (UT) consists of two ureters, the urinary bladder and the urethra. The ureters are about 30cm long and enter the bladder at an oblique angle, preventing backflow of urine by forming a 'valve' in the bladder wall. They consist of an inner lining of mucous membrane, a mid layer of muscle tissue and a fibrous outer layer.

The urinary bladder is a sac situated behind the symphysis pubis, and acts as a temporary reservoir for urine which is eliminated from the body at intervals. It is composed of four layers of tissue, the outer being the peritoneum which covers the superior bladder surface and continues upwards to become the parietal peritoneum lining the anterior abdominal wall. The peritoneum covers a layer of smooth muscle tissue which is itself composed of three layers. The inner is arranged longitudinally, the middle circularly, and the outer again longitudinally. These layers give the impression of a single mass of interlacing smooth muscle fibres which are collectively referred to as the detrusor muscle.

A submucous coat links the inner lining and the detrusor muscle, consisting of blood vessels, lymph vessels and sympathetic and parasympathetic nerve fibres. Mucous membrane lines the bladder and this is arranged in folds (rugae) when it is empty or contracted – except in the area of the trigone.

As its name suggests, the trigone has the appearance of a triangle and is formed by the openings of the ureters in the posterior wall of the bladder and the opening of the bladder neck. It has two muscle layers, the deep layer, which is the same as the muscle of the rest of the bladder, and the superficial layer, which recent research (Hilton, 1986) suggests may play a part in controlling the ureterovesical junction during micturition by preventing vesico-ureteric reflux.

The bladder neck, the opening leading to the urethra, is constructed of longitudinally arranged smooth muscle fibre. This appears to have little or no sphincteric action, not seeming to act in the maintenance of continence, but facilitating micturition by shortening and widening the bladder neck during voiding.

Urethral construction is important to continence and it is

approximately 4cm of remarkably complex tissue. Basically, the urethra is a tube which extends forwards and downwards from the bladder neck, behind the symphysis pubis, opening exteriorly at the urinary meatus. The external urinary meatus (in front of the vagina), is protected by sphincter muscle under the voluntary control of the cerebral cortex.

The urethra has three layers of tissue: mucous membrane lines the upper layer which is continuous with that of the bladder proximally, whilst distally it is lined with stratified squamous epithelium, which carries on externally with the vulva. The next layer is a vascular plexus whose composition alters with age. The recent identification of arterio-venous anastomoses suggests vascularity plays a major role in the urethral closure in young women (Hilton, 1987). Beneath this is a layer of smooth muscle which shortens and opens the urethra when contracted.

If the urethra may be visualised as divided into thirds, the mid third is circled by a striated muscle (rhabdosphincter). This causes it to close at rest and contributes to maintenance of urethral resting pressure. The levator ani muscle, where the middle and lower thirds of the urethra meet, aids the fast closure of the urethra when physical effort occurs.

Micturition

Micturition is controlled by nerve supply, urethral sphincter mechanism and detrusor activity; for this purpose the bladder, urethra and pelvic floor act together. The smooth muscle wall of the bladder is supplied by nerves from the sympathetic and parasympathetic systems. Activity of the bladder involves autonomic and voluntary nervous impulses and results from a sacral spinal reflex governed by the cerebral cortex, the cerebellum, subcortical areas of the brain and the brain stem.

A simple reflex arc is required for bladder filling and emptying. Filling is passive, and when approximately 300ml of urine has collected, stretch receptors in the bladder wall pass this information through the sacral spinal cord and into the brain stem. This in turn triggers impulses which travel back down the same route to cause the detrusor muscle to contract, the internal sphincter to relax and urine to flow out.

Control over this function is usually gained by three years of age, the reflex motor activity being suppressed by unconscious inhibition. The cerebral cortex via the pontine reticular formation, inhibits voiding until the time is appropriate.

Continence is maintained provided the bladder pressure remains lower than the sphincter pressure. There is a rise in bladder pressure as the detrusor contracts – a fall in the urethral pressure as the sphincter relaxes to allow urine to pass from the bladder and voiding to occur.

If there is a problem with the urethral closure mechanism, urine may leak even if the detrusor muscle fails to contract. Leakage is likely when the intravesicle pressure exceeds the pressure in the urethra. It was formerly believed that a major component in the maintenance of continence was the angle between the posterior wall of the bladder and the urethra. The main continence mechanism appears to be the 'pressure profile' as outlined above (McCarthy, 1980). There are many types of urinary incontinence – Table 1 explains each.

Stress incontinence, more accurately known as urethral sphincter incompetence. Occurs when urinary leakage is provoked as a direct result of physical activity. It may result from pelvic floor laxity, damage to the nerve supply from trauma, childbirth or disease; or descent of the bladder neck.

It is caused by the rise in abdominal pressure generated by a stimulus eg, sneezing, not reaching the proximal urethra. This allows the urethral pressure gradient to become reversed and urine is leaked despite all efforts to prevent it.

Urge incontinence relates to instability of the detrusor muscle and means that an urgent desire to void is felt just before involuntary loss of urine due to detrusor muscle contraction.

Sensory-urgency is an involuntary loss of urine accompanying a strong desire to void that is not accompanied by detrusor muscle contraction (ICS, 1988).

Continuous incontinence may be a result of overflow (due to retention caused by obstruction) or to a bladder that does not react to nerve stimulus (becomes large and hypotonic). The latter is indicated if a residual urine in excess of 200ml can be obtained.

Functional incontinence is a term used when a person has become socially unaware of the constraints that accompany micturition – the generally accepted requirement to void in privacy.

Table 1. Types of incontinence.

Incontinence

Since the cause of urinary incontinence is lowered intraurethral pressure, it may be helpful to look at the influencing factors of nerve supply, mechanical damage, hormonal influence, drug therapy and infection.

Damage to the nerve supply to the bladder or to the spinal cord may inhibit impulses from bladder to brain, while damage to the brain may prevent a response to bladder stimuli. Whatever the reason for this damage, be it trauma or disease process, the result is likely to be incontinence. Mechanical damage is damage to the actual structures involved, such as congenital bladder or urethral malformation, direct traumatic impact, or disease eg, cancer.

Other causes may be due to drug therapy eg, tranquillisers that may have been prescribed for a different condition. These may have alpha blockade or beta stimulation effects, which, by acting on the urethral smooth muscle, will produce incontinence. If a woman contracts an acute or chronic infection of the urethra or bladder, particular strains of *E. coli* cause an endotoxicity which inhibits the alpha adrenergic receptor property of the lower urinary tract.

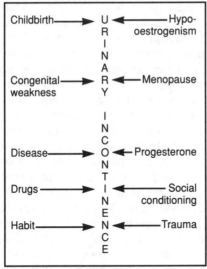

Figure 2. Influencing factors.

Many women experience incontinence for the first time when pregnant, and this may resolve itself during the postpartum. It is thought to be caused by elevated progesterone levels experienced during pregnancy – progesterone acts as a beta adrenergic stimulator and the urethral response to beta stimulation is by relaxation, creating a lowered intraurethral pressure. Similarly, during the menopause, low oestrogen levels cause periurethral vascularity to decrease, mucosal wasting and muscular hypotonia in the urethra and trigone, incontinence may be caused by a combination of one or all of these conditions.

Coping strategies
There are many facets to the problem of urinary incontinence, so how can HCPs maximise the help they can give? As has been seen, there are at least seven types of incontinence and the method of management will vary with each of them as well as with the individual's needs.

Apart from surgery and drug therapy there are several positive approaches the HCP may choose to use. In cases of stress incontinence, pelvic floor exercises (PFE), whereby weak pelvic floor muscles (levator ani) are encouraged to regain tone, contracting and relaxing gently, building up to 15 minutes four times a day. This will help control to be maintained over the urethral sphincter even when physical effort is undertaken. A similar effect can be obtained by interrupting the urinary stream when voiding.

A problem with PFE is that some women seem to have difficulty locating the pelvic floor muscles – objective physiotherapy measurement may show an increase in intra-abdominal pressure achieved by tightening the abdominal muscles and not by contracting those of the pelvic floor. To avoid this problem the concept of vaginal cones (set of nine cones, of equal shape and volume but weighing between 20 and 100g – they are made of perspex and stainless steel with a nylon thread to make them easy to remove) were developed (Peattie, 1980). Attempts are made to retain a cone in the vagina beginning with the heaviest weight that can be kept in place while walking. Once successful for two consecutive occasions in retaining the cone for a 15 minute period twice a day, a lighter weight is tried. This enables successful location of the pelvic floor muscles, which, if strengthened by regular exercise help ease the problem. Once these muscles have been found and contraction proved possible, the cones will no longer be required. However, motivation is crucial as the pelvic floor contractions should be continued throughout life to retain muscle tone.

Urge incontinence and sensory-urgency may be helped by behaviour modification techniques and drug therapy. The anticholenergic drugs will inhibit bladder contractions, while behaviour modifications centre on 're-learning' voluntary control over bladder contraction. The method often used is bladder drill – the use of frequency and volume diaries to allow self-monitoring: the woman attempts to increase the time between each felt need to void. Biofeedback and hypnotherapy have also been employed and produce an initial symptomatic improvement of about 80 per cent (Cardozo, 1978).

In cases of continuous incontinence, when the patient has a large residual urine, if dexterity, mental ability and an intact urethra permit, intermittent self-catheterisation (ISC) may be an answer. This involves a fine non-retaining catheter being inserted into the bladder at regular intervals to keep the bladder empty. Some cases of continuous incontinence may be due to retention of urine by a large mass in the pelvic area eg, constipation or tumour. The incontinence is an overflow of urine as the mass may prevent much of the urine being voided.

Functional incontinence in mentally frail people is less likely to occur if a reality orientated environment is maintained. The nursing process should be used to provide individual care and attention. Incontinence should never be regarded as 'normal', especially in elderly people.

Given that the nursing goal is continence, or, failing that, for the individual to be able to control the effects of incontinence to allow them to lead a full and active life, can anything else be done?

Continence advisor

Liaison can be carried out with the continence advisor, who will be aware of the many aspects of urinary incontinence and be able to help the patient select the equipment most suitable for her needs.

Pads and pants may be helpful when the patient is waiting for treatment, investigations, or surgery, or where surgery is refused or treatment is not feasible. Some devices may be inserted into the vagina which appear to be effective by exerting gentle pressure on the urethra, causing an increase in outflow plus an improvement in the transmission of raised intra-abdominal pressure to the mid-urethra. An example of this device is the Edwards pubovaginal spring, whose success rate is 95 per cent, decreasing to 87.5 per cent between 61-70 years (Edwards, 1973). However, these devices should be used with caution, since they may damage the urethra, due to the pressure they have to exert to remain effective.

Collection bottles and pans help the patient who experiences urge incontinence and whose movements are limited. Examples are the female urinal which is adapted to suit the female vulva. The bottom resembles the usual urinary bottle. The 'Feminal' is a type of female urinal, where the urine drains into a disposable plastic bag.

Apart from self-catheterisation, long-term urethral catheterisation may be used to control continuous incontinence. The silicone or silicone coated latex rubber catheters only should be considered for long-term use (latex may cause irritation) since they remain patent in approximately 70 per cent of people after a two month period (Blannin and Hebden, 1980).

If mentally able, patients should be taught how to care for their catheter, to ensure they play an active part in the caring process (the patient is too often seen as passive with little 'say' in the selection of treatment). They may need basic instruction in hygiene principles, and to be shown how to position the catheter to gain the maximum drainage, and should be aware of how much they need to drink to lessen the risk of infection.

Many people find urinary incontinence a most distressing experience, and may delay seeking treatment for years. The HCP can help by explaining that people do not have to suffer the indignity of leakage, because it is frequently curable and certainly containable and should not lead to a reduced quality of life. The HCP has a vital part to play in helping patients to see themselves as worthy of respect (low self-esteem correlates with sufferers of urinary incontinence), not to delay in seeking information because of family commitments or embarrassment (Norton, 1988); to seek help if the condition occurs at menopause and not to be satisfied with the explanation that it must be expected with ageing.

With improvement in the quality of life being the primary objective, the HCP must be aware of the multi-faceted nature of incontinence. Should sufferers of urinary incontinence be offered anything else?

References

Bewley, S. (1988) Who defaults after treatment for gonorrhoea? Randomised controlled study of effect of an educational leaflet. *Genitourinary Med*, **64**, 241–44.

Blannin, J.P. and Hebden, J. (1980) The catheter of choice. *Nursing Times*, **76**, 48, 2092–93.

Cardozo, L., Stanton, S.L., Hofner, J., Allan, V. (19790 Biofeedback in the treatment of detrusor instability,. *British Journal of Urology*, **50**, 3, 250–54.

Edwards, L. and Malvern, J. (1973) Long-term follow-up results with the pubovaginal spring device with incontinence of urine in women; comparison with electronic methods of control. *British Journal of Urology*, **45**, 2, 103–08.

Hilton, p. (1986) Mechanism of continence. In: Surgery of Female Incontinence. Stanton, S.L. and Tanagho, E. (Eds). Springer-Verlag, Heidelberg.

Hilton, P. (1987) Anatomy and physiology of the female lower urinary tract. Practical Urodynamics Conference organised by Royal College Obstetricians and Gynaecologists and Institute of Urology, 8–9 June 1987.

International Continence Society (1988) The standardisation of terminology of lower urinary tract function. *Scand. Journal Urology Nephrology*, **22**, Supp. 114, 5–19.

McCarthy, T.A. (1980) The differential diagnosis of urinary incontinence. *Gynaecologic Urology and Urodynamics*, 223–28.

Norton, P.A., MacDonald, L.D., Sedgwick P.M., Stanton, S.L. (1988). Distress and delay associated with urinary incontinence, frequency, and urgency in women. *British Medical Journal*, **297**, 1187–89.

Peattie, A.B., Plevnik, S., Stanton, S.L. (1988) Vaginal Cones: a conservative method of treating genuine stress incontinence. *British Journal Obstetrics and Gynaecology*, **95**, 1049–53.

Townsend, J. (1988) Costs of incontinence. *Community Medicine*, **10**, 3, 235–39.

Wilson-Barnett, J. (1978) Factors influencing patients' emotional reactions to hospitalisation. *Journal of Advanced Nursing*, **3**, 211–29.

35

Nursing care of catheterised patients

Petra M. Britton, RGN
Formerly Hospital Continence Advisor, Bloomsbury HA

Elizabeth S. Wright, RGN, DipN, CHSM
Senior Nurse, Surgical Unit, The Royal London Hospital, Whitechapel, London

Catheters are only used as a last resort in patients for whom they are absolutely necessary. In hospital, however, this can mean 10–12 per cent of those admitted. Once a catheter has been selected, the real nursing begins. There is a range of potential complications to be avoided, and the patient's psychological reaction to consider.

Encrustation, blockage, bypassing and spasm

Blockage is often caused by debris within the urine, which occurs particularly in immobile patients who may also suffer from urinary tract infection. Infected urine provides a higher incidence of encrustation (Srinvasan and Clark, 1972), and this was found by Bruce et al (1974) to reduce the rate of urine flow through the catheter lumen and often obstruct it completely.

Most urinary catheters will become encrusted to a certain extent, although catheter materials such as silicone may lessen the incidence. Encrustation occurs particularly in cases of *Klebsiella*, *Pseudomonas* or *Proteus* urinary tract infections, which produce an enzyme called urease, that breaks down the urea in the urine to release ammonia and free hydrogen ions. These can precipitate ammonium phosphate, calcium

Nurses can prevent or reduce bypassing and bladder spasm by:
- Inserting the smallest catheter possible ie, 14Ch or 16Ch.
- Using catheters with small balloons.
- If bypassing does occur:
  a. Check catheter is not blocked.
  b. Reassure and explain to the patient why this is happening.
  c. In contemporary practice one agent is particularly useful, namely Oxybutinin. Oxybutinin has a short half life but is rapidly active when administered, the therapeutic dose being 5mg tds. Unfortunately, Oxybutinin is not yet available on the British Formulary but can be obtained on named patient basis by application to the manufacturers Smith + Nephew Pharmaceuticals or Tillott's Laboratories.
  d. Question as to whether the catheter is really necessary, and remove it if possible.

phosphate or magnesium phosphate, so stones form around colonies of bacteria, or encrustation may occur on the tip and eyes of the catheter and balloon area (Hukins, Hickey and Kennedy, 1983). The encrustation around the catheter may make the balloon difficult to deflate, or block the eyes of the catheter and obstruct drainage.

According to Kennedy et al (1983), 40 per cent of all catheterised patients experience the bypassing of urine around the catheter. This can often lead to recatheterisation in an effort to reduce the problem, which is caused by the bladder being irritated by the catheter, particularly in cases of bladder instability. Kennedy et al (1983) conducted a study to examine the incidence of bypassing in patients catheterised with various sizes of catheter. Those with larger lumen catheters experienced more bypassing than those with a small Charriere size. Catheters with smaller balloons allow the catheter tip to rest lower in the bladder, resulting in less residual urine below the eye level that can leak out by bypassing.

Urinary tract infection

Urinary infection (UTI) as a result of catheterisation, particularly in the long term, is virtually unavoidable, but is usually asymptomatic (Brocklehurst and Brocklehurst, 1978). The incidence of bacteriuria ranges between 14-44 per cent on recent studies of catheterised patients (Burke et al, 1986; Crow et al, 1986), and this is further influenced by other host-determined factors, including age, sex, underlying pathology and susceptibility (immunosuppression, length of stay in hospital etc) (Garibaldi et al, 1980). It has been long established that a closed system of drainage reduces the incidence of catheter-acquired UTI quite dramatically (Dukes, 1929; Kunin, 1980).

Any section of the urinary tract may be affected by bacteriuria and spread throughout the rest of the system (Kunin, 1979), and an infection is defined by the presence of 100,000 organisms per ml of urine, or if the patient is symptomatic. The long-term effects of UTI include a higher rate of renal pathology in elderly people (Carty et al, 1981), and there is a three times greater mortality rate associated with bacteriuria during catheterisation (Platt et al, 1982). Infection may invade the 'closed system' of drainage through a number of portals, which have been well documented. Essentially, it is the proper management of this 'closed system', the aseptic catheterisation procedure initially and the early removal of the catheter. The risk of acquiring a UTI increases linearly (Garibaldi et al, 1974), so early removal will reduce the risks considerably. Catheter associated urinary tract infections can lengthen the patient's stay in hospital postoperatively by two to four days – causing considerable discomfort and inconvenience to the patient and cost to the health service (Givens and Wenzel, 1980).

Urethral strictures and pressure necrosis

The traumatic insertion of a cystoscope or catheter into the urethra is currently the most common reason for urethral stricture formation. This can result from the use of too large a catheter, forcing the catheter on insertion against a resistance, or inflating the balloon in the urethra instead of the bladder. Traumatic removal of the catheter, usually by the patient (either while disorientated or intentionally) with the balloon still inflated, may cause sufficient trauma to result in scarring and stricture formation.

Difficulty in deflating balloons

If the full amount of water can not be aspirated (other than the water within the lumen of the inflation channel) using a syringe from the balloon luer lock port, do not panic. Try these solutions:

● Jam the syringe into the port tightly and try again, after pushing the catheter a little further into the bladder.

● Check the medical and nursing notes for a record of the volume of water used to inflate the balloon.

● The balloon channel port can be cut off, and a wire stylet or fine ureteric catheter can be passed up the lumen to the balloon to prick the balloon from the inside (Browning, Bar, Harsburgh, 1984).

Although there are other methods of deflating balloons, the latter method is the method of choice and the safest for medical staff to

---

The use of large catheters and large balloons may cause traction on the bladder neck – particularly if they are not secured to relieve traction – and cause pressure necrosis. However, if the catheter is adhered to the thigh, the site should be checked at least twice daily and meatal toilet performed to ensure pressure sores do not develop on the urethral meatus. Pressure necrosis can reach such an extent in male patients, due to poor nursing and medical care, that almost the entire length of the penile shaft becomes necrosed, with the catheter exiting half way up the side of the penis.

Inflammation of the urethra may also occur in response to the materials used to manufacture the catheter, particularly if the catheter has been *in situ* for some weeks. This urethritis may develop in response to the chemical irritants, infection or ischaemia. Latex catheters have been demonstrated to bring about epithelial loss and a moderate inflamatory infiltrate (in rat urethrae). Plastic catheters produce less reaction, and silicone virtually no reaction at all (Edwards et al, 1983). An antioxidant in latex catheters and a cytotoxic organo-tin compound in plastic (PVC) catheters have been suggested as causes of urethral irritation and strictures (Wilksch et al, 1983; Ruutu et al, 1985).

Localised ischaemia within the urethra may cause stricture formation, particularly after urethral catheterisation following cardiac surgery. If the circulation via the internal pudendal arteries is compromised, the distal urethra may become ischaemic (Abdel-Hakim et al 1983, 1984; Elhali et al, 1986). Various factors may contribute ultimately to stricture formation, but the trauma caused by a catheter brings about the formation of granulation tissue which eventually fibroses, shrinks and reduces the urethral lumen.

Paraurethral abscess

This usually occurs in cases where a large sized catheter has been used and has caused obstruction to the paraurethral ducts. Bacteria then accumulate and result in abcess formation. This may then lead to cutaneous fistula formation as the erosion of the healthy tissue surrounding the urethra develops. Prostatitis, prostatic abcesses and epididymitis may occur for the same reasons.

Paraphimosis

Although not directly related to catheterisation, this condition does occur following catheterisation or meatal toilet if the professional giving the care fails to pull forward the foreskin after retracting it for the procedure. Over a period of time, in the uncircumcised patient, a retracted foreskin can become grossly oedematous and painful, requiring 'reduction' by an experienced member of staff as soon as possible. If the condition is allowed to worsen, it may not be possible to reduce the swelling and pull the foreskin forward; and will require a doral slit circumcision under anaesthetic. Staff must always ensure the foreskin is pulled over the glans following these procedures.

Other risks and problems

Febrile conditions and septicaemia have been associated with instrumentation on catheterisation of the urinary tract since 1800, while UTI is the most prevalent of all nosocomial infections, contributing to 30.3 per cent in 2.8 per cent of all patients (Meers, 1981); 34 per cent of Gram-negative bacteraemias can result from UTI, and these can ultimately lead to septicaemic conditions. The fatality rate for this is between 25 and 30 per cent.

The Report on The National Survey on Infection in Hospitals (Meers, 1981) offers some interesting results concerning nosocomial urinary tract infection in the UK. Within this survey, 8.6 per cent of patients had indwelling urinary catheters, and their presence correlated highly with the incidence of urinary tract infection: 19.4 per cent in male patients and 22.7 per cent in female patients. Control results from non-catheterised patients revealed an incidence of urinary tract infection of 1.7 per cent and 3.7 per cent respectively, while 21 per cent of catheterised patients had infected urine, and 41 per cent of all those who were infected were catheterised.

While most patients who have catheters do so only for a short time, some people do need them in the long term. This can be difficult to cope with psychologically, and nurses should ensure they offer emotional support as well as practical advice about catheter care in these cases.

Sex is a major cause of concern for some people with long-term catheters. They are unsure whether they can continue to be sexually active, and need reassurance and practical advice. Roe and Brocklehurst (1987) found in their study that no professionals had voluntarily discussed sex with any catheterised patients – surely the sexual aspects of being catheterised should be automatically discussed with patients for whom this is appropriate? The following points may be mentioned, as appropriate.

• Catheters do not have to be removed before making love.

• In men, the catheter can be taped back along the penis once an erection is achieved, and this should cause no irritation to his partner. It can, however, be traumatic to the urethra, and lead to stricture formation (Norton, 1986), and suprapubic catheters may be more appropriate in sexually active people.

• Women's catheters can be strapped down on to the abdomen.

• Nurses should tactfully ensure catheterised women are aware that the catheter is not in the vagina, but a separate orifice.

• The 'missionary' position can cause tension on catheters – a comfortable position can usually be found by trial and error.

• KY Jelly can be used to increase lubrication.

• Catheterised people can be shown how to remove their catheter before intercourse and reinsert it afterwards if they prefer.

• It is a good idea to give the patient information on what counselling is available, such as sexual counsellors, or SPOD (The Association to aid the Sexual and Personal relationships of people with a Disability) who are at 286 Camden Road, London N7 0BJ.

References

Abdel-Hakim, A. et al (1983) Urethral stricture after cardio-vascular surgery; a retrospective and prospective study. *Journal of Urology*, **130**, 1100–02.

Abdel-Hakim, A. et al (1986) Role of urethral ischaemia in the development of urethral strictures after cardio-vascular surgery; a preliminary report. *Journal of Urology*, **135**, 275–77.

Browning, G.G.P., Barr, L., Horsburgh, A.G. (9184) Management of obstructed balloon catheters. *British Medical Journal*, **289**, 89–91.

Bruce, A.W., Sira, S.S., Clark, A.F., Awad, S.A. (1974) The problems of catheter encrustation. *Canadian Med. Ass. Journal*, **111**, 238–41.

Burke, J.P., Larson, R.A., Stevens, L.E. (1986) Nosocomial bacteriurea: estimating the potential for prevention by closed sterile urinary drainage. *Infection Control*, , 2 suppl. 96–99.

Carty, M., Brocklehurst, J.C., Carty, J. (1981) Bacteriuria and its correlates to old age. *Gerontology*, **27**, 72–75.

Dukes, c. (1929) Urinary infections after excision of the rectum. *Proc. Roy. Soc. Med*, **22**, 259–69.

Elhalali, M.M. et l (196) Urethral stricture following cardiovascular surgery: role of urethral ischaemia. *Journal of Urology,* **135,** 275–77.

Garibaldi, R.A. et al (1974) Factors predisposing a bacterium during indwelling urethral catheterisation. *New Eng. J. Med,* **291,** 216–19.

Garibaldi, R.A. et al (1980) Meatal colonisation of catheter associated bacteriuria. *New Eng. J. Med,* **303,** 316–18.

Givens, C.D. and Wenzel, R.P. (1980) Catheter associated urinary tract infections in surgical patients: A controlled study in the excess morbidity and costs. *Journal of Urology,* **124,** 646–18.

Hukins, D.W.L. et al (1983) Catheter encrustation by struvite. *British Journal of Urology,* **55,** 304–05.

Kunin, C.M. (1980) Urinary tract infections. In symposium on surgical infection. *Surg. Clinicians of America,,* **60,** 223–31.

Meers, P. et al (1981) Report on the National Survey on Infections in hospitals. *J. of Hosp. Infection,* **2,** suppl, 1–39.

Norton, C. (1986) Nursing for continence. Beaconsfield Publishers, Beaconsfield.

Platt, R. et al (1982) Morbidity associated with nosocomial urinary tract infection. *New Eng. J. Med,* **307,** 637–42.

Roe, B. and Brocklehurst, J.C. (1987) Study of patients with indwelling catheters. *Journal of Advanced Nursing,* **12,** 713–18.

Ruutu, M. et al (1985) Cytoxicity of latex urinary catheter. *British Journal of Urology,* **57,** 82–87.

Sririvasan, V. and Clark, S.S. (1972) Encrustation of catheter materials *un vitro.. Journal of Urology,* **108,** 473.

Wilksch, J. et al (1983) The role of catheter surface morphology & extractable cytotoxic material in tissue reactions to urethral catheters. *Br. J. Urol;* **55,** 48–52.

Acknowledgements

Mr E.J.G. Milroy, Consultant Urologist, The Middlesex Hospital, and Mr C. Chapple, Senior Registrar, Urology, The Middlesex Hospital.

36

Assessment, observation, and measurement of pain

Jane Latham, SRN, DN
Freelance Nurse Consultant in Pain Management, London

Assessment, observation, and measurement of pain are all closely interlinked. It is impossible to measure and observe pain effectively without having made an accurate in-depth assessment of the pain at the time of referral for care. The original assessment can then be used as a baseline for all further assessments, observations, and measurements.

Undoubtedly, all pain problems have both physical and psychological components. It is extremely important to try and ascertain what part each component plays in the pain problem. For example, has the physical pain caused any psychological or social problems, or have social or psychological problems perhaps initiated the physical pain? There is often an overlap on these two essential questions, but whatever the primary cause of the pain it is a very real problem, and it has to be dealt with effectively and sympathetically whenever making assessments, measurements, and observations.

Assessment of a pain history
Physical aspects
1. The initial onset of the pain should be documented; eg trauma, illness, surgery, or unknown cause. Both previous medical histories and the patient's recollection of events and experiences are useful in building up a pain history.
2. The anatomical position of the primary site of the pain and any pain referring from this area should be documented (see the KCH Pain Clinic Chart; Figure 1).
3. A description of the pain itself should be documented, so that the cause can be accurately diagnosed; eg "burning" suggests nerve involvement, "dull ache" suggests visceral pain, and "recurring intermittent" or "continuous" pain indicates the pain pattern. A carefully constructed questionnaire (such as the McGill Pain Questionnaire; Figure 2) can be useful in gaining a more objective appreciation of the patient's description. Objective information is gained by using a system of "blind scoring", to analyse the completed questionnaire.
4. Factors that make the pain better or worse should be documented;

eg time of day, activity, position, food, stress, anxiety, or isolation. Although the patient will be asked this directly, many other points not thought important by the patient may be highlighted throughout the assessment. Thus, the patient and the assessor may conclude that different factors affect the pain.

5. The effectiveness of previous medication and therapies should be documented. This will be useful in assessing the most "patient acceptable" effective form of treatment.

6. Any medical or other history seen as relevant by either the assessor or the patient should be documented for reference.

Social and environmental aspects

1. The pattern of pain over time can be influenced by events and attitudes within the family and this should be documented; eg a patient in hospital may be worried about a dependant at home, marital problems

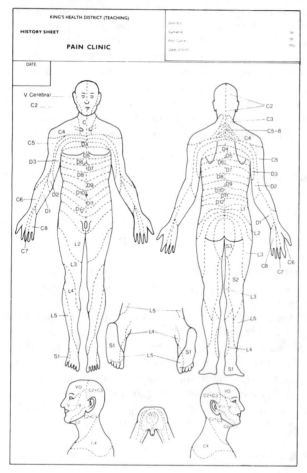

Figure 1a

between a patient and their spouse may be exacerbating or changing a pain syndrome, bereavement could be causing loneliness or depression, or the pain could be giving secondary gain to the patient from other members of the family or friends.

2. Housing and environmental factors that can have an effect on perception of pain should be documented; eg whether the patient lives alone or shares with other members of the family or friends, if the housing is up to standard or whether there are maintenance problems, the area the home is in, and changes in the home situation over the relevant period of time.

3. The work status should be documented; eg the type of work involved, any change or loss of job over the relevant period — either prior to the onset of pain or as a result of the pain.

4. Interests and hobbies should be documented, and any changes in habit noted.

Figures 1a and 1b. The King's College Hospital Pain Clinic Chart for documenting the anatomical position of the primary site of the pain and any pain referring from this area. (Reproduced by kind permission of the Pain Clinic.)

Figure 1b

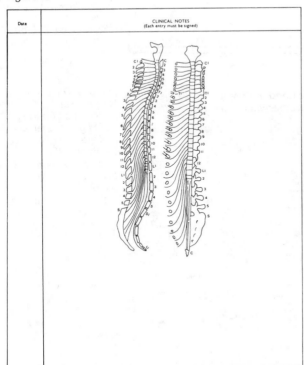

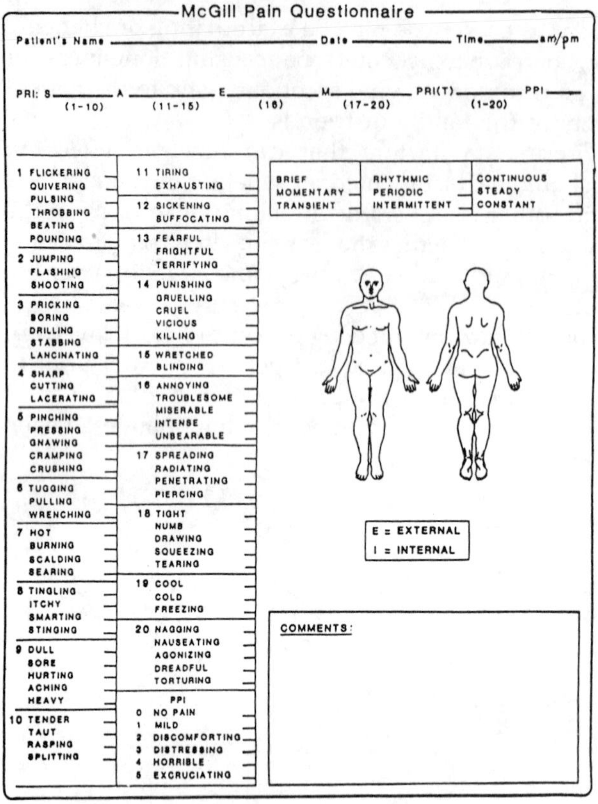

McGill Pain Questionnaire

Patient's Name ______ Date ______ Time ______ am/pm

PRI: S ______ (1-10) A ______ (11-15) E ______ (16) M ______ (17-20) PRI(T) ______ (1-20) PPI ______

1 FLICKERING, QUIVERING, PULSING, THROBBING, BEATING, POUNDING
2 JUMPING, FLASHING, SHOOTING
3 PRICKING, BORING, DRILLING, STABBING, LANCINATING
4 SHARP, CUTTING, LACERATING
5 PINCHING, PRESSING, GNAWING, CRAMPING, CRUSHING
6 TUGGING, PULLING, WRENCHING
7 HOT, BURNING, SCALDING, SEARING
8 TINGLING, ITCHY, SMARTING, STINGING
9 DULL, SORE, HURTING, ACHING, HEAVY
10 TENDER, TAUT, RASPING, SPLITTING
11 TIRING, EXHAUSTING
12 SICKENING, SUFFOCATING
13 FEARFUL, FRIGHTFUL, TERRIFYING
14 PUNISHING, GRUELLING, CRUEL, VICIOUS, KILLING
15 WRETCHED, BLINDING
16 ANNOYING, TROUBLESOME, MISERABLE, INTENSE, UNBEARABLE
17 SPREADING, RADIATING, PENETRATING, PIERCING
18 TIGHT, NUMB, DRAWING, SQUEEZING, TEARING
19 COOL, COLD, FREEZING
20 NAGGING, NAUSEATING, AGONIZING, DREADFUL, TORTURING

PPI
0 NO PAIN
1 MILD
2 DISCOMFORTING
3 DISTRESSING
4 HORRIBLE
5 EXCRUCIATING

BRIEF	RHYTHMIC	CONTINUOUS
MOMENTARY	PERIODIC	STEADY
TRANSIENT	INTERMITTENT	CONSTANT

E = EXTERNAL
I = INTERNAL

COMMENTS:

Figure 2. The McGill Pain Questionnaire can be used to document the patient's description of the pain. (Reproduced by kind permission of Elseviere; Melzack, 1975.)

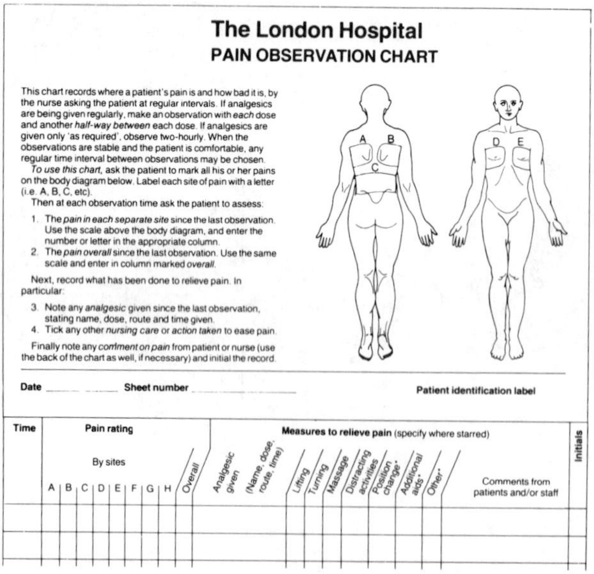

The London Hospital
PAIN OBSERVATION CHART

This chart records where a patient's pain is and how bad it is, by the nurse asking the patient at regular intervals. If analgesics are being given regularly, make an observation with *each* dose and another *half-way between* each dose. If analgesics are given only 'as required', observe two-hourly. When the observations are stable and the patient is comfortable, any regular time interval between observations may be chosen.

To use this chart, ask the patient to mark all his or her pains on the body diagram below. Label each site of pain with a letter (i.e. A, B, C, etc).

Then at each observation time ask the patient to assess:

1. The *pain in each separate site* since the last observation. Use the scale above the body diagram, and enter the number or letter in the appropriate column.
2. The *pain overall* since the last observation. Use the same scale and enter in column marked *overall*.

Next, record what has been done to relieve pain. In particular:

3. Note any *analgesic* given since the last observation, stating name, dose, route and time given.
4. Tick any other *nursing care* or *action taken* to ease pain.

Finally note any *comment on pain* from patient or nurse (use the back of the chart as well, if necessary) and initial the record.

Date ______ Sheet number ______ Patient identification label

Time	Pain rating: By sites A	B	C	D	E	F	G	H	Overall	Measures to relieve pain (specify where starred): Analgesic given	(Name, dose, route, time)	Lifting	Turning	Massage	Distracting activities	Position change*	Additional aids*	Other*	Comments from patients and/or staff	Initials

Figure 3. The London Hospital Pain Observation Chart is used by both staff and patients. It can be used to measure the effectiveness of recent treatment and to prompt appropriate action. (Reproduced by kind permission of The London Hospital.)

Psychological/psychiatric aspects

Following the assessment of the pain history, and with the agreement of the patient, it may be felt that a more in-depth psychological/psychiatric assessment may be needed; for instance, obsessive personality, stress, tension, or changes in life style, which may be an indication of depression or psychological problems. As well as the subjective assessment of these patients, questionnaires that are open to more objective analysis (such as McGill's) are useful to assess how the patient feels about themself and their illness. The questionnaires can be lengthy, but do provide an opportunity for patients to talk about the way they feel. Examples of questions which require a yes/no answer are:

- Are you upset by the way people take your illness?
- Do you frequently try to explain to others how you are feeling?
- Do you find your illness affects your sexual relations?
- Would all your worries be over if you were physically healthy?
- Are you more sensitive to pain than other people?
- Do you think there is something seriously wrong with your body?

Observation and measurement

Informal observations It is in circumstances where the patient is unaware that they are being observed that the most natural reactions are seen. Therefore it is extremely useful to learn the art of being able to observe the patient in pain informally as well as more formally.

The most important observations to note when the patient is alone or interacting with relatives, doctors, nurses, or other patients are:

- Physical movement; eg mobility, positional changes, or restriction of movement.
- Facial expressions; eg relaxed or screwed up with pain.
- Mood; eg depressed, happy, or stoical.

Interactions with different groups may give rise to different reactions, eg a patient may react "normally" for their complaint with a nurse, put on a stoical noncomplaining attitude to a doctor, and make the most of their situation in front of relatives.

Formal observation and measurement

Any observation or measurement that requires some form of documentation is a *formal* assessment. The most appropriate system should be chosen, depending upon the nature of the patient's illness. Several systems are outlined below.

1. Figure 3 shows the London Hospital Pain Observation Chart, which is used to monitor and record physical and psychological aspects of pain over a period of time, and incorporates sites and intensities of pain and actions taken, such as analgesia, physiotherapy, and nursing care. This illustrates the need to combine routine observations such as pulse, blood pressure, and temperature, with more specific observations of pain and by the patient.

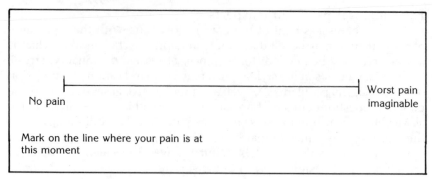

Figure 4. The Visual Analogue Scale is a popular and simple method for the patient to use to measure his pain.

2. There are several charts available to measure pain, although some of them are rather complicated and misleading for the patient. One of the most popular measurement charts is the Visual Analogue Scale (VAS; see Figure 4). The patient marks on the line the intensity of the pain between ''No pain'' and ''Worst pain imaginable''. Some charts divide the line into numbers 1-10, and the choice is very much a matter of preference.

3. For outpatients, pain diaries are a useful form of combining measurements at a set time each day with the patient's description of the pain every day, how it may have changed, and how (if at all) it may have affected their life.

4. Mechanical pain recorders, whereby the patient presses a button at regular intervals throughout the 24-hour period, are a useful method of pain measurement. The more firmly the patient presses, the more intense is the pain. The pain recorder is useful for research purposes, since it allows a continuous 24-hour period of assessment, which one person would find it extremely difficult to cover, and more than one person assessing leads to questions of consistency of observation. It is important to remember that should the patient be asleep, no pain is recorded.

Follow-up to assessments

It is essential that all assessments are documented and reported to the appropriate people. There are, however, many ways in which nurses can become actively involved in further patient care.

It may be found that following assessment the patient's needs are those of basic nursing care. For example, regular repositioning of a patient in bed may lessen discomfort, or noticing that a patient experiences pain before the next dose of analgesia means reassessing the analgesia prescription.

Treatments may be needed following assessment, which can be carried out by nurses on an inpatient or outpatient basis, for instance continuous syringe pump top-ups or transcutaneous nerve stimulation. This provides the ideal situation in which to combine carrying out a treatment while allowing time for support, counselling, and reassessment.

Nurses can become involved in other disciplines or therapies through patients in pain and learn basic but invaluable skills, for example the psychologist teaches relaxation, which can then be used by the nurse in conjunction with other treatments.

Should invasive medical techniques such as nerve blocks be necessary, the nurse should have adequate knowledge to support and follow up the patient with appropriate counselling or teaching and observations to measure and assess the pain and any changes.

Referral may be needed to other disciplines, for instance if there are problems relating to family or housing then social workers may be the most appropriate people to become involved, and a nurse is often the most obvious liaison person in these cases.

References
Hasking, J., and Welchew, E. (1985) Post-Operative Pain – Understanding its Nature and How to Treat it. Faber & Faber Ltd., London. pp73 and 150
Melzack, R. (1975) The McGill Pain Questionnaire: Major properties and scoring methods. *Pain*, **1**, 275
Raiman, J.A. (1981) Responding to Pain. *Nursing*, **Nov., 1362**

37
Setting standards for pain control

Jo Hockley, RGN, SCM

Formerly Senior Nurse, Support Care Team, St Bartholomew's Hospital, London; currently studying MSc in Nursing and Health, Edinburgh University

Over the last 20 years hospices have been established as places of excellence in the control of distressing symptoms. The hospice movement has alerted attention to the control of chronic pain and played a large part in influencing the current interest in pain control per se. However, Lunt and Hillier's research (1982), shows that in fact only 10 per cent of cancer deaths occur in hospices and 60 per cent in hospitals. Therefore, it is important that the knowledge of pain control taught by the hospice movement infiltrates the acute setting.

Working in a teaching hospital now for the last few years, but having been a ward sister for four years at St Christopher's Hospice, London, the author has had first hand experience of what can be achieved in a hospice, and the problems of pain control in the acute setting (Table 1).

Convincing colleagues
1. Acute vs chronic pain
2. Lack of teaching
3. Lack of assertiveness
4. Lack of continuity.
In assessment, plan and evaluation of care
1. **Assessment:**
(a) In hospital – tendency to miss pain because it is not 'visible'
(b) Individual experience of pain
2. **Planning:**
(a) Factors which foil nurses' plans
3. **Evaluating:**
(a) Lack of time
(b) Lack of routine recordings
(c) Lack of continuity of nursing staff

Table 1. Problems of pain control in the acute setting.

It is of paramount importance that these problems are identified and faced if patients are to get adequate pain relief. This article does not address how one actually controls pain, nor does it discuss pain assessment; rather it focuses on the problems that prevent nurses from achieving the ideal.

It is important to recognise that one difficulty is created when people hold the wrong values. These values generate 'wrong' standards and lead to nurses having difficulty in convincing those colleagues – medical and nursing – whose standards generate suboptimal plans of care.

Convincing colleagues

There are four points that influence the problem of convincing colleagues.

1. Acute pain vs chronic pain   This includes recognising the subtle differences between them. The major experience that medical staff and nurses have with pain on both a personal and a professional level, is that of acute pain – pain acting in its natural sense as a 'warning', eg, appendicitis, burns. However, chronic pain – whether that of cancer or arthritis – must be called a 'useless' pain. The basic cause is known, but cannot be cured, so nurses must try to prevent pain breaking through.

Table 2 gives a comparison of analgesic use in acute and chronic pain.

	Acute	**Chronic**
Aim	Pain relief	Pain relief
Sedation	Often desirable	Undesirable
Duration	2-4 hours	As long as possible
Timing	On demand	In anticipation
Dose	Standard	Individually determined
Route	Injection	By mouth
Adjuvent medication	Uncommon	Common

Table 2. Comparison of analgesic use in acute and chronic pain.

2. Lack of teaching   The lack of adequate teaching on pain control, and therefore the lack of confidence in dealing with a patient in pain, can be an extremely demoralising situation for nurses in the acute setting. Too often they recognise that the patient's pain is not adequately controlled, but feel powerless to change the situation.

Some comments from the nurses interviewed in the author's research (Hockley, 1989) regarding patient's pain control were as follows:

"Generally, by 'the end' the patient is comfortable, but it takes quite a long time to get him that way . . ."

"I would say that 50 per cent of the terminally ill patients that I have looked after have some degree of pain when they are dying."

Both situations show that the nurses felt that patients' pain control could have been better.

Within the hospice, all nurses working on the wards, particularly the trained nurses (who make up 50 per cent of the staff), are totally 'tuned in' to maximum relief of pain, both from an educational and a clinical point of view. Unfortunately, in many acute hospitals, not only is there a lack of teaching, but there are also rarely more than two trained nurses on duty together to provide the support and experience needed.

Since the Support Care Team has been running at St Bartholomew's Hospital, London, it has concentrated on teaching the principles of pain control both directly within the school of nursing and indirectly by example within the clinical setting on the wards. Nurses are encouraged to learn new skills; the team does not 'take over' the work. For instance, if a patient needs a 24-hour syringe driver, the team specialist stands by while the nurse loads the driver for the first time. They do not do it for her.

3. Lack of assertiveness   The nurse often sees herself as a lesser individual in understanding pain control because of a lack of teaching on the subject. However, many nurses are very good at perceiving and assessing pain at a basic level, but perhaps lack the confidence to put the problem across when faced with medical staff – especially if the medical staff are unsure of how to improve the situation.

This perceived inferior status hinders assertiveness and in itself can expose student nurses to possible indifference if the lack of recognition of a patient's analgesia is allowed to fester. Faced with such a situation, a student nurse may become deeply frustrated and stressed. She may even be tempted to give up the battle for good pain control by adopting the value that pain does not need controlling, or she may just opt out of the job. Either way, she becomes ineffective in any future challenge. Thus the Support Care Team aims to become an advocate for nurses trying to convince colleagues regarding analgesia. The team will work alongside them, confirming that the patient is in pain. In this way, the advocacy role enables nurses to grow in assertiveness.

Ensuring that trained nurses have a good knowledge of pain control, that they see pain taken seriously and acted upon, has to be the best atmosphere in which student nurses will grow in confidence and assertiveness in the recognition, assessment and relief of a patient's pain.

4. Lack of continuity   This has to be one of the main difficulties with working in the acute setting. The house officers are only on a ward for a maximum of six months – and sometimes only three. The ward sister and trained nurses no sooner get the doctor 'tuned in' to their way of thinking about pain control, than he or she moves on.

The same problems are also present at a nursing level. The most cohesive ward at our hospital regarding pain control is one where there has been little change in trained staff and where the ward sister has been a committed member of the team for the last five years.

Problems regarding the nursing process
Creating a nursing process model for patients in pain is not hard, once the 'wrong' values have been readjusted. However, there are difficulties in the acute setting that can interfere with the process of assessing, planning and evaluating the care of patients in pain that are not usually a problem in the hospice.

Assessment In hospitals – probably because of the hustle and bustle of different things going on there is a tendency to make observations purely on visible evidence. This came out in the author's research (Hockley, 1989) when the communication of symptoms between patient, nurse and doctor was examined. It is easy to miss pain because it is not always a visible problem, unlike vomiting or oedema (Table 3).

Symptom	No. of people Patient	Nurse	Doctor
Effectively communicated			
Malaise	23	23	23
Constipation	14	14	14
Oedema	11	11	11
Vomiting	7	7	7
Ineffectively communicated			
Insomnia	23	21	18
Sore mouth	21	15	15
Pain	18	15	15
Nausea	14	11	10

Table 3. Communication of symptoms.

We all know that the experience of pain is *individual* – different cultures, personalities, previous exposure to pain, coping mechanisms and so on, all go to make up a patient's level of pain control and different factors that raise and lower this threshold (Table 4). The problems faced on the busy, acute wards often compound to increase patient's experience of pain. Particularly important aspects are sleeplessness, fear, lack of explanation and isolation and nurses must take account of these when assessing pain.

> The nurse needs to sit down and ask the patient:
> **1. *Where* is the pain?** She must also remember that of the two-thirds of patients with cancer who experience pain as many as 80 per cent will have more than one pain, and 30 per cent will have four or more pains.
> **2. *What* does it feel like?**
> **3. *How* long does it last?**
> We simply cannot 'see' these things.

Plan for care   Some emphasis has to be given to the general management of the planned care. However well drugs have been prescribed, if the patient is not able to *get* the medication, the pain remains a burden.

Factors that increase experience of pain	Factors that decrease experience of pain
Discomfort	Relief of symptoms
Insomnia	Sleep
Fatigue	Rest
Anxiety	Sympathy
Fear	Understanding
Anger	Diversion
Sadness	Elevation of mood
Depression	Security
Isolation	Analgesics
Introversion	Anxiolytics
(Past experience)	Antidepressants

Table 4. Factors which modify pain (Twycross and Lack, 1983)

Again, the author's research highlighted many of these issues, such as prescription boards being in the pharmacy when four-hourly morphine was due. Nurses might well remember to collect the board from the pharmacy when an important new drug is involved, but may easily forget if it has gone down for aperients for a patient who also happens to be having regular morphine elixir.

One patient explained that she had to wait until the night sedation round had finished before she got her medication, as her morphine elixir was kept in a special cupboard. During the night, analgesia can be delayed while waiting for a second trained nurse to check an opiate.

In the hospice setting the organisation is somewhat different. Prescription boards are always available (there are no pharmacies); a drug round is performed every four hours, unlike in the acute setting where a regular round is done six-hourly. Also, the drug trolleys have a locked cupboard within them so that nurses do not have to return to a separate cupboard for the opiates – which are therefore given at the same time as the patient's other medications.

Nurses might not be able to change how a busy teaching hospital is managed, but they do need to be aware of these potential hazards.

Evaluation   Difficulties in achieving the ideal standard of care for patients in pain are created by the lack of time to spend in evaluating how well the medication is working. Ideally, pain should be assessed half an hour after any given medication, four-hourly prior to the next opiate dose, and then evaluated daily. Often it is only a 'rough' daily assumption that is recorded. There is definitely a lack of simple routine recording charts which could guide the student nurse, but even if these were more widely available, nothing will take the place of a conscientious nurse who has been taught properly to make time to assess and record pain regularly on a care plan.

The lack of continuity of nursing staff – especially with student nurses changing wards and going onto night duty – interrupts the continuity of being able to stabilise standards.

These are just a few problems highlighting the need to set standards for pain control, whether it is postoperative pain or chronic cancer pain.

Setting the standards

Nurses begin their training with idealistic standards of what they believe is important in the care of patients. Unfortunately, these values or beliefs often become altered as the nurse encounters more experienced people with different standards – perhaps nurses are tempted to think their own values are wrong when faced with opposition. So how can nurses set the right standards, particularly with the patient who has pain?

Standards are statements of quality which serve as a model to facilitate and evaluate the delivery of optimal nursing care. The standards of care can be divided into structure, process and outcome (AACN, 1981).

Structure   This is the working environment of the system under review, including:
1. Organisational and managerial characteristics.
2. Physical facilities and equipment.
3. Staffing patterns, grades of staff, specialist qualifications and educational attainment.
4. Aspects may be decided upon internally or 'imposed'.

Process   A series of actions, changes or functions that bring about an end or result.

Outcome   This is the result to be achieved.

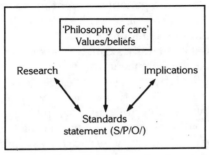

Figure 1. Relation of philosophy of care to standard setting (Boyes, 1987).

Figure 1 shows that the nurse's *values* about care can be put into a standard statement which enables her to apply research, see 'gaps' where more research needs to be done, and look at the implications of the standard set to enable her to carry out and meet the objective of care.

For example, should there be more teaching; more staff; more equipment or a change in routine?

In this way, the Support Care Team has been able to set standards for terminally ill patients in pain, as follows.

Structure standard

The trained nurse:

1. Will have received instruction in teaching techniques.
2. Will have developed a perception of pain in malignant disease. She will be able to assess acute and chronic pain.
3. Will have knowledge of analgesics and their actions, side-effects and contraindications.
4. Will have knowledge of non-pharmacological methods of controlling pain, including positioning, pressure relieving devices.
5. Will have knowledge of the palliative role of hormone therapy, chemotherapy and radiotherapy.
6. Will function as a participating member of the multidisciplinary team and be fully cognisant of the roles of each of the health professionals in the team, particularly with regard to their roles in relieving pain.
7. Will have access to a full range of teaching aids.
8. Will have access to current articles/books on the treatment of acute and chronic pain.
9. Nurse staffing levels will take into account the time needed to enquire into and accomplish the patient's/family's education about pain problems and their alleviation.
10. The ward will be equipped with appropriate analgesic equipment, furniture and bedding.

Process standard

The trained nurse:

1. Will assess regularly the patient's current management of pain.
2. Will teach the correct use of prescribed medications and encourage efficient self-medication techniques.
3. Will facilitate patient's/family's concerns about opiate analgesics.
4. Will demonstrate competence in the use of non-pharmacologic aids to pain control, particularly the use of syringe drivers.
5. Will discuss the patient's activities of daily living and leisure time and suggest priority planning to enable rest periods to be taken.
6. Will collaborate with the clinical nurse specialist/support team, pain clinic, and oncology/radiotherapy services. Will discuss with medical staff the need to review uncontrolled pain.
7. Will arrange for adequate pain control to be continued at home.

Outcome standards

The patient/family:

1. Will be able to discuss any fear about pain in terminal disease.

2. Will be able to recognise factors and activities which increase pain. They will discuss steps to remove or reduce these factors.

3. Will be able to demonstrate the use of analgesia over a period of four days and will describe the appropriate use of analgesic drugs.

4. Will be able to know when the patient has been started on opiates and will discuss fears about opiate medication.

5. Will be able to demonstrate the need to continue and modify regular aperients when on opiates.

6. Will be familiar with non-pharmacological aids for pain control and the reason for commencing them.

7. Will be able to demonstrate their knowledge of a crisis plan for relieving breakthrough pain, including the contact numbers of professionals who can provide back-up if necessary.

Hospice and hospital

My time at St Bartholomew's has been an invaluable learning situation – seeing the differences between the two settings of a hospice and teaching hospital. It should not be any more difficult to control pain in a hospital setting, as long as nurses are aware of some of the problems faced, and are prepared to re-evaluate their standards.

The Support Care Team is invaluable because it can be an advocate for the nurse trying to convince the powers-that-be about a patient's pain and can assist the efforts to train new housemen and nurses by providing a concrete model with experience to back up ward sisters' aims.

References

AACN – American Association for Critical Care Nurses. (1981) Standards for Nursing Care of the Critically Ill. Reston Publishing Company, Inc. Reston, Virginia USA.

Boyes, M. (1987) Setting Standards for nursing care. Presented at Challenge of Choice conference. St. Bartholomew's Hospital, London EC1.

Hockley, J., Dunlop, R. and Davies R. (1988) Symptoms of distress in the terminally ill patient and his family and the response to setting up a Hospital Support Team. *British Medical Journal*, **296**, 1715-1717.

Hockley, J. (1989) Caring for the dying in acute hospitals. *Nursing Times*, **85**, 47-50.

Lunt, B. and Hillier, R. (1981) Terminal care: present services and future priorities. Hospital support teams rather than in-patient services. *British Medical Journal*, **283**, 595-598.

Twycross, R.G. and Lack, S.A. (1983) Symptom Control in Advanced Cancer. Pitman, London.

38

A case for accuracy: monitoring blood pressure

David Wells, RGN, DPSN
Senior Charge Nurse, Victoria Hospital, Blackpool

Blood pressure monitoring is probably one of the most frequent 'observations' made by nurses (Brylan, 1985). Arterial blood pressure recording by auscultation is usually taught to 'learner' nurses in introductory blocks, supporting the contention that British student nurses learn arterial blood pressure measurement techniques at "an early point in their professional education" (Draper, 1987). According to information supplied by nurse teachers in several schools of nursing, this training consists of up to three hours of lectures and practice, with no learning packages or refresher courses for learners (or trained staff) available to back it up. Practice for learners would seem to consist of testing each other's blood pressure with binaural stethoscopes, while once in the ward, blood pressure measurements taken by learners are used as a basis for treatment.

Errors in recording

If we consider the studies which suggest the potential sources of error from equipment, observer and patients are legion and statements such as O'Brien's (1979) that "many doctors and nurses are unaware of the potential errors of technique and fail to appreciate the limits of blood pressure measurement", perhaps we should question the suitability of training in this area and the wisdom of relying on measurements made by inexperienced learners, untrained staff and nurses who may have received little updating since their first year of training.

Examination of the literature published over the last 10 years appears to support concern over the lack of published British studies into the evaluation of accurate blood pressure recording techniques in practice (Draper, 1987). Many British nursing textbooks appear to encompass only a basic outline of the practicalities of taking and recording arterial blood pressure, and despite the current trend for textbooks to have a research base, the majority appear to show little evidence of this as far as blood pressure monitoring is concerned. It would, therefore, seem possible to question the knowledge base on which nurses establish their criteria for evaluating their competence in this technique, and there could be difficulties in accepting the legitimacy of their results in some cases. Given that blood pressure recordings form an important database on which decisions about patient care are made, this is a daunting prospect.

Research needs

There appear to be many areas requiring further enquiry with the field of sphygmomanometry:

- The adequacy of preparation learner nurses receive to record blood pressure.
- The usefulness of results of blood pressure recordings obtained by learner nurses.
- Evaluation of the effectiveness of teaching methods for practical procedures, such as blood pressure recordings.
- A further evaluation into the adequacy of the blood pressure recording equipment currently available.
- The usefulness of blood pressure recordings obtained in stressful areas such as outpatient clinics in comparison to results obtained from GP surgeries.
- An overall evaluation of the ability of both trained and trainee staff to record accurate blood pressure.

Quality nursing care requires informed observation and accurate reporting of information (Brylan, 1975), and blood pressure recording appears to be regarded as an observation of minor importance in that it is often designated to inexperienced nurses, to those who have not received updating in this practice and even, in some hospitals, to auxiliaries. Research seems to indicate that the average blood pressure recording may be, at best, inaccurate.

Recording a blood pressure

1. Allow sufficient time for the procedure eg, five minutes for each recording (O'Brien, 1979).

2. Ensure the patient is well rested and relaxed. In most cases, the position is not important if the arm is supported at the same level as the heart.

3. The arm used should be recorded - otherwise variances may occur (Bruya, 1985).

4. Choose a cuff with a width 20 per cent greater than the diameter of the limb and of a suitable length to encircle the arm.

5. Wrap the cuff securely around the upper arm.

6. Attach an adequately maintained manometer (Conceirao, 1976) to the cuff and place on a level surface at nurse's eye level (Thompson, 1981).

7. Place the bell of the stethoscope (O'Brien, 1979) over the brachial artery just below the cuff.

8. Inflate the cuff quickly until the artery is occluded.

9. Release the pressure immediately, allowing a controlled, slow, steady fall of the mercury meniscus.

10. Listen for the Korotokoff sounds (Table 1) of blood flow - phase 1, phase 4 and phase 5, recording them to the nearest 2mm of mercury. The systolic blood pressure is assumed to relate to the onset of phase 1 and the diastolic blood pressure to the onset of phase 4, although many writers suggest phase 5 must also be recorded.

Phase 1. A loud clear snapping tone.
Phase 2. A succession of murmurs.
Phase 3. The disappearance of murmurs and the appearance of a tone resembling the first phase.
Phase 4. The tone becomes less clear or dull.
Phase 5. The disappearance of all sounds.

Table 1. Korotokoff sounds.

If it is necessary to reinflate the cuff (a series of recordings will be required if the heart rhythm is unstable), the cuff must be completely deflated and a few seconds allowed before reinflation.

Accuracy
Nurses who are up-to-date on the potential sources of inaccuracies (eg, from the observer, technique, the equipment or the patient's psychological or physiological status) are best equipped to take accurate measurements, teach others and ensure that the correct working equipment is available. High priority should be given to obtaining valid recordings in the light of its role in, for example, the treatment of hypertension. Educators, authors, managers, researchers and clinical practitioners must, therefore, be aware of the importance of both this clinical skill and their role in ensuring that future generations of nurses are competent and safe practitioners in this vital task.

References
Bruya, M. (1985) Nursing decision making. *Nursing Administration Quarterly*, 9, 4, 19-31.
Brylan, A. (1985) Doing the obs. *Nursing Times*, 8, 7, 24-25.
Conceircao, S. (1976) Defects in sphygmomanometers. *British Medical Journal*, 1, 469-471.
Draper, P. (1987) Not a job for juniors. *Nursing Times*, 83, 10, 58-62.
Hahn, G.D. (1985) Clinical monitoring in anaesthasesia. *JAAN*, A 53, 149-61.
O'Brien, E.T. (1979) ABC of blood pressure measurement. *BMI*, 2, 775-6, 920-21.
Thompson, D.R. (1981) Recording patients' blood pressure. *Journal of Advanced Nursing*, 6, 283-90.

39

Central venous pressure monitoring

Sandra Haynes, RGN, DipN
Research Nurse, Glenfield Hospital, Leicester

The central venous pressure (CVP) is a measure of the pressure in the right atrium of the heart or the great veins within the thorax. It serves as a guide for the assessment of right sided cardiac function, and the objectives of monitoring the CVP are to:
- serve as a guide for fluid replacement in seriously ill patients;
- estimate blood volume deficits;
- determine pressures in the right atrium and central veins;
- evaluate a patient for circulatory failure (in context with the total clinical picture).

Indications for measuring CVP
Central venous pressure may be measured in the following circumstances:
- when the patient is experiencing cardiac failure;
- when there is difficulty in stabilising the circulatory system;
- post-surgery to detect postoperative complications, such as shock or haemorrhage;
- in cases where the patient has undergone massive trauma;
- to generally monitor a patient's condition.

Inserting the catheter
In order to measure the CVP, a long intravenous catheter is inserted into either the subclavian, internal or external jugular, or the median basilic vein. It is then threaded through to the superior vena cava until it lies just before the entrance to the right atrium (Figure 1). If the catheter tip lies outside the chest, the pressure measurements will be artificially high (Hanning and Calman, 1984). It may be necessary in some circumstances to insert the catheter under a general anaesthetic, but the procedure is often carried out at the bedside using local anaesthetic. The nurse has a number of responsibilities during the procedure. It is important to ensure the patient receives a full explanation of what is to happen and the reasons why it is necessary.

The necessary equipment should also be assembled. This may vary with particular doctors' preferences, but the basic equipment is:

- a central venous catheter;
- infusion solution and infusion set;
- cutdown tray; skin cleansing solution;
- spirit level;
- local anaesthetic, syringes and needles;
- dressing materials for the site.

Positioning of the patient is an important nursing duty during the procedure, and will help ensure the catheter is passed easily, with the minimum of trauma. If the subclavian vein is to be used, the patient should ideally be helped into the supine position with the head turned to the opposite side to the insertion point. The foot of the bed may be elevated to encourage dilation of the vein and to prevent the risk of air embolism. The positioning is similar if the internal jugular vein is used.

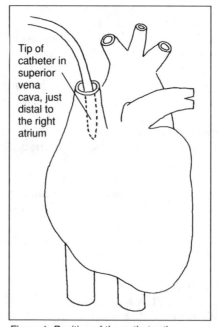

Tip of
catheter in
superior
vena
cava, just
distal to
the right
atrium

Figure 1. Position of the catheter tip.

Nurses should remain with the patient throughout the procedure, providing both physical and psychological support as necessary; while no pain should be felt, having a catheter inserted 'into the heart' can be extremely stressful. Once the catheter is in position, the nurse should ensure that no fluid is infused until the position of the catheter has been checked by an X-ray. It may be appropriate at this stage to ascertain the point from which the CVP reading will take place (usually the sternal angle or mid axilla). The point to be used should be marked and recorded in the care plan - it is important that CVP is always read from the same point, as the sternal angle reading is approximately 5cm water higher than that at the mid axilla.

Once the catheter is in position it can be attached to a manometer and giving set so that the CVP can be monitored (Figure 2). A manometer with a three way stopcock is normally used so that three separate systems are created by manipulating the stopcock (Figure 3).

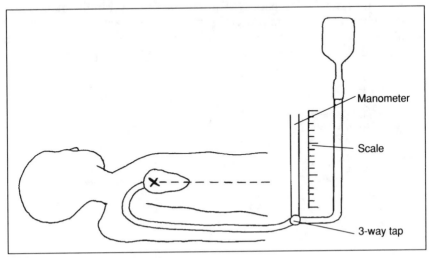

Figure 2. The catheter is attached to a manometer.

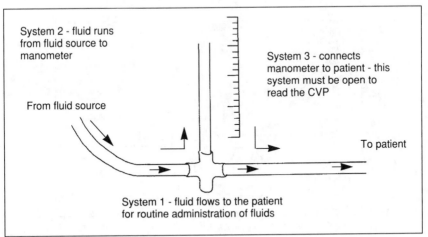

Figure 3. The three systems.

Interpreting the CVP

Before the CVP measurement is taken, it is important to ensure the catheter is patent by observing the gentle oscillations that occur in the fluid level of the manometer with respirations. The patient should be placed in a baseline position which should be noted and should remain the same for subsequent readings. The zero point on the manometer should be adjusted to the same level as the zero reference point on the patient. This is done with the use of a spirit level. The manometer is then filled from the reservoir by manipulating the stopcock (Figure 4a). The stopcock should again be manipulated so that the fluid from the manometer flows to the patient (Figure 4b). The fluid in the manometer should now fall with inspiration. When it has stopped falling, it should continue to oscillate gently with inspiration. The value for the CVP can then be taken as the mean value between the oscillating points.

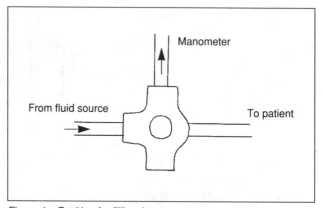

Figure 4a. Position for filling the manometer.

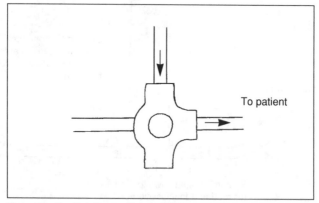

Figure 4b. Position for reading the CVP.

Measuring the CVP

Centimetres of water are used for reading a CVP; a normal CVP is taken to be within the range of 5-12cm of water. Normal values may, however, change from patient to patient, so the management of a patient should not rest on one CVP reading alone, but on a series of readings. The CVP reading should also be interpreted in context of other observations, such as urine output, pulse, respirations and blood pressure. A CVP near to zero may indicate hypovolaemia, while a CVP above 15-20cm water may indicate hypervolaemia, pneumothorax, poor cardiac contractability or cardiac tamponade (Brunner and Suddarth, 1980).

Sometimes the amount of fluid replacement needed is calculated according to the CVP readings together with the urinary output. As long as the urine output remains satisfactory and the CVP readings do not change significantly, this is an indication that the body can cope with the amount of fluid being given. If, however, the CVP begins to rise accompanied by a drop in urine output, this indicates that there is decreased cardiac output to perfuse the kidneys and the patient may be developing circulatory overload.

Care of the central venous catheter

Most catheters in use will be made of either polytetrafluoethylene or Teflon, both of which have good biological resistant properties. Radio-opaque catheters are usually preferred so they can be seen on X-ray. Central venous catheters provide ideal entry sites for bacteria, so strict aseptic technique should be used whenever dealing with the catheter or catheter site to minimise any contamination. Once in place, the catheter should be manipulated as little as possible and it is often advantageous to combine changes of dressings with changes of the giving sets, blood sampling and giving of any medications via this route. The catheter site should be inspected regularly for signs of inflammation or sepsis. Dressings should generally be changed between one and three times a week, and this provides an ideal time to inspect the catheter site. Occlusive dressings appear to the best type for dressing the site: OpSite, which is translucent, semipermeable and contours to the body shape, often proves to be the most comfortable (McCannon, 1986). One of the most common problems experienced with catheters is blockage. This can be avoided by maintaining the flow of fluid with a flow control device, such as an Ivac or Imed pump. The administration set should be changed every 24 hours, or in accordance with local policy, using an aseptic technique.

The patient's vital signs should be monitored closely, and in the event of persistent pyrexia and tachycardia, contamination of the catheter tip should be suspected. Under these circumstances it will be necessary for blood cultures to be taken both from a peripheral vein and the catheter, to determine the site of infection. Swabs of the catheter site should also be taken. Contamination is not the only risk involved in inserting the catheter. The choice of vein is important - there is a higher risk of complications in subclavian vein catheterisation eg, pneumothorax has been shown to occur in 1.5-5 per cent of patients even when the catheter is inserted by an experienced clinician. Good technique and careful monitoring, however, minimise the risks presented by CVP monitoring, while the benefits to be gained from the procedure can be substantial.

References
Atkins, S. (1989) Parenteral nutrition - the nurse's role. *Surgical Nurse*, February, 13-18.
Brunner, L. and Suddarth, D. (1980) Textbook of Medical-Surgical Nursing. Harper and Row, London.
Hanning, C. and Calman, K. (1984) Basic Skills in Clinical Medicine. Churchill Livingstone, London.
McCannon, G. (1986) Dressing subclavian catheters. *Nursing Times*, **82,** 12, 40.

Bibliography
Huddak, C., Gallo, B., Lohr, T. (1986) Critical Care Nursing - A Holistic Approach. J.B. Lippincott Company, Philadelphia.
Gives general advice on the care of patients with central lines and care of the catheters.
Yates, A., Moorhead, P., Adams, A. (1984) Intensive Care. Hodder and Stoughton, London.
Gives general guidance on the care of CVP lines.

40

A reassessment of oral healthcare

Jane Barnett, RGN
Clinical Nurse Specialist, Infection Control, Acute Unit, Mid-Staffordshire Health Authority

The structures of the oral cavity must remain healthy to ensure comfort, maintenance of nutrition, protection from infection and a sense of wellbeing (Perry and Potter, 1986). Even a minor alteration in the health of the oral cavity can have a significant effect on a person's wellbeing. Shepherd *et al* (1987) define the healthy mouth as one which can masticate food properly, has an adequate saliva flow and is cleaned by mechanical means two or three times daily. Gibbons (1983) suggests a healthy mouth can be assessed by the absence of plaque and debris, although even the healthiest mouths usually have some degree of this.

Control of plaque may be possible and made easier with the aid of disclosing tablets, but nurses will require education and practice to identify the plaque accurately and to implement oral care accordingly. Block (1976) suggests it takes only 24 hours for plaque to form on the teeth, which implies that unless patients are assisted in performing rigorous mouthcare, they are almost immediately being placed at risk of dental decay or gum disease on admission to hospital.

Although the physiological effects of poor oral hygiene are readily recognised and identified, the psychosocial importance is frequently overlooked. Trenter-Roth and Creason (1986) suggest these factors can be far-reaching due to the role the mouth plays in speech and the physical expression of intimate affection. A patient with a dry mouth will experience speech difficulty, dry, cracked lips will make smiling painful, and halitosis lead to mutual avoidance between a patient and others.

Assessment of the mouth

Many nursing forms allow little, if any, room for a detailed assessment of a patient's mouth on admission to a ward and during his or her stay in hospital. Even if more emphasis were to be placed on assessment, it does not necessarily follow that better mouthcare would result.

Schweigner *et al* (1980) describe a detailed form of assessment which may uncover invaluable diagnostic information concerning a patient's general health. Although these methods appear complex and extensive, they found that nurses who were taught basic oral assessment techniques were able to complete a thorough inspection in 10 minutes. De Walt (1975) devised an 'oral assessment guide' designed to examine these nine areas (Table 1), which were given a range of scores from one to three, one being the lowest rating. Both forms of assessment are complex, however, and require expert teaching at an early stage in nurse training to ensure the practice is learned and carried out.

- Salivation
- Tongue moisture
- Tongue colouring
- Moisture of palates
- Condition of gingival tissue
- Colour of membranes
- Lip texture
- Lip moisture
- Soft tooth debris

Table 1. The nine areas of the oral assessment guide (De Walt, 1975).

Education

Although mouthcare is part of every introductory nursing programme, it is rarely taught by experts in the field, and it is often the most junior nurse who is asked to undertake mouthcare (Wallace and Freeman, 1978). At the Nightingale School of Nursing at St Thomas' Hospital, London, the Department of Community Dental Health was requested to provide the dental health education input into the six week introductory block for student nurses (Munday and Gelbier, 1984). An evaluating questionnaire from the students showed that three quarters felt the nurse's role was important in maintaining patients' oral hygiene. This study showed that if relevant information is provided on the role of dental plaque in dental caries and periodontal disease and the importance of maintaining good oral hygiene of hospitalised patients, nurses will develop a more positive attitude towards dental health. A study in the Crewe district highlighted the need for further education among health professionals to enable them to present correct dental health messages to the public so that the benefits of preventive dental service can be fully appreciated (O'Hara, 1988). Howarth (1977) and Lewis (1984) suggest it would be useful if nurses were taught oral care by dental hygienists to enable them to correctly assess the mouth and give appropriate care. The cost implications of this educational input and the nursing time were not, however, discussed.

Factors affecting oral hygiene

There are many factors which can directly or indirectly affect the normal healthy mouth and its structures. It is not always patients who are 'nil by mouth' who are at greatest risk of poor mouthcare, as alternative methods of hydration are available and nurses are more aware of the potential problems associated with dehydration (Howarth, 1977). More commonly, it is people who are reluctant to eat or drink who become dehydrated and, therefore, develop a dry, crusted mouth.

De Walt and Haines (1969) studied the effects of four stressors on the healthy mouth of a volunteer. These were: oral breathing, continuous oxygen via a nasal cannula, intermittent suctioning and 'nil by mouth'. After five hours with only two applications of oral hygiene during the last hour, various after-effects were experienced (Table 2). Immediate relief was achieved when mouthcare was given using a toothbrush and dentifrice followed by lemon and glycerine swabs to the mucosa, tongue and lips. An increase in the acidity of the oral saliva occurred after three hours, as did changes in the oral mucosa.

• Extreme dryness of the mouth with numbness of the roof of the mouth and tongue • A burning sensation of the tip of the tongue • Red and inflamed lips with cracks • Every tooth surface coated in debris • Difficulty in speaking • Some blistering of the oral mucosa

Table 2. Effects of stressors on oral hygiene.

The ageing process

Many elderly people have problems with their mouths, which can have a debilitating effect on their wellbeing. The physical action of chewing promotes saliva and gastric secretions and facilitates digestion, which in turn makes the chewing and tasting of food pleasurable (Ettinger and Manderson, 1975). These authors consider dental care an important part of elderly patients' rehabilitation.

Due to the ageing process salivary flow decreases, making elderly people more susceptible to dental problems, especially those associated with the trauma of ill-fitting dentures (Geissler and McCord, 1986). Many elderly people expect dentures to last them their lifetime, so self-referral for ill-fitting dentures is low. There is an increased incidence of oral carcinoma with age, which in some cases may be related to wearing ill-fitting dentures (Ettinger and Manderson, 1975). In this study, 53 per cent of people wearing dentures had some form of denture associated or induced pathology which required treatment.

Many elderly people have reduced neuromuscular control, and find it difficult to use a normal toothbrush (Ettinger and Manderson, 1975). There are, however, many modifications which can enable people with physical disabilities to clean their teeth, and in certain circumstances, automatic toothbrushes may be a valuable aid for elderly people.

Many of the oral problems associated with ageing are drug-related. Lamy and Lamy (1985) suggest that xerostomia (dryness of the mouth due to lack of normal secretions) is probably one of the most common undesirable effects of drugs on the oral health of older adults. Many different types of drugs cause ·xerostomia (Table 3). Howarth (1977) suggests that the elderly drugged person may also lose the thirst reflex.

Blaney (1986) includes antibiotics in her list of problem-associated drugs, as these can destroy the normal flora in the mouth, and may lead to *Candida albicans* infections, which can have devastating effects on a person's ability to eat and drink normally.

- Anticholinergics
- Antihypertensives
- Antihistamines
- Antipsychotics
- Anorectics
- Narcotic analgesics
- Anticonvulsants
- Antineoplastics
- Sympathomimetics
- Antidepressants
- Diuretics

Table 3. Types of drugs which cause xerostomia.

Cytotoxic chemotherapy

Most cytotoxic drugs act by interfering with the reproductive cycle of the tumour cell, causing the cell to die. The drugs are, however, relatively non-specific in action, and can attack normal as well as cancer cells (Allbright, 1984). Stomatitis or inflammation of the oral mucosa is a common problem associated with certain chemotherapeutic agents (Allbright, 1984). While careful attention to oral hygiene will not avoid stomatitis, it will help to minimise the problem. The indirect effects of chemotherapy on oral epithelial cells result from the drugs' myelo-suppressive action. This causes generalised immunosuppression, mani-fested by neutropenia, lymphocytopenia and thrombocytopenia, which makes the mouth susceptible to infection and bleeding (Ostchega, 1980). The effect of daily trauma on the patient's already thinned mucosa, combined with the drug induced immunosuppression makes the mouth susceptible to ulceration, haemorrhage and infection. Any such infection may be potentially harmful as the damaged mucosa may enable entry to the bloodstream, which can result in septicaemia (Allbright, 1984).

Children are apparently even more susceptible to complications from chemotherapy. Oral complications in children during or following chemotherapy appear more quickly than in adult patients (Ostchega, 1980). Sonis and Sonis (1979) state oral complications in younger patients is three times that observed in adults, with an overall rate greater than 90 per cent, which may be due to the factors listed in Table 4.

Oral thrush caused by the fungus *Candida albicans* affects many people with advanced cancer (Pople and Oliver, 1986). Although present in the mouths of many healthy people, candidiasis or moniliasis is seen in most patients with white blood cell counts below 200/cumm, which may occur as a result of chemotherapy (Ostchega, 1980).

- Radiation therapy being used more frequently in combination with chemotherapy than in the adult population
- Acute lymphocytic leukaemia and acute monocytic leukaemia may represent more frequent leukaemias in children, which require treatment with chemotherapy regimens not commonly used in the management of adults
- Oral developmental changes, such as tooth eruption and exfoliation in children may predispose them to secondary oral infections not usually occurring in adults

Table 4. Factors contributing to the high rate of oral complications in children undergoing chemotherapy.

Besides bacterial and fungal infections, people undergoing immunosuppressive therapy are susceptible to viral infections such as herpes simplex. Chemotherapy may activate the virus, causing eruptions on the patient's lips (Ostchega, 1980), and particular care is therefore needed to ensure that nurses do not risk infecting themselves or others.

Although it is generally obvious to the carer when an oral infection is present, it may be undetectable at first. Burnie *et al* (1985) reported how *Candida albicans* was transmitted between patients on the hands of staff in an intensive care unit, which resulted in an outbreak of systemic infection. It is important, therefore, that nursing staff protect themselves and other patients by adhering to good infection control practices. This involves good hand hygiene before and after delivering oral care and wearing well-fitting non-sterile gloves for contact with oral mucosa.

Radiotherapy
Oral changes which occur as a result of radiation therapy for head and neck tumours manifest themselves in the form of dryness or xerostomia and consolidation of the remaining saliva into mucous and viscous matter, making swallowing difficult. The small volume of saliva remaining after therapy gradually loses its detergent and lubricating qualities, and the pH falls from about 7 to 5.5 or less. This altered pH may no longer buffer the lactic acid produced by bacteria in the mouth, and can result in dissolution of tooth enamel instead (Bersani and Carl, 1983).

Another side-effect of exposure to high energy beams is mucocitosis, which usually appears in the first week following a dosage of about 1,000rads. The surface of the lips' mucous membranes and lateral borders of the tongue become denuded, and a pseudomembrane forms, which eventually peels off, resulting in difficulty in speaking, and pain while eating and drinking (Bersani and Carl, 1983). Campbell (1987) describes oral problems of children who undergo radiotherapy to the head and neck, and these include radiation induced caries, osteo-radionecrosis of the jaw, trismus, xerostomia, parotitis and loss of taste.

Methods of providing oral care
Howarth (1977) carried out a study to determine whether or not standard mouthcare procedures were effective and left patients feeling

comfortable. Her study of 50 patients indicated that formal mouthcare procedure using foamsticks has little effect: four hourly care provided only a transient refreshing effect, and the swabbing procedure was mechanically ineffective at removing debris from the teeth, thus exposing patients to proliferation of pathogenic organisms in the debris. Harris (1980) studied 20 nurses caring for 22 elderly patients and recorded that foamsticks were chosen for use in 44 per cent of 79 oral hygiene treatments, although only 20 per cent of the patients preferred it. Toothbrushes were prejudged by several nurses to be unsuitable for an edentulous mouth, despite the fact that it has been shown to be necessary in maintaining healthy gums and tongue (Ettinger and Manderson, 1975). Trenter-Roth and Creason (1986) suggest that convenience and lack of trauma potential may influence which tool nurses choose for mouthcare, as will lack of provision of toothbrushes and toothpaste in ward store cupboards.

It is widely accepted that the toothbrush is the most efficient method of removing plaque and, therefore, of preventing gum disease and tooth decay (Gooch, 1985). Some degree of control for toothbrush trauma occurs when the brusher is providing self-care, but is undermined in nurse-administered oral care - if the patient is unable to speak, the only feedback may be the subsequent development of oral lesions (Trenter-Roth and Creason, 1986). De Walt (1975) found that when a group of elderly patients undergoing mouthcare with a medium-firm toothbrush were compared with another undergoing care with a foamstick, the plaque and gingival subscores were more improved in the toothbrushing group than the foamstick group. Although these findings suggest foam-sticks are less effective for plaque removal than toothbrushes, the medium toothbrush resulted in deterioration of soft tissues four times more often than in those receiving care with a foamstick, suggesting a medium-firm toothbrush is too traumatic for some elderly mouths. Howarth (1977) suggests that if soft baby toothbrushes were available for patient use, nurses would be more inclined to use them. Ideally, toothbrushes should have a small head with soft multitufted nylon bristles, and an abrasive toothpaste should be avoided (Alderman, 1988).

Harris (1980) advocates that an automatic toothbrush is even more effective for patient use. During a study involving patients with blood dyscrasias, Wallace and Freeman (1978) observed a dramatic improvement in mouthcare following use of an automatic toothbrush, with a lower incidence and severity of mouth ulcers and few patients suffering from bleeding gums; incidence of thrush which descended into the respiratory tract was almost non-existent. It would be advisable, however, to clean the holder thoroughly after each use, and to provide separate toothbrush attachments for individual patients, which should be disposed of at regular intervals, as with normal toothbrushes.

Dental floss is an efficient method of removing plaque, but requires nurses to be educated on how to use it correctly without causing people gum trauma. Forceps are another method of administering oral care, but are big and clumsy (Howarth, 1977). They are also no longer cheap so there does not appear to be a valid reason for their use. Harris (1980) found that 66 per cent of nurses who use forceps and swab regarded it as tolerable or satisfactory, although the same percentage also regarded it as being difficult to manipulate and having a potential for trauma. No nurse cited it as a preferred tool. The swabbed finger and foamstick were the two most popular methods of oral cleansing in Howarth's study. Although Harris (1980) suggests there are occasions when a swabbed finger is a useful adjunct to mouthcare, Shepherd *et al* (1987) consider it ineffective as rather than removing debris and plaque, it has the potential to compress them into the crevices and gaps in the teeth. Wallace and Freeman (1978) suggest swabbing should only be used for people who do not have their natural teeth.

Solutions
In a study on antimicrobial chemicals Passos and Brand (1966) compared the effectiveness of alkaline mouthwash containing alcohol with hydrogen peroxide and Milk of Magnesia; a numerical rating for the condition of the mouth was given using a standard form of assess-ment. Milk of Magnesia, although not having any antimicrobial activities, was believed to be beneficial in cleansing and reducing the acidity related to microbial glycolysis. Hydrogen peroxide was ranked as most effective, and alkaline mouthwash the least. The validity of this result, however, is questionable, as different mechanical techniques were used with each chemical. Sodium bicarbonate is frequently used for oral care and is an effective cleansing agent, especially if sores are present (Howarth, 1977), although unpleasant to taste (Howarth, 1977; Gooch, 1985). It also creates an alkaline environment which is not recommended as the mouth has a normal pH of 6 to 7, and which if altered may have adverse effects on the normal oral mucosa (De Walt and Haines, 1969).

Glycothymoline has a refreshing action, but no lasting effect and can be unpleasant to taste (Howarth, 1977; Gooch, 1985). No mention of dilution of glycerin appears on procedure sheets of nursing texts, although there are warnings about its astringent properties in early nursing books (Howarth, 1977). Glycerin combined with lemon in the form of swabs is another frequently used aid to oral care, but care must be taken as lemon is a salivary stimulant and will result in reflex exhaustion due to over-stimulation if used too frequently (Howarth, 1977; Shepherd *et al*, 1987). Following a study involving tests on 15 college students, lemon juice and glycerol did not meet the criteria for a safe, effective oral hygiene agent (Wiley, 1969). The pH of the combinations of lemon and glycerol used ranged from 2.2 to 3.9, well below the normal pH of between 6 and 7 of the oral cavity, and this acidity would make the suspension chemically, if not mechanically, decalcifying to teeth. Wiley also suggests that the moistening effect of glycerol would be counteracted by the drying effect of lemon. One controlled study which used a lemon and glycerol solution for the treatment group and saline as a control substance was carried out using elderly patients (Van Drimmelin and Rollins, 1969), and the differences in mouth scores after five days of treatment were not statistically significant. Oral moisture declined in both groups, and was lower in the lemon and glycerol group until the fifth day of treatment. The significance of this study is questionable, however, as oral fluids were not restricted prior to assessment.

Gooch (1985) suggests that tap water, which is the cheapest fluid available and has a pH of 7, is an ideal mouth rinse and should be the most frequent choice. Chlorhexidine is a popular choice, as it is widely believed to inhibit bacterial growth and control plaque development (Shepherd *et al*, 1987). Users need to be aware of the potential for black staining of teeth, although this is usually only associated with long-term use. Little research has been done on the microbiological effects of antibacterial mouthwashes on the mouth organisms, but an *in vivo* study by Richards and McCague (1988) comparing mouth rinses, found that a chlorhexidine-based substance (Corsodyl) had marked antibacterial activity and would, therefore, be effective in combating bacterial infections in the mouth and throat. Corsodyl was also shown in laboratory tests to be effective in curbing microbial growth (Grenby and Saldanha, 1984). Fine (1985) compared a chlorhexidine antiseptic with a povidine-iodine solution and physical hygiene treatment to assess its capacity for plaque control; in terms of reducing gingival inflammation, the plaque control achieved with the two chemicals was equivalent to descaling in the dental surgery and self-use of dental floss or wood points, while povidine-iodine also caused less staining of teeth than chlorhexidine. Care is needed not to overuse oral antiseptics, as this may lead to disruption of the normal flora of the mouth. Evidence to support use as a prophylactic agent in immunosuppressed patients is lacking.

Toothpastes
Although toothbrushing is widely discussed in the literature, toothpastes are rarely mentioned. Alderman (1988) suggests a non-abrasive tooth-paste should be used, and Gooch (1985) points out that toothpaste left in a mouth can have a drying effect, so care should be taken to ensure it is all removed, either by mouthwash, a foamstick or a nurse's swabbed finger. Shepherd *et al* (1987) consider chlorhexidine so useful for mouth-care that they suggest it be incorporated into a toothpaste.

Further research
There has been little change in oral care procedures for many years, and mouthcare is not given high priority among nursing duties. Much of the research on oral care is now dated, and if further research is to be

performed, an accurate rating scale must be employed to remove the many variants in oral conditions between patients or subject groups.

When delivering oral care, different goals require different approaches. If relief for a dry mouth is all that is needed, then frequent mouth rinses may suffice; if plaque control is needed, then more active intervention is required. It is important, therefore, that nursing goals are defined so the effectiveness of the care delivered can be evaluated. More controlled studies are required to update nurses on the appropriate clinical practice for oral care. However, sufficient information is available which can help nurses improve procedures instead of relying on ritualistic care.

References
Allbright, A. (1984) Oral care for the cancer chemotherapy patient. *Nursing Times*, **80**, 40-42.
Alderman, C. (1988) Oral hygiene. *Nursing Standard*, **40**, 2, 24.
Bersani, G. and Carl, W. (1983) Oral care for cancer patients. *AJN*, **4**, 533-36.
Blaney, G.M. (1986) Mouthcare 1 - basic and essential. *Geriatric Nursing*, **7**, 5, 242-47.
Block, P.L. (1976) Dental health in hospitalised patients. *AJN*, **76**, 1162.
Burnie, J. *et al* (1985) Control of an outbreak of *Candida albicans. BMJ*, **291**, 1092-93.
Campbell, S. (1987) Mouthcare in cancer patients. *Nursing Times*, **83**, 29, 59-60.
De Walt, E. and Haines, A.K. (1969) The effects of specified stressors on health oral mucosa. *Nr. Research*, **18**, 1, 22-27.
DeWalt, E. (1975) Effect of timed hygiene measures on oral mucosa in a group of elderly subjects. *Nr. Research*, **24**, 104-08.
Ettinger, R.L. and Manderson, R.D. (1975) Dental care of the elderly. *Nursing Times*, **71**, 1003-06.
Fine, P.D. (1985) A clinical trial to compare the effect of two antiseptic mouthwashes on gingival inflammation. *Journal of Hospital Infection*, **6**, (Supplement), 189-93.
Geissler, P. and McCord, F. (1986) Dental care for the elderly. *Nursing Times*, **82**, 53-54.
Gooch, J. (1985) Mouthcare. *Professional Nurse*, **1**, 3, 77-78.
Grenby, T.H. and Sladanha, M.G. (1984) The antimicrobial activity of modern mouthwashes. *Brit. Dent. J.*, **157**, 7, 239-42.
Harris, M.D. (1980) Basic Principles of Nursing Care. International Council of Nurses, London.
Howarth, H. (1977) Mouthcare procedures for the very ill. *Nursing Times*, **73**, 354-55.
Lamy, M.L. and Lamy, P.P. (1985) Drugs, older adults and oral health. *Journal of Gerontological Nursing*, **11**, 10, 36-37.
Lewis, I.A. (1984) Developing a research based curriculum: an exercise in relation to oral care. *Nr. Ed. Today*, **3**, 6, 143-44.
Miller, R. and Rubinstein, L. (1987) Oral health care for hospitalised patients: the nurse's role. *J. of Nr. Edu.*, **26**, 9, 362-66.
Munday, P. and Gelbier, S. (1984) Provision of dental health education in nursing training. *Nr. Edu. Today*, **3**, 6, 124-25.
O'Hara, A. (1988) Open wide. *J. of Dist. Nr.*, **6**, 8, 8-9.
Ostchega, Y. (1980) Preventing and treating cancer chemotherapy's oral complications. *Nursing*, **80**, 47-51.
Passos, J.Y. and Brand, L.M. (1966) Effects of agents used for oral hygiene. *Nursing Research*, **15**, 3, 196-202.
Perry, A.G. and Potter P.A. (1986) Clinical Nursing Skills and Techniques - Basic, Intermediate and Advanced. Mosby-Year Book, St Louis.
Pople, J. and Oliver, D. (1986) Oral thrush in hospice patients. *Nursing Times*, **82**, 45, 34-35.
Richards, R.M.E. and G.J. (1988) *In vivo* estimation of the antimicrobial activity of proprietary mouthwashes. *The Pharma-ceutical Journal*, **241** (Supplement)
Schweiger, J.L. *et al* (1980) Oral assessment: how to do it. *AJN*, **80**, 654-57.
Shepherd, G. *et al* (1987) The mouthtrap. *Nursing Times*, **83**, 19, 25-27.

Sonis, A.T. and Sonis, S.T. (1979) Oral complications of cancer chemotherapy in paediatric patients. *Journal of Pedodontics*, **3**, 122-28.

Trenter-Roth, P. and Creason, N.S. (1986) Nurse administered oral hygiene: Is there a scientific basis? *Journal of Advanced Nursing*, **11**, 323-31.

Van Drimmelin, J. and Rollins, H.F. (1969) Evaluation of a commonly used oral hygiene agent. *Nursing Research*, **18**, 327-32.

Wallace, J. and Freeman, P.A. (1978) Mouthcare in patients with blood dyscrasias. *Nursing Times*, **74**, 22, 921-22.

Wiley, S.B. (1969) Why glycerol and lemon juice? *AJN*, **69**, 342-44.

41

A policy that protects: the Waterlow Pressure Sore Prevention/Treatment Policy

Judith Waterlow, RGN, RCNT

Council Member, Tissue Viability Society: Member, Wound Care Society; Lecturer and Study Day Organiser

As the cost of treating pressure sores rises, many hospitals have formed groups to produce a pressure sore prevention and treatment policy. The cost of treating pressure sores is known to be £1-1.5 million per health authority, and is increasing at a rate of 13 per cent per annum. Another £100,000 to £1,000,000 could be added to this should the authority be sued as a result of patients developing pressure sores during hospital stays. Assessment should be at the heart of a policy for the prevention of pressure sores if it is to be successful (Livesley, 1989).

The Waterlow card

The Waterlow Pressure Sore Prevention/Treatment Policy started life as the Waterlow Pressure Sore Risk Assessment card (Waterlow, 1985). Its name was changed to encourage users to see it as an aid to both prevention and treatment of pressure sores. The card was developed in its original form in medical areas such as coronary and intensive care, surgical, orthopaedic and geriatric wards, using 650 patients who had been admitted for longer than three days. Each patient was assessed on admission and then every third day until discharge or death. When the card was well established, a questionnaire was sent to all participants, and results showed that the card was quick, simple to use and stimulated interest in the prevention and treatment of pressure sores among the nursing staff.

The assessment side of the card (Figure 1) was formulated as a result of reading all available research on pressure sores and endeavouring to put the information on a card in the most simple and comprehensive way possible. Scores are allocated to headings on the card: these are build/weight for height, continence, skin type (visual risk areas), mobility, sex, age, appetite and special risks (subdivided into tissue malnutrition, neurological deficit, major surgery/trauma and medication). The user assesses the patient and selects the appropriate heading with its score; the patient can then be categorised as 'not at risk', 'at risk', 'high risk', or 'very high risk' depending on the total score.

WATERLOW PRESSURE SORE PREVENTION/TREATMENT POLICY
RING SCORES IN TABLE, ADD TOTAL.   SEVERAL SCORES PER CATEGORY CAN BE USED

BUILD/WEIGHT FOR HEIGHT	★	SKIN TYPE VISUAL RISK AREAS	★	SEX AGE	★	SPECIAL RISKS	★
AVERAGE	0	HEALTHY	0	MALE	1	TISSUE MALNUTRITION	★
ABOVE AVERAGE	1	TISSUE PAPER	1	FEMALE	2		
OBESE	2	DRY	1	14 - 49	1		
BELOW AVERAGE	3	OEDEMATOUS	1	50 - 64	2	e.g.: TERMINAL CACHEXIA	8
		CLAMMY (TEMP ↑)	1	65 - 74	3	CARDIAC FAILURE	5
CONTINENCE	★	DISCOLOURED	2	75 - 80	4	PERIPHERAL VASCULAR DISEASE	5
		BROKEN/SPOT	3	81+	5	ANAEMIA	2
COMPLETE/ CATHETERISED	0					SMOKING	1
OCCASION INCONT.	1	MOBILITY	★	APPETITE	★		
CATH/INCONTINENT OF FAECES	2	FULLY	0	AVERAGE	0	NEUROLOGICAL DEFICIT	★
DOUBLY INCONT.	3	RESTLESS/FIDGETY	1	POOR	1	eg: DIABETES, M.S., CVA, MOTOR/SENSORY, PARAPLEGIA	4-6
		APATHETIC	2	N.G. TUBE/			
		RESTRICTED	3	FLUIDS ONLY	2		
		INERT/TRACTION	4	NBM/ANOREXIC	3	MAJOR SURGERY/TRAUMA	★
		CHAIRBOUND	5				
© J. Waterlow 1988						ORTHOPAEDIC - BELOW WAIST, SPINAL ON TABLE > 2 HOURS	5 5
						MEDICATION	★
SCORE:	10+ AT RISK					STEROIDS, CYTOTOXICS, HIGH DOSE ANTI-INFLAMMATORY	4

OBTAINABLE FROM: NEWTONS, CURLAND, TAUNTON, TA3 5SG

Figure 1. Assessment side of the Waterlow card.

The importance of assessing all patients (except perhaps some short stay cases) cannot be over emphasised. The assessment rating should be entered in the notes together with any preventative measures taken, and patients should be reassessed according to the degree of risk or any change in their condition. By keeping records over a period of time it is possible to establish the proportion of patients falling into the various risk categories. With this evidence, cost-effective allocation of aids can be made. In view of potential litigation, the fact that the patient has been assessed, the score written down and appropriate preventive measures taken can only help the health authority's case. Assessment and documentaton carried out with the card can be used as a record for research or to persuade management to buy the necessary preventive aids (Richardson, 1990).

Prevention and treatment
The three stages of 'risk' on the Waterlow card enable the carer to select appropriate preventive aids for each patient (Figure 2). The assessment ratings may be returned to a hospital manager who could use the three stages to review staffing needs.

The card may also be used for the allocation of patients to primary care teams. By keeping a running total score of the risk factors of each team's patients, the overall loading of the teams can be balanced. Records can be kept on a NOBO board to allow all staff and supervisors to be kept up to date with the current situation on the ward.

The top of the card, contains a reminder that tissue damage often starts before admission, as patients may spend many hours on hard surfaces such as the ground, hard ambulance stretchers or in casualty (Verslysen, 1988). It should not be forgotten that patients may be shocked and therefore at even greater risk from tissue damage due to hypertension causing deformation and compression of tissues against hard surfaces.

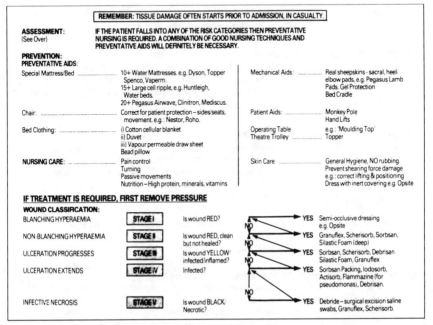

Figure 2. Treatment policy suggested by the Waterlow card.

Below the 'reminder' on the card it is stated that "if the patient falls into any of the risk categories then preventive nursing is required. A combination of good nursing techniques and preventive aids will definitely be necessary". This statement is followed by a selection of beds and mattresses which are divided into the three risk categories.

The original survey of the card showed that 50 per cent of patients did not come within any of the risk categories, and no special preventive aids were required. Of the study population, 26 per cent came within the 'at risk' area, 16 per cent at 'high risk' and 8 per cent in the 'very high' category, and results showed an increasing number of patients in each area of risk developed pressure sores (Waterlow, 1985). By having three bands of risk the correct preventive mattress/bed may be allocated to each patient - it is not widely known that pressure sore reducing abilities vary greatly with different surfaces (Clark, 1987).

Prevention   This area of the card suggests a variety of preventive aids, from mattresses to mechanical and patient aids. All are intended as an 'aide memoir' for staff to enable them to investigate the numerous appliances available on the market. Care must be taken when selecting aids so that they meet the needs of the type of patients for whom they are being purchased, and are not just chosen because they are the cheapest - cost-effectiveness is all important.

Classification of pressure sores

Stage i   Blanching hyperaemia
Reactive hyperaemia causes a distinct erythema after pressure is released. Light finger pressure will cause blanching of this erythema, indicating the microcirculation is intact.

Stage ii   Non-blanching hyperaemia
Erythema remains after release of pressure. A degree of microcirculatory disruption and inflammation, oedema and thickening occurs. Superficial, swelling, induration, blistering, epidermal ulceration may be present.
If sensory innervation is intact, pain will be present.

Stage iii   Ulceration progresses through to the subcutaneous tissue
Ulcer edges are distinct, but surrounded by erythema and induration. At this stage, damage is still reversible.

Stage iv   Lesion extends into the subcutaneous fat
Small vessel thrombosis and infection compound fat necrosis. Distinct ulcer margin, but lateral extension of necrosis continues under the skin. Deep fascia temporarily impedes downward progress.

Stage v   Infective necrosis
Necrosis penetrates deep fascia and muscle induration proceeds rapidly. Joints and body cavities can become involved. Multiple sores may communicate.

Closed pressure sores
Deep extensive damage to tissues, but the surface presents as a small ulcer.

Healing stages of a clean incision

Stage i   The phase of traumatic inflammation - 0 to 3 days
Stage ii   The destructive phase - 1 to 6 days
Stage iii   The proliferative phase - 3 to 20 days
Stage iv   The maturation phases - 20 days to 1 year.

Wound healing and repair is a continuous process so naturally these stages overlap to some extent.

It should be noted that nutrition is repeated in the section of the card devoted to nursing care (it also appears as appetite on the assessment side of the card). The nutritional status of patients throughout hospitals has been found to be poor (Dickerson, 1986).

Treatment The lower third of the card is devoted to five stages of wound classification (Table 1) (Hibbs, 1988). During the survey, each ward had a full description of the stages displayed in the treatment room (Figure 3). Having identified the stage of wound, suggestions for treatment for each stage are listed (Versluysen, 1988).

Future development
The Waterlow Pressure Sore Prevention/Treatment Policy is intended to help staff in all clinical areas. Hospital, A&E and ambulance trolleys should have increased pressure reducing abilities. People admitted to accident centres should be assessed for risk and appropriate measures taken to prevent compression of tissues. All patients admitted for longer than three days should be assessed, with the assessment rating and appropriate measures taken recorded in the nursing notes. Patients should be reassessed according to the degree of risk - the higher the risk the more frequent the reassessment - and if their condition changes. If the patient develops a pressure sore - 95 per cent of all sores are preventable (Hibbs, 1988) - the stage of wound, position, size and treatment should all be entered in the patient's nursing notes.

The card should be considered as a 'live' document. Over 80,000 cards have now been distributed, and it is up to the users to improve the accuracy of the scoring system by providing feedback. This could generate a wealth of invaluable empirical evidence for reassessing how much weight should be attributed to the various factors.

By allocating a negative score to a variety of types of pressure relieving aids, it should be possible to keep patients below 'at risk' levels. It is unlikely there will ever be sufficient money to buy all the aids that could be used, but if all aspects of pressure sores are documented and allocated a weighting factor, judgements can be made as to where the resources would best be deployed and on easily assessed numbers.

An assessment card cannot satisfy everyone, and some nurses may argue that certain factors should or should not be included; a score is too high or low; the risk levels are too high or low. To all these people I would say the card belongs to the user, and is intended to benefit patients, not to win prizes for the author. It should not be considered as a tablet of stone to be followed or rejected slavishly, and I would be delighted to receive information from users which will help further develop and refine the card. Evidence which indicates modification is necessary is just as welcome as that which confirms the present scoring system. We are all different, and there are many factors, which it would be impossible to quantify, that influence patients' susceptibility to tissue damage. By all the laws of statistics, the more empirical evidence that is made available the more accurate the scoring system will become.

References

Clark, M. (1987) Tissue viability conference Durham, following two years research for the DHSS.

Dealey, C. Regional Study Days for The Society for Tissue Viability.

Dickerson, J.W.T. (1986) Hospital induced malnutrition: prevention and treatment. *The Professional Nurse*, **1**, 12, 314-16.

Hibbs, P.J. (1987) Strategies for the elimination of pressure scores. *Care-Science and Practice*, **5**, 4, 15-19.

Hibbs, P.J. (1988) Pressure Area Care For The City and Hackney Health Authority. Prevention plan for patients at risk from developing pressure sores. Policy for the management of pressure sores. City and Hackney Health Authority, London.

Livesley, B. (1989) Hard cost of soft sores. *Health Service Journal*, **99**, 5139,231.

Richardson, B. (1990) Clinical and Financial Implication. Paper delivered at conference on pressure sore prevention sponsored by Pegasus Airwave Ltd.

Versluysen, M.C. (1988) Pressure sores in an orthopaedic population: an epidemiological survey. *Journal of Bone and Joint Surgery*, March.

Waterlow, J.A. (1985)A risk assessment card. *Nursing Times*, **89**, 27, 49-51.

Waterlow, J.A. (1988) The Waterlow card for the prevention and management of pressure sores: towards a pocket policy. *Care-Science and Practice*, **6**, 1, 8-12.

42

Managing pressure sores: local treatment

Moya J. Morison, BSc, MSc, BA, RGN
Clinical Audit Co-ordinator, Stirling Royal Infirmary

Local problems which can delay the healing of pressure sores include the presence of necrotic tissue, excess slough and wound infection, and this chapter discusses priorities in the local management of these chronic open wounds. Wider aspects of care, such as providing appropriate patient support, improving mobility and nutritional status and providing psychological support will be discussed in the next chapter.

A local wound management policy

The aim of local wound management is to provide the optimum micro-environment for healing. Where the skin's integrity is breached, a dressing is usually required which will take over some of the functions of the missing tissue, protecting the underlying cells from the harmful effects of dehydration, fall in temperature, further mechanical damage and infection. No single dressing is suitable for all wounds (Turner, 1983; 1985), indeed each wound may require several different types of dressing as priorities change during the healing process.

Over the last 10 years a bewildering variety of new wound care products have come on the market, and it is very difficult for nurses to know how to choose *one* product from within a particular category. Many of the products have not been subjected to extensive, comparative clinical trials. Although products may *look* alike, their physical and chemical properties may be significantly different (Thomas, 1990). To overcome this problem many health authorities are now developing a wound management policy, enabling them to rationalise their stocking and use of products.

The selection of products to be included in a local policy document is normally undertaken by the local Drugs and Therapeutics Committee, and it is valuable to have representation from all members of the healthcare team who have a special interest in, and responsibility for, wound management – including representatives from the community. As well as deciding which dressings to make *readily available*, it is helpful if the committee indicates those wound care products which should be *avoided*, or used with extreme caution, with the restriction that they can only be used when *formally prescribed* by the doctor on the drug prescription sheet. The action that should be taken by a nurse who feels that a *harmful* substance is being prescribed has been explained in the UKCC advisory document 'Exercising Accountability'.

Particularly where a local wound care policy does not exist, readers may find it helpful to refer to Morgan (1990), Morison (1992a, b) and Thomas (1990).

These sources provide further information on the advantages and disadvantages of a number of wound care products and how to choose between them. The section which follows should also be of assistance. As a general principle:

Before using *any* wound care product for the first time ALWAYS consult the manufacturer's recommendations, contraindications, precautions and warnings. If there is still any doubt about the suitability of a dressing, the pharmacist or the doctor should be consulted, so that the material selected is a team decision.

Priorities

After assessing the wound (Morison, 1989a), what are the priorities in the *local* management of pressure sores? Essentially, the priorities are the same as for any chronic open wound.

Debridement   The first priority is to remove all debris such as any foreign material, devitalised soft tissue, excess slough and necrotic tissue which can delay healing and encourage infection. Methods for removing necrotic tissue and excess slough include:

- **Surgical excision** – the quickest method of achieving a 'clean' wound bed, but not a realistic option for some patients, especially the severely debilitated.
- **Enzymatic treatment, eg, by Varidase** – a gentle, effective method at a physiological pH.
- **Hydrocolloid dressings, eg, Granuflex Comfeel and Tegasorb or hydrogels, eg, Scherisorb** which rehydrate necrotic tissue and create conditions that encourage the body's natural debriding processes.
- **Acid creams or solutions, eg, Aserbine** – effective debriding agents, but care is needed to protect surrounding skin from possible irritation or maceration.
- **Hypochlorite and other chlorinated solutions, eg, Eusol, Milton, Dakin's solution** – their possible toxicity to living tissues with prolonged use strongly militates against their use (Brennan et al, 1985, 1986; Leaper and Simpson, 1986; Thomas, 1990).

Wound infection   There is a risk of a wound becoming clinically infected at *any* stage during the healing process. Until the epidermis is completely restored, there is no effective mechanical barrier to the entry of micro-organisms when the wound is exposed. Whether or not an infection develops depends upon:

- the dose of any contaminating organism;

• its virulence;
• the resistance of the host to infection.

Many micro-organisms are, however, commensal – living on the surface of a wound without causing an acute inflammatory tissue response. This is especially true for chronic open wounds such as pressure sores and leg ulcers. It is therefore only necessary to take a wound swab for culture and antibiotic sensitivity testing if a **clinical infection** is suspected, for instance if there is inflammation, localised heat, oedema of the wound margins, pain, copious cream, grey or green exudate or offensive odour.

A systemic antibiotic may be prescribed where cellulitis is present, or where a very virulent micro-organism such as B-haemolytic *Streptococcus* is isolated in a debilitated patient. However, the routine topical use of antibiotics, such as fucidin or cicatrin is unwise as their injudicious use can encourage the emergence of multiple antibiotic-resistant strains of bacteria. In a heavily infected pressure sore extending into the dermis or deeper, Iodosorb or Debrisan can be effective treatments. Consult the manufacturer's recommendations for methods of application which aid subsequent removal. For shallow, open infected wounds, alternatives include Actisorb Plus, a charcoal dressing which also reduces odour, or non-adherent dressings impregnated with antiseptics such as Inadine or Bactigras.

There is increasing evidence that the wound exudate produced as part of the body's own defence against infection contains many bactericidal components (Hohn et al, 1977). Antiseptics should therefore only be required for severely debilitated patients or where wounds are extensive and there is a high risk of contamination. Superficial infected wounds can also be dressed with an alginate dressing, changed daily and used in conjunction with a systemic antibiotic.

Odour Malodorous wounds can be very distressing for patients, and can lead to self-imposed social isolation, loss of appetite and depression. Treating the infection that leads to the malodorous exudate is important. The odour itself can be controlled by the use of an activated charcoal dressing such as Actisorb Plus. If there is a moderate amount of exudate present, an absorbent foam dressing which has a charcoal dressing backing, such as Lyofoam C, is helpful. Flagyl, when prescribed and given systemically or topically can also have a deodorising effect. While the problem of infection is being tackled, other simple remedies should not be forgotten, such as changing bed linen and clothing as it becomes contaminated, changing the dressing if 'strike through' occurs, offering the patient a single room if possible, providing fresh air, using perfume and encouraging relatives to bring in scented plants. There is more to providing 'the ideal environment' for wound healing than choosing the most appropriate dressing, as the next chapter will demonstrate.

Excess exudate   Even when necrotic tissue and excess slough have been removed and a pressure sore is no longer clinically infected, it may still produce a moderate amount of exudate which can strike through non-occlusive dressings. This increases the risk of wound infection, or of macerating the wound margins if the surrounding tissues become waterlogged. The volume of exudate should lessen in time, but until this stage is reached an absorbent, non-adherent dressing is needed. There is a number of options including:

- Alginate dressings, eg, Kaltostat and Sorbsan – biodegradable dressings useful for packing pressure sores where tracking is present. The wound should be lightly packed to prevent skin flaps from growing over cavities and encouraging the wound to granulate from beneath.
- Polyurethane foam sheets, eg, Lyofoam, Allevyn – for relatively shallow, medium-to-heavily exuding pressure sores, eg, Allevyn cavity wound dressing for deeper wounds.
- Hydrocolloids, eg, Granuflex E and Comfeel. Paste or beads are especially helpful in deep wounds with no tracking. When applied to patients with a sacral sore, consider the use of a specially shaped hydrocolloidal dressing.

Your choice of dressing will be affected by such practical considerations as the site and size of the wound, the volume of exudate, comfort and cosmetic acceptability to the patient and, of course, the cost of the dressing (preferably calculated on a weekly basis, as this overcomes the bias against a product with a high unit cost if it requires less frequent dressing changes than a lower cost product.).

Clean superficial pressure sores   The aim here is to continue to provide a moist environment for healing and to protect the surface of the wound from further mechanical damage and from contamination. A film dressing such as OpSite, Flexigrid or Tegaderm, or a hydrocolloid sheet dressing is recommended. Alternatively an alginate dressing such as Kaltoclude can be used.

The catalogue of substances used to treat pressure sores in the distant past (Forrest, 1982) and the present (David et al, 1983) makes depressing reading, and the more 'way out' solutions require no further comment here. Hyperbaric oxygen therapy, the use of ultrasound or ultraviolet light by the physiotherapist, should be considered. An account of methods for surgically closing pressure sores is given by Morison (1992a).

No matter how appropriate a wound dressing regime is selected, if the underlying causes of the pressure sore are not alleviated, delayed healing is inevitable. Wider issues such as providing the most appropriate patient support system, improving mobility and nutritional status, and providing psychological support will be discussed in the next chapter.

References
Brennan, S.S. and Leaper, D.J. (1985) The effect of antiseptics on the healing wound: a study using rabbit ear chamber. *British Journal of Surgery*, **72**, 10, 780–82.

Brennan, S.S. Foster, M.E., Leaper, D.J. (1986) Antiseptics toxicity in wounds healing by secondary intention. *Journal of Hospital Infection*, **8**, 3, 263–67.

David, J.A. et al (1983) An investigation of the current methods used in nursing for the care of patients with established pressure sores. Nursing Practice Research Unit, Harrow.

Forrest, R.D. (1982) Early history of wound treatment. *Journal of the Royal Society of Medicine*, **75**, 198–205.

Hohn, D.C. et al (1977) Antimicrobial systems of the surgical wound. *American Journal of Surgery*, **133**, 5, 597–600.

Leaper, D.J. and Simpson, R.A. (1986) The effect of antiseptics and topical antimicrobials on wound healing, *Journal of Antimicrobial Chemotherapy*, **17**, 2, 135–37.

Morgan, D.A. (1990) Formulary of Wound Management Products 4th edn. Clwyd Health Authority.

Morison M.J. (1992a) A Colour Guide to the Nursing Management of Wounds. Wolfe Publishing, London.

Morison, M.J. (1992b) Which Wound Care Product? *Professional Nurse*, **7**, 4 (wallchart).

Morison M.J. (1989a) Pressure sores: assessing the wound. *Professional Nurse*, **4**, 11, 532–35.

Thomas, S. (1990) Wound Management and Dressings. Pharmaceutical Press, London.

Turner, T.D. (1983) Absorbents and wound dressings. *Nursing*, **2**, 12, Supplement.

Turner, T.D. (1985) Which dressing and why? In: Westaby, S. (ed). Wound Care. Heineman, London.

Bibliography
Morison, M.J. (1992) A Colour Guide to the Nursing Management of Wounds. Wolfe Publishing, London.

43

Pressure sores: removing the causes of the wound

Moya J. Morison, BSc, MSC, BA, RGN
Clinical Audit Co-ordinator, Stirling Royal Infirmary

Articles in the nursing press on the prevention and management of pressure sores probably outnumber any other single topic. This is perhaps not only a reflection of the size of the problem, but also of many nurses' feelings that more could be done to prevent pressure sores from developing and to improve their management. The last chapter discussed priorities in the local management of pressure sores. This chapter explores more general issues and outlines a very simple 10 point action plan aimed at preventing pressure sores in high-risk patients and managing them appropriately when tissue breakdown occurs. The general principles are the same.

General treatment aims

In the past, considerable research attention has been focused on the prevention of pressure sores, but relatively little on the effectiveness of the most commonly used treatment methods (Chapman and Chapman, 1986). Certainly, no definitive treatment for pressure sores has yet emerged but the general principles are clear:

- to remove the *extrinsic* factors significant in the development and delayed healing of pressure sores such as: unrelieved pressure, shearing and frictional forces;

- to alleviate the effects of the *intrinsic* factors that can contribute to tissue breakdown and delayed healing such as malnutrition, incontinence and debilitating concurrent illness;

- to provide the optimum *local* environment for healing at the wound site.

The 10 point plan (Table 1) reflects these principles.

Since almost any patient problem can lead directly or indirectly to delayed wound healing it would be far too simplistic to suppose that all aspects of the care of a patient with a pressure sore could be adequately covered in one chapter. Ways of providing the optimum local environment for healing were described in the previous chapter. There is

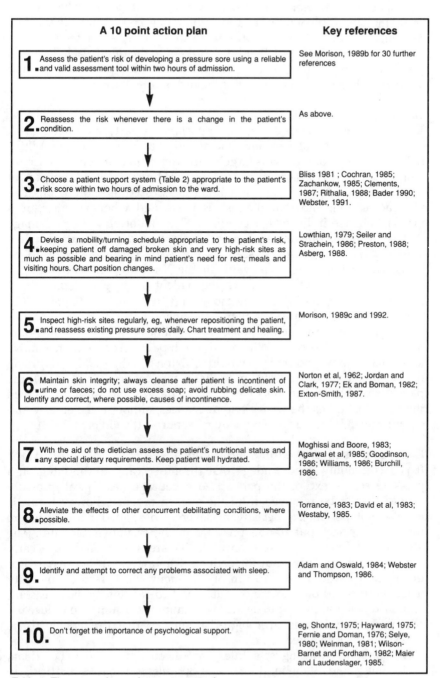

A 10 point action plan	Key references
1. Assess the patient's risk of developing a pressure sore using a reliable and valid assessment tool within two hours of admission.	See Morison, 1989b for 30 further references
2. Reassess the risk whenever there is a change in the patient's condition.	As above.
3. Choose a patient support system (Table 2) appropriate to the patient's risk score within two hours of admission to the ward.	Bliss 1981 ; Cochran, 1985; Zachankow, 1985; Clements, 1987; Rithalia, 1988; Bader 1990; Webster, 1991.
4. Devise a mobility/turning schedule appropriate to the patient's risk, keeping patient off damaged broken skin and very high-risk sites as much as possible and bearing in mind patient's need for rest, meals and visiting hours. Chart position changes.	Lowthian, 1979; Seiler and Strachein, 1986; Preston, 1988; Asberg, 1988.
5. Inspect high-risk sites regularly, eg, whenever repositioning the patient, and reassess existing pressure sores daily. Chart treatment and healing.	Morison, 1989c and 1992.
6. Maintain skin integrity; always cleanse after patient is incontinent of urine or faeces; do not use excess soap; avoid rubbing delicate skin. Identify and correct, where possible, causes of incontinence.	Norton et al, 1962; Jordan and Clark, 1977; Ek and Boman, 1982; Exton-Smith, 1987.
7. With the aid of the dietician assess the patient's nutritional status and any special dietary requirements. Keep patient well hydrated.	Moghissi and Boore, 1983; Agarwal et al, 1985; Goodinson, 1986; Williams, 1986; Burchill, 1986.
8. Alleviate the effects of other concurrent debilitating conditions, where possible.	Torrance, 1983; David et al, 1983; Westaby, 1985.
9. Identify and attempt to correct any problems associated with sleep.	Adam and Oswald, 1984; Webster and Thompson, 1986.
10. Don't forget the importance of psychological support.	eg, Shontz, 1975; Hayward, 1975; Fernie and Doman, 1976; Selye, 1980; Weinman, 1981; Wilson-Barnet and Fordham, 1982; Maier and Laudenslager, 1985.

Table 1. The prevention and management of pressure sores.

only space here to refer to ways of alleviating the *intrinsic* problems such as malnutrition, incontinence, and debilitating concurrent illness. Key references to these problems are given in Table 1, so that nurses can follow up particular topics that interest them in the depth each deserves. Ways of removing the *extrinsic* factors that can cause pressure sores and delay their healing, is the subject of the rest of this chapter.

Ongoing assessment

The plan in Table 1 emphasises the importance of early and ongoing risk assessment – even for a patient who already has a pressure sore. Which risk assessment tool to use is largely a matter of personal preference, so long as the user is aware of its limitations (Morison, 1989b), but it is of paramount importance that the patient is assessed as soon as possible after admission, and that the risk is reassessed whenever there is a material change in his or her condition. The underlying tissue damage that can lead to a pressure sore can occur very rapidly, for example when a patient is waiting to be seen in the A&E Department, or to be transferred from there to a ward; in the X-ray department during a special procedure which requires the patient to be placed on a hard surface; or on operating theatre tables and trolleys (Nightingale, 1978; Stewart and Magnano, 1988). Some patients are at risk for only part of the day, during the acute phase of an illness or for a few hours immediately post-surgery. Whether through pain or sedation, they move less than they normally would (Exton-Smith, 1987). Nursing interventions need to keep pace with the changing nature of the patient's problems. Patients of *all* ages can develop pressure sores given the right (or rather the wrong) circumstances, although the elderly and chronically debilitated are obviously most at risk (David et al, 1983).

Relief of pressure, shearing and friction

It is a commonly quoted adage that the nurse can put anything on a pressure sore – except the patient. To encourage healing, all pressure should ideally be removed from the site. In practice, however, this is usually not possible, especially in severely deformed patients where repositioning can put undue pressure on other vulnerable sites. The ideal way to reduce pressure on high-risk areas is to encourage early mobility (Asberg, 1988), but for patients who are paralysed, sedated or unconscious, who are on a form of treatment which restricts mobility (such as traction) or who are on enforced bed-rest for medical reasons, regular repositioning by nurses will be required. The aim is to reduce the pressure per unit time over high-risk sites so that irreversible tissue breakdown is prevented.

A number of turning schedules have been devised (eg, Lowthian, 1979; Seiler and Stahelin, 1988). The *30° tilt technique* is particularly effective since the pressure is transferred to low-risk 'soft' sites such as the gluteal muscles, which can tolerate pressures up to three-and-a-half times higher than those tolerated over bony prominences (Preston, 1988). This makes four hourly turning feasible for many patients. Extended periods of eight hours or more without turning are possible for some, allowing a complete night's sleep. As sleep favours the anabolic healing processes (Adam and Oswald, 1984) wound healing should be greatly facilitated.

The ideal support system
The actual surface that a patient rests on is also very important (Bliss, 1981; Cochran, 1985; Zacharkow, 1985). An ideal support system should:
- distribute pressure evenly, or provide frequent relief of pressure by varying the areas under pressure.
- minimise friction and shearing forces;
- provide a comfortable, well ventilated patient support interface which does not restrict movement unduly;
- be acceptable to the patient;
- not impede nursing procedures;
- be easily maintained;
- be inexpensive.

Those most effective at providing pressure relief are expensive, while the cheaper devices are less effective in pressure distribution. The advantages and disadvantages of a number of commonly available beds, mattresses and overlays, and the principles behind their use are given in Table 2. For further information on this complex subject nurses are referred to Bader (1990) and Webster (1991).

The beneficial effects of even the most sophisticated support systems can be counteracted if nurses handle patients carelessly, and it is nurses' responsibility to understand when a support system is not functioning properly so that it can be reported for repair. The value of inexpensive and well-tried alternatives should not be underestimated. Sheepskin fleeces under the buttocks and heels can reduce frictional forces, paraplegic patients can be taught to relieve pressure from the sacral area while in bed by using monkey poles and rope ladders. Bed cradles should be used to remove the pressure of bedclothes from the lower limbs of vulnerable patients, especially those with peripheral vascular problems who are particularly susceptible to trauma, and where the consequences of a pressure induced wound could be severe enough to precipitate amputation. It seems unlikely that there will ever be enough high-technology beds for all our high-risk patients, so it is important to make the best use of existing resources, matching those at highest need to the best pressure relieving aids. It is also important to prolong the useful life of even the humblest equipment, as Larcombe (1988) explains for the basic hospital mattress.

Developing a pressure sore policy
If relevant research into the prevention and management of pressure

Table 2. Some pressure relieving beds, mattresses and overlays (Morison, 1992).

Type	Examples (Manufacturers)	Description and principles behind use	Uses and advantages
I Devices to alternate the area of the body under pressure			
Alternating pressure mattresses and overlays.	Nimbus Dynamic flotation system (Huntleigh Health Care).	A low-pressure system with figure-of-eight shaped cells to achieve a pressure rating below 20 mm Hg for over 60% of the 10 min cycle. Can be used in dynamic or static mode for certain procedures. Sensor pad ensures that patient is automatically supported at optimum pressures, regardless of weight distribution or position.	1. Very high risk, critically ill patients; patients with severe burns; following major surgery; and patients with existing grade 4–5 pressure sores. 2. A high-performance, low-pressure system at relatively low cost. 3. Fits on top of all standard hospital beds and most domestic beds. 4. Useful for transporting patients to and from X-ray and theatre; mattress can be isolated from pump and will stay inflated for over 24 h.
	Pegasus Airwave System (Pegasus Airwave).	Two layers of air cells; produces a deep rhythmic wave effect from feet to head by deflating every third cell in a 7.5 min cycle. A continuous air flow ventilates the mattress and reduces problems caused by sweat and urine.	1. For very high risk patients; the critically ill; patients for whom normal lifting is contra-indicated; and patients with existing pressure sores. 2. Regular zero skin pressure, for about 2 min in every 7.5 min cycle, which allows blood re-circulation and prevents local ischaemia over high-risk sites. 3. Low interface pressures minimise forward slide and hammocking. 4. Feet-to-head airwave effect aids venous return. 5. Reliable, durable, and easy to clean.

Alpha Xcell (Huntleigh Health Care) Double Bubble and Alphacare Plus Pump (Huntleigh Health Care).	Alternates the area of the body under pressure. The mattress consists of air cells, which are alternately inflated and deflated by means of an electric pump, controlled on a time switch.	1. Can be very effective in preventing pressure sores in moderate-risk patients; also useful for patients with existing sores, even where positional change is restricted, e.g., traction; large-cell mattresses more effective than medium- or small-cell types. 2. Inexpensive, durable, reliable, and easy to use. 3. Degree of support can be altered according to patient weight and size.

II *Devices to reduce and distribute pressure more evenly*

1. Water beds	Beaufort–Winchester (Paraglide).	Patient's weight is evenly distributed in a controlled volume of water (based on Pascal's law) so that there are no pressure gradients and tissue distortion does not occur. Only in deep-tank models is there a sufficient volume to displace the patient's mass without developing tension on the enveloping membrane.	1. Good systems are capable of providing the total hydrostatic support needed for very high-risk patients; for patients with existing pressure sores; and for patients with severe burns. 2. Patients find them comfortable. 3. Pain relief often reported.

(cont.)

256

Table 2. (cont.)

Type	Examples (Manufacturers)	Description and principles behind use	Uses and advantages
2. *Air-fluidised beds*	Clinitron (Support Systems International).	Uses dry flotation to provide hydrostatic support. A flow of warm air is pumped through fine particles, e.g., sand or glass microspheres, to provide fluid-like support characteristics.	1. Provides true hydrostatic support, suitable for intensive care, e.g., a patient with severe burns, multiple trauma, or a critically ill patient who cannot tolerate manual lifting. 2. Air temperature can be controlled. 3. System can absorb exudate, so providing a healthy skin environment. 4. Air fluidisation can be continuous or intermittent; patient handling is easier when fluidisation is switched off. 5. Fluidisation can be stopped instantly in case of cardiac arrest.
3. *Low air-loss bed systems* (LALBS)	Mediscus (Mediscus).	The LALBS consists of waterproof, but vapour permeable, sacks arranged in groups, with pressure valves controlling each group to suit body contours. The bed is hinged, and bellows at the head and foot control posture. There is automatic deformation of the bed to accommodate body form.	1. Uniform pressure on maximum body surface area; therefore suitable for very high-risk patients and patients with existing sores. 2. Low shear stresses. 3. Water can evaporate from the support surface. 4. Temperature and humidity are controllable. 5. Air sacks are easily removable for washing/disinfection. 6. Minimum lifting of patient; variable positions possible. 7. Mobile.

4. Low pressure air bed	Simpson–Edinburgh (Kellie).	Consists of two standard air beds placed one on top of the other on a wooden base and with padded sides. An air pump inflates the mattresses to a pre-set pressure and, when the patient is placed on the bed, air is discharged to keep the pressure constant.	1. Low- to moderate-risk patients. 2. Prevents the patient from grounding. 3. Adjustable pressure control ensures the bed is not over-inflated. 4. Relatively inexpensive.
5. Cut foam mattress	Polyfloat (Talley).	Consists of two layers of foam bonded together with the upper layer cut into almost independent blocks to reduce the hammock effect from the tension in the otherwise solid foam mattresses.	1. Low-risk patients. 2. Inexpensive, light, and easy to use. 3. Considerable improvement on solid foam mattresses, reducing shearing, but effectiveness is greatly reduced if sheets are tucked in.

257

(cont.)

Table 2. (cont.)

Type	Examples (Manufacturers)	Description and principles behind use	Uses and advantages
6. *Bead Pillow overlays*	Beaufort Bead Pillow Support System (Paraglide).	Patient sinks into the transverse pillows and the beads conform to the patient's shape, instantly adjusting to movement and repositioning.	1. For low-risk patients, and patients with arthritic, rheumatic, and muscular pain. 2. Suitable for both home and hospital use. 3. Very easy to use and adaptable for patients with deformities. 4. Comfortable. 5. Machine washable.
7. *Silicone fibre overlays*	Spenco (Spenco Medical). Superdown (Huntleigh Health Care).	Made up of horizontal fibre-filled compartments.	1. Low-risk patients. 2. Easy to use and maintain, machine washable (with care). 3. Comfortable.
III *Devices to aid turning* Net Suspension beds	Mecabed (Arjo-Mecanaids).	Patient is supported on a slightly elastic open-mesh net suspended from a frame, which fits over the bed. Operated by two winding handles.	1. Moderate- to high-risk patients, especially those unable to tolerate physical handling for turning. 2. Bed conforms to body contours. 3. Provides a ventilated skin environment. 4. One nurse can easily turn even heavy patients.

sores is to be put into practice, its results must be made available to nurses at ward level by nurse educators (Morison, 1989a). The role of management in ensuring theory is put into practice should not be underestimated – it is, after all, the budget-holders who ultimately determine how much is spent on pressure sore prevention and care.

It helps where a health authority has a pressure sore prevention and treatment policy, based on the latest research, which is known and carried out by all staff and which includes monitoring equipment in use, planning equipment acquisition and deciding on priorities (Livesley, 1987; Hibbs, 1988).

References

Adam, K. and Oswald, I. (1984) Sleep helps healing. *British Medical Journal*, **289**, 24 Nov. 1400-01, (letters section).

Agarwal, N. et al (1985) The role of nutrition in the management of pressure sores. In: Lee, B.K. (Ed) Chronic Ulcers of the skin. McGraw-Hill, New York.

Asberg, K.H. (1988) Early activation for elderly patients in acute medical wards. *Care: Science and Practice*, **6**, 3, 69-73.

Bader, D.L. (Ed) (1990) Pressure Sores: Clinical Practice and Scientific Approach. MacMillan, London.

Bliss, M.R. (1981) Clinical Research in patient support systems. *Care: Science and Practice*, **1**, 17-36.

Burchill, P. (1986) Bodybuilders. *Community Outlook*, August, 19-22.

Chapman, E.J. and Chapman, R. (1986) Treatment of pressure sores: the state of the art. In: Tierney, A.J. Clinical Nursing Practice. Churchill Livingstone, Edinburgh.

Clements, S. (1987) And so to beds. *Community Outlook*, September, 16-17.

Cochran, G.V.B. (1985) Measurement of pressure and other environmental factors at the patient – cushion interface. In: Lee, B.K. (Ed) Chronic Ulcers of the Skin. McGraw-Hill, New York.

David, J.A. et al (1983) An investigation of the Currrent Methods Used in Nursing for the Care of Patients with Established Pressure Sores. Nursing Practice Research Unit, Harrow.

Ek, A.C. and Boman, G. (1982) A descriptive study of pressure sores: the prevalence of pressure sores and the characteristics of the patients. *Journal of Advanced Nursing*, **7**, 51-57.

Exton-Smith, N. (1987) The patient's not for turning. *Nursing Times*, **83**, 42, 42-44.

Fernie, G.R. and Dornan, J. (1976) The problems of clinical trials with new systems for preventing or healing decubiti. In: Kenedi et al (Eds) Bedsore Biomechanics. Macmillan, London.

Goodinson, S.M. (1986) Assessment of nutritional status. *Nursing*, **3**, 7, 252-57.

Hayward, J. (1975) Information: a prescription against pain. Royal College of Nursing, London.

Hibbs, P. (1988) Action against pressure sores. *Nursing Times*, **84**, 13, 68-73.

Jordan, M.M. and Clark, M.O. (1977) Report on the incidence of pressure sores in the patient community of the Greater Glasgow Health Board Area on 21 January 1976. University of Strathclyde Bioengineering Unit and The Greater Glasgow Health Board, Glasgow.

Larcombe, J. (1988) One good turn deserves another. *Nursing Times*, **84**, 11, 36-38.

Livesley, B. (1987) An expensive epidemic. *Nursing Times*, **83**, 79.

Lowthian, P. (1979) Turning clocks system to prevent pressure sores. *Nursing Mirror*, **148**, 21, 30-31.

Maier, S.F. and Laudenslager, M. (1985) Stress and health: exploring the links. *Psychology Today*, **19**, 8, 44-49.

Moghissi, K. and Boore, J. (1983) Parenteral and Enteral Nutrition for Nurses. Heinemann Medical Books, London.

Morison, M.J. (1989a) Delayed pressure sore healing can be prevented. *The Professional Nurse*, **4**, 7, 332-36.

Morison, M.J. (1989b) Early assessment of pressure sore risk. *The Professional Nurse*, **4**, 9, 428-31.

Morison, M.J. (1989c) Pressure sores: assessing the wound. *The Professional Nurse*, **4**, 11, 532-35.

Morison, M.J. (1992) A Colour Guide to the Nursing Management of Wounds. Wolfe Publishing, London.

Nightingale, K.M. (1978) Out of sight: out of mind: an enquiry into the incidence of pressure injuries in the operating department. *NAT News*, August, 22-26.

Norton, D. et al (1962) An Investigation of Geriatric Nursing Problems in Hospital. National Corporation for the Care of Old People, London.

Preston, K.W. (1988) Positioning for comfort and pressure relief: the 30 degree alternative. *Care: Sci. and Pract*, **6**, 4, 116-19.

Rithalia, S.V.S. (1988) What inflation pressure and which air mattress? *Care: Science and practice*, **6**, 2, 45-47.

Seiler, W.O. and Stahelin, H.B. (1985) Decubitus ulcers: preventive techniques for the elderly patient. *Geriatrics*, **40**, 7, 53-60.

Selye, H. (Ed) (1980) Selye's Guide to Stress Research, 1. Van Nostrand Reinhold, London.

Shontz, F.C. (1975) The Psychological Aspects of Physical Illness and Disability. MacMillan, New York.

Stewart, T.P. and Magnano, S.J. (1988) Burns or pressure ulcers in the surgical patient? *Decubitus*, **1**, 1, 36-40.

Torrance, C. (1983) Pressure Sores: Aetiology, Treatment and Prevention. Croom Helm, Beckenham.

Webster, J.G. (Ed) (1991) Prevention of Pressure Sores: Engineering and Clinical Aspects. Adam Hilger, Bristol.

Webster, R.A. and Thompson, D.R. (1986) Sleep in hospital. *Journal of Advanced Nursing*, **11**, 4, 447-57.

Weinman, J. (1981) An Outline of Psychology as Applied to Medicine. John Wright, Bristol.

Westaby, S. (Ed) (1985) Wound Care. Heinemann Medical Books Ltd, London.

Williams, C.M. (1986) Wound healing: a nutritional perspective. *Nursing*, **3**, 7, 249-51.

Wilson-Barnett, J. and Fordham, M. (1982) Recovery From Illness. John Wiley, Chichester.

Zacharkow, D. (1985) Wheelchair Posture and Pressure Sores. Charles C. Thomas, Springfield.

Bibliography
Morison, M.J. (1992) A Colour Guide to the Nursing Management of Wounds. Wolfe Publishing, London.

44

A holistic approach and the ideal dressing: cavity wound management in the 1990s

Sue Bale, BA, RGN, NGN, HV, DipN
Director Nursing Research, Wound Healing Research Unit, University of Wales College of Medicine, Cardiff

The 1980s saw the advent of a range of products specifically designed for the treatment of cavity wounds. Not only were these materials becoming widely available, but, more importantly, interest in wounds was growing throughout the nursing profession. Apart from the dearth of dressing materials preceding the 1980s, lack of interest and apathy towards the subject of wounds existed. Nurses involved in wound care were left to manage as best they could with little available advice or information.

In the early 1980s, however, small groups of nurses and individuals became increasingly aware that their problems were shared by others. Patients with wounds, especially those with problems, encountered a number of healthcare professionals for treatment, including nurses, GPs, surgeons, dermatologists, plastic surgeons, pharmacists and occasionally physiotherapists. One local multidisciplinary group formed into the Wessex Rehabilitation Association, which expanded and later became the Tissue Viability Society. In its earliest days it gave probably the only plat-form for members of all disciplines to discuss wound care. With the help of this group the Wound Care Society was able to develop into its present form. The Wound Care Society is run by nurses for nurses. It organises an annual conference and publishes a quarterly newsletter, information and educational packs, and its membership is over 1,000 and rising.

In the light of these developments, nurses have been seeking to improve the wound care given to their patients. This chapter attempts to help address that need.

Holistic care for patients with cavity wounds
Good wound care requires a holistic approach to patients with cavity wounds. Nurses also need to be reasonably knowledgeable about the range of dressing materials available both for patients cared for at home and in hospital.

When confronted with a cavity wound, no matter how large or small, the first instinct is to make a snap decision on which treatment or dressing to use. This temptation should be resisted in favour of briefly reviewing the patient's medical history. A number of factors can delay healing and these should be identified as a matter of priority. It may not be possible to improve or reverse these factors in many cases, but their presence should be recognised and a delay in healing anticipated.

Assessing individual needs

A patient with diabetes had amputation of toes and metatarsal heads, which took many months for the wound to heal, regardless of the local wound care given. The patient's diabetes first needed to be stabilised following surgery and readjusted as the wound healed. Healing in people with diabetes is inevitably slow, but the poor blood supply to the lower limb only increases the delay in healing. A care plan for the management of this wound can only begin after these factors have been taken into consideration

A sacral pressure sore can measure only 4 x 4 cm, yet take 18 months to heal. Again it is not the local wound care that is the issue, but the patient's physical condition. An 86-year-old lady had severe rheumatoid arthritis, which required high doses of steroids. Her mobility was also impaired. Several factors are at work here - she is elderly, has a systemic, inflammatory disease, is not very mobile and takes steroids. Healing could be expected to be slow, and this was reflected in the prolonged healing phase. Although small, a care plan for the management of this wound would plan for such a delay in healing.

These case histories also illustrate how the theory of wound healing (the theoretical factors which delay healing) had a practical bearing on our every day experiences.

Assessment

Wound size   In general the larger the wound, the longer it takes to heal, so wound size can be used to calculate probable healing time. The healing rates of some wound types, such as pilonidal sinus excisions and abdominal wall wounds have been carefully measured, and it is often possible to predict with some accuracy how long they take to heal (Marks, 1983). Wound size may also influence the choice of dressing - while a number of products can be used for small cavities, the choice for larger wounds is more limited to products which provide the required bulk with just one or two packs.

Wound measurement   Changes in the size of the wound must be monitored to assess the effectiveness of a particular treatment. Surgically created cavities usually have even contours and depth, and their length and breadth is generally easy to measure. Weekly measurement is sufficient, and should show progress. Wound volume is more difficult to assess and offers no real advantage over the measurement of linear dimensions. Chronic wounds such as pressure sores are often more difficult to measure, because they may extend under the skin edge. The simplest way to assess their extent is to insert a probe under the edge of the cavity and mark the boundary on the skin with an ink marker. Remeasurement may only be necessary every two to three weeks, because these wounds generally heal much more slowly.

Wound shape It is important to recognise the significance of wound shape in good wound healing. Ideally, surgically created cavities should be boat or saucer shaped, with evenly sloping sides. Pockets, tracts or sinuses within a cavity can mean that drainage of exudate is inadequate, which may greatly delay healing. Poor wound shape also restricts the range of materials that can be used. A long narrow cavity, for example, will require a dressing which can be comfortably inserted into the space available but can also be easily removed from the depth of the wound without leaving behind fibres and particles which could become a focus for infection. Where wound shape is so poor that progress towards healing is unacceptably slow, the wound may require surgical revision to give it more regular contours: this is occasionally necessary when wounds which have undergone primary closure subsequently breakdown. Occasionally wounds which have been sutured primarily breakdown in part, and often the district or practice nurse encounters this situation and makes the first assessment of the extent of the problem. The wound must be gently probed to reveal the extent of wound breakdown: where the cavity extends under the skin edge further than 5cm, wound drainage may not be sufficient to allow sound healing, and surgical revision may be needed to improve the wound's shape.

Pressure sores are particularly prone to develop into poorly shaped wounds and as surgical revision is not always possible or advisable, it is essential that dressing materials are chosen carefully.

Age
Advancing age results in a slower rate of healing.

Nutrition (Vitamin C, Zinc)
Poorly nourished patients or those lacking the vitamins and minerals needed for tissue repair can have impaired healing.

Diabetes mellitus; renal failure; jaundice ; inflammatory diseases
A range of systemic diseases can be linked with poor healing.

Drug treatments
A range of steroids and anti-inflammatory drugs slow down healing.

Table 1. Some factors which can affect healing.

Exudate The amount of exudate produced varies enormously between cavities: new surgical wounds can exude heavily, while some pressure sores produce very little fluid. This variation affects the choice of dressing - some products are highly absorbent and able to deal with copious discharge, whereas others have a limited absorbent capacity. Use of inappropriate dressings can sometimes have serious consequences; for example, if a product is unable to cope with the exudate produced by a wound, the surrounding skin may become macerated, while a highly hydrophilic product applied to a lightly exuding wound may cause the wound surface to dry excessively, which can delay healing and sometimes even cause pain.

The following questions need to be addressed:-
1. Does the shape allow free drainage?
2. Is there a foreign body such as a piece of suture material present?
3. Is there any slough or necrotic tissue present which needs to be removed?
4. Is the wound infected?

Table 2. Assessing whether surgical revision is necessary.

Slough or necrotic tissue   When slough or necrotic material is present on the wound surface, healing will be delayed or prevented. In the past, a range of solutions and lotions including Eusol and Aserbine™ were used to remove such tissue, but they can also damage the surrounding skin and impair wound healing (Leaper, 1986). Fortunately, dressings such as hydrogels and hydrocolloids are now available which encourage natural debridement without causing unnecessary damage (Bale, 1990). When sloughy or necrotic tissue has become softened or loosened, it may be possible to remove it surgically without anaesthesia but the practitioner must be experienced in this field.

1. Bright red or raw looking granulation tissue.
2. Superficial bridging.
3. Bleeds easily on light contact.
4. The patient complains of pain or discomfort.

Table 3. Clinical signs of infection.

The wound bed   In the pregranulation stage, cavity wounds often appear red-raw with an uneven surface of adipose tissue; this is normal for this early stage of healing. Within 10-14 days, however, the appearance of the wound will change as granulation tissue is formed. A healthy wound should be pale pink (sometimes covered with a pale yellow membrane), pain-free and should not bleed easily if touched. However, infection will alter the appearance of the wound; the tissue may change from pale pink to deep red and the wound may bleed easily on light contact and become uncomfortable or painful. Superficial bridging may also occur. Since infection can delay healing, prompt treatment is needed. For deep seated infections a wound swab followed by a course of the appropriate antibiotic is generally indicated, but more superficial infections can sometimes be treated topically. No dressing will be effective until the infection is cleared.

Excessive granulation   From time to time, re-epithelialisation fails to take place due to excessive granulation or 'proud flesh'. The simplest treatment is application of 75 per cent silver nitrate sticks which cauterises the tissue, but the use of a cream containing a corticosteroid is less traumatic, although this should only be applied under medical supervision.

Social situation and personal needs

When planning wound care do you ever ask yourself - "What does the patient want?" Although the importance of patient compliance has long been recognised by district nurses, it is often not translated to the care of patients with other wound types. Unless patients are happy with the treatment chosen, they are unlikely to support it, so dressing should be selected with the patient, either first in hospital or by the district nurse in the patient's home. The following factors may need to be considered.

1. Does the patient want to go back to work/school? If so could a dressing be chosen which the patient could manage him or herself with supervision? Otherwise, can dressing changes be easily undertaken (with the chosen dressing) early in the morning or in the evening to allow an uninterrupted day? Do the relatives also need some teaching in order to support the patient?

2. Do any other aspects of care need to be considered? Patients with stoma and fistula appliances or prostheses may need more time and attention to be devoted to these aspects of care than to the wound care.
3. Is the district nurse the best person to carry out wound care? Some patients, such as the very young or handicapped may prefer the person they know best caring for the wound, which is often a parent.

4. Are the home conditions conducive to the chosen treatment? Where home conditions are dirty or there is a lack of basic facilities, wound care which requires strict asepsis is not appropriate. A compromise, as an alternative, would best suit these situations.

The following case histories illustrate where these need to be taken into consideration. A young mother with an older child had to run her home and look after her family. Her small axillary wound was expected to heal within two weeks, but she did not want to wait for a daily visit from the district nurse or to go to the health centre for treatment - she simply wanted to manage the wound herself under a nurse's supervision. Her wishes were complied with and she managed the wound without difficulty until it healed 12 days later.

A little girl had had an emergency appendicectomy which neces-sitated leaving the wound open to heal by granulation. She was only happy to have her mother touching the wound area, so a dressing was selected which Mum could manage. Again, the district nurse supervised the wound care and healing was achieved to the satisfaction of all.

A patient who recently had formation of a stoma was being looked after by relatives. They were happy to give most of the wound care, leaving the district nurse free to spend her time teaching them to manage the stoma - a priority, since the stoma will always need to be managed, while the wound healed within a matter of weeks.

---

1. Maintains high humidity between wound and dressing.
2. Removes excess exudate and toxic components.
3. Allows gaseous exchange.
4. Provides thermal insulation.
5. Impermeable to bacteria.
6. Free from particles and toxic wound components.
7. Allows removal without causing trauma during dressing change.

Table 4. Characteristics of an ideal dressing.

Decisions about wound care should be tailored to suit each individual patient. A holistic approach is essential for delivery of good wound care. The characteristics of an ideal dressing (Table 4) were identified by Turner (1979). It is important for nurses to be able to view dressing products in terms of how they perform and how close each comes to the criteria for an ideal dressing. At present the materials available for managing cavity wounds can be considered in these groups: gauze, dextranomers, hydrogels, hydrocolloids, foams, alginates.

Granulating wounds

The traditional principles for the management of cavity wounds requiring strict aseptic technique and the use of forceps and gauze dressings are very much out-of-date (Table 5).

- Uncomfortable.
- Requires frequent dressing changes (daily or twice daily).
- Adheres to the granulating surface of the wound.
- Requires aseptic technique which is time consuming.
- Requires dexterity and skill to apply properly.
- Is often used in conjunction with antiseptics which have been found to be toxic to granulation tissue.

Table 5. Disadvantages of gauze packing.

Gauze packing With extensive wounds, packing can be painful and traumatic at dressing changes. Gauze is also unlikely to be able to cope with large amounts of wound exudate and is likely to leak.

Dextranomers (Debrisan, Iodosorb) These are available in beads, in a medicated form, in paste and in pads and ointment. They are cleansing and debriding dressings designed for infected, purulent, sloughing and necrotic wounds.

Hydrogels (Vigilon, Geliperm, Scherisorb) Available in wet or dry sheets or granulated gels. The flat sheets of hydrogel are designed for flat areas of granulating wounds such as burns, dry wounds, fungating lesions and skin graft donor sites. The granulated gels are used for cavities and for the removal of slough and necrotic tissue (Bale, 1990).

No one of these products for cavity wounds is universally suitable for all situations, but the holistic assessment outlined here should indicate the type of material needed. It is essential that a dressing material is only chosen after a comprehensive patient assessment. The process requires some knowledge of what environment each dressing can provide, which should then be matched to the physical characteristics of the wound. This process should help ensure the right dressing is put on the right wound at the right stage of healing.

The Drug Tariff

Provision of dressing materials in the community currently comes via the GP on a FP10 prescription. The GP is allowed to prescribe from a restricted list of products on the Drug Tariff, and where dressings are concerned not all the materials available to patients treated in hospitals are available on the list (Bale, 1989). (It is generally accepted that although availability varies between health authorities, hospital patients generally have access to all materials in an adequate range of sizes).

Until July 1988, a range of traditional materials were available for the treatment of cavity wounds. The Drug Tariff listed few modern materials, which included: boil dressings; dressing packs (sterile/ multiple); perforated film dressing (Melolin); semipermeable adhesive film (Opsite, Tegaderm, Bioclusive); semipermeable waterproof plastic wound dressing (Elastoplast); sterile knitted viscose dressings (NA, Tricotex); gauze (cotton, cotton and viscose, impregnated, Capsium, cellulose wadding); polysaccharide (Debrisan, Iodosorb). However, in July 1988 a number of newer products for granulating wounds were added to the Tariff including alginate, foam and hydrocolloid material. By the summer of 1990 the range of materials had been extended to include Inadine, Comfeel and Scherisorb gel, and at last at least one dressing from each of the main groups was available.

For the first time district nurses had direct access to modern materials, but, after the initial euphoria, it was quickly realised that the product sizes available were too small to deal with the wounds encountered in the community (Bale, 1989). In response, the problem of dressing sizes and the range of sizes of materials available on Drug Tariff is being increased to meet the needs of patients being managed in the community.

References

Bale, S. (1989) Cost-effective wound management in the community. *Professional Nurse*, **4**, 12, 598-601.

Bale, S. (1989) Community nurses' awareness of dressing materials. *Care: Science and Practice*, **7**, 4.

Bale S. (1990) Using modern dressings to effect debridement. *Professional Nurse*, **5**, 4, 244-48.

Leaper, D.J. (1986) Antiseptics and their effects on healing tissue. *Nursing Times*, **82**, 23, 45-47.

Marks, J. (1985), Pilonidal sites excision - healing by open granulation. *B. J. Surg.*, **72**, 637-40.

Marks, J. *et al* (1983) Prediction of healing times and an aid to the management of open granulating wounds. *World J. Surg.*, **7**, 641-45.

Note

Sorban 10 x 10cm dressing has recently been added to the Drug Tariff.

45

Consider the mind as well as the body: nursing care and support in multiple sclerosis

Susan A. Banks, RGN, RMN
Special Projects Officer for The Disablement Income Group

Nurses working on neurological units will undoubtedly regularly encounter patients with multiple sclerosis (MS), unlike those on general wards who are unlikely to nurse many. There appear to be two main groups of patients concerned with MS in acute hospitals: those who are in for neurological testing, who may as a result be given a diagnosis of MS (Group 1) and those who have previously been diagnosed and are in for assessment and treatment of an MS relapse or for treatment of an unrelated condition (Group 2).

Diagnosis

In Group 1, patients will most likely have suffered an episode of neurological deficit from which they may or may not have recovered. Any neurological symptomatology, be it impairment of vision, weakness or paralysis in an arm or leg, or vertigo is frightening, and is probably made worse by not knowing the cause. Patients admitted for neurological investigation will therefore be apprehensive, and this may be compounded by uncertainty about what the tests involve. They will overtly or covertly be looking to the nurse for explanations and reassurance of symptomatology and the tests they are to undergo.

Obviously, nurses cannot comment on the cause of patients' complaints until the tests have been completed, but if they are totally conversant with all the procedures for neurological testing, such as clinical examination, evoke responses, MRI scans, balance tests and lumbar puncture, explanation will help to allay patients' fear of the unknown. Clearly nurses can play a supportive role in listening to patients' account of what has happened to them leading up to admission, and this may well indicate patients' opinion of what is wrong with them and their innermost fears. Talking to a nurse may be the first opportunity patients have to talk in depth about their symptoms and resulting day-to-day problems. These may range from coping with work or a young family to specific problems such as difficulties with mobility or bladder. While they will have been seen by a neurologist, consultations are often brief, and it can be a great relief to talk to someone outside the home.

If a diagnosis of MS is made there may be little time to talk about it, because the patient may be discharged soon after the tests are completed. Individuals show different responses to the diagnosis, so it is difficult to generalise about the emotional response people show to the knowledge that they are suffering from a chronic, possibly disabling disease of the nervous system. There are, however, certain common responses. Some people who have suspected they had MS for some time experience a great sense of relief, while others may have had no idea and are consequently stunned and shocked by the news. Whatever the initial response, people have to 'work through' different emotions, of which there are many, including denial, anger and fear of not knowing what course the disease will take. Connell (1983) and Ginther (1978) both suggest that patients with MS grieve and mourn the loss of their identity as healthy people. Sensitive evaluation is needed in assessing how much information the patient wants on learning the diagnosis, as emotional support and accurate information in the early stages is known to help people with MS and their families (Burnfield and Burnfield, 1982; Segal, 1987).

Established diagnosis

Group 2 patients may well have had MS for some time, but nurses should remember they have not always been suffering from MS. Many individuals have previously been supremely fit people, and have had to cross the psychological and physical divide from being able-bodied to becoming 'disabled'. One patient related a conversation with her brother-in-law in which she mentioned she had been a county hockey player, to which he replied: "But Jennifer, I've always thought of you as a crockery-smashing, ataxic, un-coordinated person."

Patients with MS frequently have build-up of neurological deficit leading up to the picture of disability the nurse sees when they are admitted to the ward. It is important to realise that in reaching this appearance over what may have been a relatively short period of time or some years, they have often suffered much heartache, despair, frustration and anger at having to adapt to the various episodes of demyelination.

In addition to dealing with multiple symptomatology, patients have often acquired a great deal of knowlege about MS, and may know more about it than the nurses and junior doctors. This can be quite intimidating, but expertise is not uniquely acquired through professional training. Patients are also experts, with a different kind of expertise, acquired due to their experience (Robinson, 1987). Sharing the patient's knowledge and experience and the nurses' knowledge, communicative skills and ability to implement resources can be of great mutual benefit.

Nurses can, therefore, learn a great deal about MS from patients, and it will be apparent how totally individual each patient is in the way that MS has affected him or her. Almost any manifestation of neurological disorder can be observed in people with MS, and extreme variability occurs not only from one person to another but also in the same person at different times (McAlpine *et al*, 1972).

Empathising

Nurses who have not experienced neurological symptoms can find it difficult to understand or empathise with some of the symptoms patients complain of. Unfortunately, neurological textbooks, when describing symptoms, frequently omit to describe what the patient feels. For example the accompanying symptom with diplopia is nausea and nystagmus, which often appears to make stationary objects move from side to side or up and down. Walking, when ataxic or with leg spacticity, is tiring and, when coupled with frequency of micturition, is exhausting for the patient. Pain is a symptom often omitted, indeed McAlpine (1985) states that well-read patients complain that it receives little mention in popular or professional accounts of MS, which is unfortunately true. In a small American study of 28 people who had had MS for an average of 28 years, 82 per cent had some form of pain (Kassiner and Osterberg, 1987). Fatigue is one of the most commonly reported symptoms (McAlpine *et al*, 1972), yet it too receives little attention in textbooks. It is extremely disabling, unlike normal healthy tiredness and is rather like tiredness associated with influenza. Fatigue accentuates other MS symptoms, such as blurred vision and clumsiness and heaviness of limbs, and may be brought on by infection, heat, exertion, hunger or for no apparent reason.

Action for Research into MS (ARMS), 4a Chapel Hill, Stansted, Essex CM24 8AG. Tel: 0279 815553	Encourages research into treatment, prevention and cure of MS, and works to improve public understanding of the disease. Runs therapy centres with physiotherapy, counselling, nutritional advice and hyperbaric treatment. Operates 24-hour counselling service to anyone suffering from MS or their family and friends: London: 071-222 3123. Midlands: 021-476 4229. Scotland: 041-945 3939.
Multiple Sclerosis Society of Great Britain and Northern Ireland 25 Effie Road, Fulham London SW6 1EE. 071-736 6267	Dual objectives of promoting research to find the cause and cure of MS and to provide a welfare and support service for people with MS and their families. Runs 'Crack' groups especially concerned with the welfare of younger sufferers, and holiday homes.

Table 1. Addresses for further information. Both charities issue information packs for patients and professionals.

In addition to living with physical disability and the uncertainty of MS, patients frequently suffer financial hardship, especially if they are unable to work. Consequently many cannot maintain a reasonable standard of living, while socialising may be out of the question. Isolation is frequently a problem and these problems culminate in loss of morale. Interpersonal relationships suffer and there is often friction within the family. Apart from the physical care people with MS receive while in hospital, which must not be understated, nurses can give no greater support than time to listen. Langton Hewer (1980) states that because of the nature of the disease, patient management requires skill, sympathy, time and patience. By listening and encouraging patients to talk about their day-to-day existence, nurses will be able to evaluate how effectively they are coping and ascertain any major problems they are currently contending with. Increased awareness of the nature of MS, and a more positive approach can help peole with MS manage their illness.

Objectives should be first, to take into account the patient's needs; second, to assess and give multidisciplinary help as appropriate to attain an optimum physical and psychological state, and third, to supply information, of which the patient may not be aware, on resources in the community. The ultimate aim should be to enable people to achieve self fulfilment and respect, alleviation of financial hardship, social integration and independence at any stage of the disease.

Teaching sessions: 1
Information for people newly diagnosed as having MS

Multiple sclerosis is a chronic disease affecting the central nervous system (CNS) (the brain and spinal cord). The insulation or protective layer around nerves, the myelin sheath (Figure 1), becomes inflamed and thins or disappears. This damage – demyelination – results in nerve impulses being delayed, causing various disabilities, such as difficulty with movement, balance and altered sensations.

It is not known why this inflammation occurs. The body attempts to repair the damage, and this results in hardened patches (sclerosis). These episodes of inflammation can occur at different times and in different places: the course of MS is unpredictable. There are two main patterns:

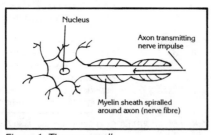

Figure 1. The nerve cell.

Relapse/remitting Most people have this pattern. In a relapse the disease is active, inflammation is occurring and nerves are being damaged, while in a remission it is quiet. However, residual symptoms may be present because of damage to the nerves. Some people have a very benign course going for many years without a relapse and never suffering severe disability.

Chronic progressive With this pattern, people experience a gradual worsening of symptoms over many years. They do not have relapses or remissions, but their symptoms fluctuate, and vary greatly, depending on the nerves affected by demyelination. These include problems with balance, bladder, double vision, weakness, clumsiness, stiffness affecting one or both legs and arms, and impairment of sensation and touch. Fatigue is common in people with MS, probably because the CNS is under attack. The disease has a bad press, and only the worst cases are highlighted, but people with MS have normal life expectancy and probably only 20 per cent eventually need a wheelchair. People with MS can and do experience life fully including love, marriage, children, work and happiness. (Reproduced with permission from ARMS).

Teaching sessions: 2
Notes to discuss with people who have been diagnosed previously Obtain an overall picture by going over the course the patient's MS has run – chronic progressive, relapsing/remitting. Query number of years, frequency of attacks and how much it has interfered with normal life. If the patient is severely disabled, ask for how long. What current problems and disabilities does the patient have? Damage done by demyelination cannot be repaired, but some symptoms may be alleviated, and help, of which the patient may be unaware, may have a range of problems.

Sessions 1 and 2 may be used in conjunction, according to the information the patient requires.

Sources of help and support
Bladder
• Incontinence, which may be due to bladder overfill or unstable detrusor muscle.
• Frequency and urgency, which may be due to bladder irritability and/or infection.
• Retention: referral to urodynamics clinic is necessary to ascertain mechanism involved. Probanthine may help bladder irritability. Once the mechanism for bladder dysfunction is determined, the patient can be referred to a continence advisor and may be taught intermittent self-catheterisation. An indwelling catheter can be helpful on outings.

Bowels Constipation is a common problem in MS. Complete loss of bowel control is rare, but if it does occur, it undoubtedly causes great distress. The continence advisor may be able to advise on protection.

Fatigue Patients usually have their own rest programme, but physiotherapy can help increase stamina and endurance. Has home assessment been carried out by an occupational therapist, who can advise on aids and appliances to make life less tiring?

Financial help and advice Disablement Income Group (DIG), Millmead Business Centre, Millmead Road, London N17 9QU. Tel: 081-801 8013. Advisory service on benefits and services. Researches the economic and social problems of disability and campaigns for a national disability income.

• Disability Rights Handbook Mentioned in Useful Reading – a valuable asset to any ward.

Muscle spasms Is patient taking Baclofen?

Mobility (outdoor) If patient can walk, how limited is his or her walking distance? Has patient had recent physiotherapy assessment? Is patient in receipt of Mobility Allowance? Application forms are available from the Department of Social Security; the allowance can help with purchase of a car or occupant-controlled powered wheelchair. The Orange Badge Scheme – details from Social Services – allows parking concessions.

Occupational therapist can assess whether aids, if used, can be improved. It is preferable for a wheelchair assessment to be performed at the patient's home.

Mobility, Boundary House, 91/3 Charter House Street, London EC1M 6BT. Tel: 071-253 1211. An organisation to ensure disabled people who wish to obtain a vehicle or electric wheelchair, using mobility allowance, may do so.

Banstead Park Mobility Centre, Park Road, Banstead, Surrey SM7 3EE. Tel: 073 73 51756. Offers information and advice on any outdoor mobility problems including provision of individual assessments.

Mobility (indoors) In an assessment at home, the occupational therapist will be able to recommend improvement grants for essential works, such as downstairs toilet, stair lift extensions.

Under the Disabled Persons (Services Consultations Representation) Act 1986, a disabled person, carer or authorised representative may request an assessment of their needs from social services for the following: home help; radio and/or television and help in using the library; lectures, games, outings and any help needed to take advantage of educational facilities; help with travelling to any of these or similar activities; home adaptation; holidays; meals at home or at a local centre; a telephone and special equipment to use it.

Aids and equipment Disabled Living Centres are being established throughout the country, where people can see the variety of aids available. Where no commercially available aid is suitable for use by a disabled person the Royal Association for Disability and Rehabilitation's (RADAR) REMAP department can often help. REMAP comprises of engineers and occupational therapists who design or adapt equipment

to suit individuals, often at no charge.
Disabled Living Foundation, 380/384 Harrow Road, London W9 2HU.
Tel: 071-289 6111.
REMAP 25 Mortimer Street, London W1N 8AB. Tel: 071-637 5400.

Intractable pain   Referral to a pain clinic.

Sexual   Impotence in men, as part of a complex of neurological symptoms, is not uncommon. In contrast, women do not often spontaneously complain of sexual dysfunction, but a history of such a problem can quite commonly be elicited on direct questioning. Emotional factors may also be a cause, and counselling may help considerably.
SPOD (Association to Promote the Sexual and Personal Relationships of People with Disabilities), 286 Camden Road, London N7 0BJ Tel: 071-607 8851/2.

Speech and swallowing   Referral to speech therapist.

Severe disability   Does the patient require a lot of help? Is he or she in receipt of Attendance Allowance? Does the patient require a care attendant? Care attendant schemes, operating in some parts of the country, are service options to enable physically disabled people between 16 and 65 years to live independently and participate in activities available in the community. The schemes also give assistance when family carers are not available. Where such schemes do not exist the Independent Living Fund can help buy in care. For information write to: PO Box 183, Nottingham NG8 3RD. It is important that patients apply to the Fund before 1993.

Vision   As well as neurological assessment, has the patient had recent ophthalmological assessment? Magnification aids may or may not help. Prism glasses can alleviate diplopia.

Other information
Work   Under the terms of the Disabled Persons (Employment) Act 1944, employers with 20 or more employees are required to employ no less than 3 per cent registered disabled people. It can therefore be useful to register as disabled at the local Job Centre. The Department of Employment can lend tools, aids or equipment to registered disabled people, and can also give a grant to employers of up to £6,000 to adapt their premises to make them suitable for disabled employees.

Assessment for work, training and rehabilitation can be carried out at a course held at an employment rehabilitation centre. An appointment can be made for assessment through the disablement resettlement officer at the Job Centre.

Organisations giving advice

Association of Disabled Professionals, The Stables, 73 Pound Lane, Banstead, Surrey SM7 2HU Tel: 07373 52366.

Opportunites for the Disabled, 1 Bank Buildings, Princes Street, London EC2R 8EU. Tel: 071-726 4963.

Royal Association for Disability and Rehabilitation (RADAR). Publishes many leaflets and books. Provides an advisory service and is also particularly active in areas of employment, mobility, access and holidays.

Homeworking   Some local authorities run homeworking schemes, and applications should be made through the DRO.

British Computer Society, 13 Mansfield Street, London W1N 0BP. Tel: 071-637 0471. A specialist group which offers specific advice on activities relating to computing and the disabled.

Holidays

Holiday Care Service, 2 Old Bank Chambers, Station Road, Horley, Surrey RH6 9HW. Tel: 0293-774535. An information service on holiday provision for disabled people.

References

Burnfield, A. and Burnfield, P. (1982) Psychological aspects of multiple sclerosis. *Physiotherapy,* **68,** 5, 149–50.

Connell, H, (1983) More than a physical illness. *Nursing Mirror,* **24,** 40–42.

Ginther, J. (1978) But You Look So Well. Nelson-Hall Inc, Chicago.

Kassiner, M.R. and Osterberg, D. (19) Pain in multiple sclerosis. *American Journal of Nursing,* **87,** 968.

Langton Hewer, R. (1980) Multiple sclerosis management and rehabilitation. *International Rehabilitation Medicine,* **2,** 116–25.

McAlpine, E. *et al* (1972) Multiple Sclerosis: A Reappraisal. (2nd Edn) Churchill Livingstone, Edinburgh.

McAlpine's Multiple Sclerosis (1985) Churchill Livingstone, Edinburgh.

Robinson, I. (9187) The Salmon James Lecture. Profitable Partnership? The profession and the patient in the management of multiple sclerosis. In: Multiple Sclerosis Immunological, Diagnostic and Therapeutic Aspects.

Segal, J.C. (1987) Emotional Reaction to Multiple Sclerosis. Action for Research into multiple sclerosis. (ARMS) Publications, London.

Useful reading

The Disability Rights Handbook – £3.50 25. Denmark Street, London WC2H 8NJ. Telephone: 071-240 0806. An invaluable guide to all benefits and services available to disabled people and their families.

Books about MS

Burnfield, A. Multiple Sclerosis – A Personal Exploration. Souvenir Press, London.

Povey, R., Dowie, R., Prett, G.) Learning to Live With Multiple Sclerosis. Sheldon Press, London.

Matthews, B. Multiple Sclerosis: The Facts. Oxford University Press, Oxford.

Forsythe, E. Multiple Sclerosis: Exploring Sickness and Health. Faber and Faber, London.

Graham, J. Multiple Sclerosis: A Self-Help Guide to its Management. (3rd ed) Thorsons, Wellingborough.

ARMS MS and Pregnancy. Research publication, available from ARMS.

Text Books

McAlpine's Multiple Sclerosis. Churchill Livingstone, Edinburgh.

Clifford-Rose, F. and Jones, R. (Eds) Multiple Sclerosis: Immunological, Diagnostic and Therapeutic Aspects. John Libbey, London.

Both these books are obtainable through a reference library.

Product Awareness

46

Catheters: making an informed choice

Petra M. Britton, RGN
Formerly Hospital Continence Adviser, Bloomsbury H.A.

Elizabeth S. Wright, RGN, Dip.N, CHSM
Senior Nurse, Surgical Unit, The Royal London Hospital, Whitechapel, London

A study by Crow et al (1986) reported that 10-12 per cent of patients admitted to hospital will have a urethral catheter inserted. They may be used to relieve anatomical or physiological obstruction of the urinary tract, facilitate postoperative repair and/or to measure urinary output. Catheters may also be used to manage urinary incontinence, but only as a last resort. This chapter is designed to give nurses the information to make an informed decision on choosing the correct catheter for a particular patient.

The right material

There is a large range of catheters, made of different materials, all designed to be used for a specific length of time. When catheterising a patient for the first time it is always best to consider short-term use – this not only prevents money being wasted on expensive long-term catheters, but also allows the nurse to identify patients who will have perpetual problems from catheters blocking or bypassing (see complications of catheter management in next month's article).

Length of use can be divided into three main categories:

- short-term – one to 14 days;
- short- to medium-term – three to six weeks.
- medium- to long-term – six weeks to three months.

Short-term catheters (Polyvinylchloride (PVC) or polyurethane or Latex rubber). Latex rubber tends to be irritant and the incidence of adverse reaction is high, so it is not used commonly, but when it is, it should be as a short-term catheter. Plastic (PVC) becomes soft at body temperature, but rigid at lower temperatures and is often found to be uncomfortable by female patients, especially when sitting. They do have good drainage lumens and are generally used postoperatively for irrigation following urological surgery, but they are prone to encrustation, and recommended by manufacturers to remain *in situ* for up to 14 days only. PVC catheters are used for intermittent catheterisation (Nelaton catheters), and at home, they can be used for a week before disposal.

Low friction catheters   This type of catheter is designed with a specially treated surface which becomes smooth and slippery after it has been kept in water for 30 seconds. They are designed to cause less trauma to the urethra and discomfort to the patient and are used for intermittent catheterisation, but can only be used once.

Short- to medium-term catheters   (Latex-Teflon coated or Silicone coated Latex). Teflon coating is claimed to make the Latex inert and give a smoother surface, allowing the catheters to be used for up to three or four weeks. They are prone to encrustation, but there is less incidence of urethritis. Silicone coated Latex catheters are dipped in Silicone Elastomer, which is claimed to be resistant to encrustation and also to cause less incidence of urethritis. These catheters are also less likely to suffer from balloon deflation and can be used for up to six weeks.

Medium- to long-term catheters   (100 per cent Silicone or Hydrogel encapsulated). As 100 per cent Silicone catheters are not coated, the lumen tends to be larger, and there is less risk of blockage. However, because Silicone permits gas diffusion, they tend to have problems with balloon deflation over time, and can fall out before their expected life is over (Studer et al, 1983). Silicone is inert, so there is less incidence of urethritis, and the catheters seldom encrust. We recommend they are used for up to three months.

Hydrogel encapsulated catheters are relatively new on the market. The material resembles living tissues more than any other synthetic biomaterial in its physical properties. In a non-hydrated state the catheters are similar to 100 per cent Silicone catheters, in that they are soft but inert. Hydrated, they become smoother, decreasing the friction in the urethra. They are also inert and resistant to infection and encrustation. Their maximum recommended use is three months.

Self-retaining or intermittent catheters

Once it has been decided a catheter is required, whoever is inserting it should be aware of the range available and their different functions, with the comfort and wellbeing of the patient in mind. There is an enormous range of catheters available which can basically be divided into three main categories:

- ballooned urethral catheters (self-retaining);
- urethral catheters without balloons;
- suprapubic catheters (also self-retaining).

Ballooned urethral catheters   The standard two-way Foley catheter is the most commonly used of these catheters. It is called two-way because it has two channels, one for urine drainage and a smaller one for balloon inflation. It can be used for any patient requiring bladder drainage for any length of time – the material is the important factor, depending on how long the catheter is to remain *in situ*.

A standard three-way catheter is often referred to as an irrigation catheter. It has three channels – one for urine drainage, one for the irrigation fluid to run into the bladder and one for balloon inflation, and is most commonly used in prostatic surgery, where continuous irrigation can be maintained without disconnecting the catheter from closed drainage.

Urethral catheter without balloons (Nelaton catheter)   This is also known as the intermittent catheter. It has only one channel to allow for urine drainage, and no balloon, and can be used to obtain a single specimen of urine, empty the bladder prior to surgery, or most commonly, for intermittent self-catheterisation in patients who are unable to empty their bladder properly.

Suprapubic catheter   The bladder may be catheterised suprapubically, and several catheters have been specially developed for this purpose. This form of catheterisation is used mainly in urological surgery, trauma to the urethra, and sometimes as a last resort in urinary incontinence.

Specialist catheters
Paediatric catheters   These are designed and produced specifically for use in infants and young children. In design they are identical to the standard two way Foley Catheter but are manufactured with a 3-5ml balloon and are available in two sizes, eight and 10 Charriere.

Tiemann tipped catheter   This has an additional feature of a coudé, or curved tip (Figure 1). There may be one or three drainage eyes in the curve at the tip to allow more drainage. It was designed to negotiate the membraneous and prostatic urethra in patients with prostatic hypertrophy.

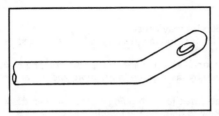

Figure 1. Tiemann tip.

Whistle tipped catheter   This provides a large drainage area, having a lateral eye in the tip, and eyes above the balloon (Figure 2). It is mainly used for postoperative urine drainage where large clots and debris may be present in the urine.

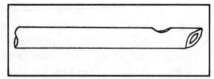

Figure 2. Whistle-tip.

Roberts catheter   This has an eye above and below the balloon (Figure 3) which assists maximum drainage of the bladder and reduces the residual volume retained. It is most effective when urine bypassing is a problem or complete preoperative drainage is required.

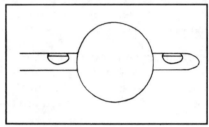

Figure 3. Roberts.

Suprapubic catheters   Malecot or Depezzer catheters are commonly used for suprapubic drainage. They are single lumen catheters with a star shaped end to prevent displacement once in the bladder, and have four drainage holes. Suprapubic catheters are introduced using a trocar needle, and often need a firm pull to remove them, as the star will cause some resistance. If a long-term suprapubic catheter is required, once a tract has formed, (after 10 days), an ordinary long-term Foley catheter can be used without the need of an introducer.

There are many other catheter variations available but they are not commonly used.

A large balloon (30ml+) may cause:

1. Irritation of the bladder trigone, leading to bypassing and/or expelling of the catheter (McGill, 1982).

2. Residual urine forms below the eye of the catheter, and cannot drain away. This can also lead to bypassing due to irritation, and urinary infections due to static urine.

3. If there is repeated traction or tugging on the catheter, the weight of a large balloon is more likely to damage the bladder neck.

4. It is commonly thought confused patients will be unable to pull larger balloons out, but it is not unknown for them to pull out a fully inflated 30ml balloon. It is infinitely better for the patient to remove a 10ml one instead. Also the patient often removes the catheter in the first place because they were experiencing discomfort from the 30ml balloon.

Table 1. Which balloon size?

Size

The diameter of a Foley catheter shaft is measured in Charriere (Ch) or French (Fr) size. One Ch is equivalent to one third of a mm of the external diameter of the catheter shaft. Thus a 12Ch catheter has a shaft measurement of 4mm.

The main rule in size is to choose the smallest catheter that will drain adequately (McGill, 1982). For adults this is normally 12, 14 or 16Ch. Except in cases where there is heavy haematuria, sizes larger than 18Ch should not normally be considered.

Common misconceptions   "When urine bypasses the catheter, the answer is to insert a larger one" (Kennedy and Brocklehurst, 1982). McGill (1982) reported that a large catheter with a large balloon is likely to stimulate inappropriate bladder contractions. Also, it is not necessary to try and occlude the urethra, the urethral folds will normally close upon themselves. Except at the sphincter there should be enough space around the catheter to allow the para-urethral glands to drain freely. Inserting a large catheter will inhibit the drainage of these glands and can lead to abcess and stricture formation (Blandy, 1981; Edwards et al, 1983). Larger catheters are in any case likely to cause more bypassing, since the urethra is a slit, and the catheter pushes the walls further apart.

Too large a catheter may also lead to blockage and infection of the ejaculatory ducts and lead to epididymitis, or to obstruction of the prostatic ducts causing prostatitis or prostatic abcess (Blandy, 1981). Where the catheter lies up against the urethral wall, it can give rise to pressure sores, which in turn lead to stricture formation (Blandy, 1981). Figure 4 shows areas at risk.

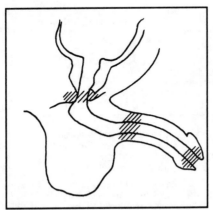

Figure 4. Areas at risk of stricture formation.

"The larger the catheter, the larger the eyes and lumen will be". A large catheter does not necessarily have larger eyes or lumen, and so will often block just as easily. Coated catheters have particularly small eyes and lumen in proportion to their size.

DOS AND DON'TS

Do select a 5ml balloon for initial catheterisation.
Do use the correct size syringe to inflate the balloon to the required capacity. Repeated opening of the valve cap by small volumes may weaken it.

Don't add sterile water to a balloon when bypassing occurs.
Don't use tap water or air to inflate the balloon. Tap water may contain small particles which could block the lumen and make further inflation or deflation of the balloon impossible. Also the water in the balloon gradually migrates into the bladder (Studer et al, 1983).

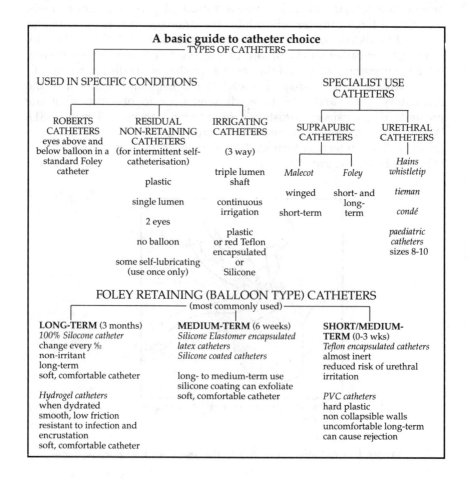

A basic guide to catheter choice
── TYPES OF CATHETERS ──

USED IN SPECIFIC CONDITIONS

SPECIALIST USE CATHETERS

ROBERTS CATHETERS
eyes above and below balloon in a standard Foley catheter

RESIDUAL NON-RETAINING CATHETERS
(for intermittent self-catheterisation)

plastic

single lumen

2 eyes

no balloon

some self-lubricating (use once only)

IRRIGATING CATHETERS

(3 way)

triple lumen shaft

continuous irrigation

plastic or red Teflon encapsulated or Silicone

SUPRAPUBIC CATHETERS

Malecot   *Foley*

winged   short- and long-
short-term   term

URETHRAL CATHETERS

Hains whistletip

tieman

condé

paediatric catheters sizes 8-10

FOLEY RETAINING (BALLOON TYPE) CATHETERS
── (most commonly used) ──

LONG-TERM (3 months)
100% Silocone catheter
change every ⁵/₁₂
non-irritant
long-term
soft, comfortable catheter

Hydrogel catheters
when dydrated
smooth, low friction
resistant to infection and encrustation
soft, comfortable catheter

MEDIUM-TERM (6 weeks)
Silicone Elastomer encapsulated latex catheters
Silicone coated catheters

long- to medium-term use
silicone coating can exfoliate
soft, comfortable catheter

SHORT/MEDIUM-TERM (0-3 wks)
Teflon encapsulated catheters
almost inert
reduced risk of urethral irritation

PVC catheters
hard plastic
non collapsible walls
uncomfortable long-term
can cause rejection

Correct balloon size
Manufacturers indicate on catheter packaging the maximum amount of fluid with which a balloon should be inflated. Stated capacities vary from 5ml to 30ml, but in fact they can frequently accommodate over 200ml (Bowles, 1980; Moisey and Williams, 1980). Very large balloons (75ml and over) are only used in postoperative prostatic surgery. Table 1 may assist in deciding on balloon size to use:

Female catheters
Many nurses use a standard male catheter for both sexes, because they are unaware of female length catheters (Norton, 1986), which are readily available in hospitals and on the Drug Tariff for those in community. The normal length of a female catheter is 20-25cm, and male 40-45cm. Using a male length catheter in women generally causes a number of problems: they are difficult to disguise under clothing and easier to pull accidentally; and if thigh drainage is used, the catheter will tend to loop, causing the urine to drain uphill before reaching the drainage bag. However, the female design does have some problems of its own: in large women, the inflation valve may rub against the skin, causing sores; and there is also more risk of traction on the bladder neck.

References
Blandy, J.P and Moors, J. (1981) Urology for Nurses, Blackwell Scientific, Oxford.
Bowles, W. (1980) When the Foley won't deflate. *Consultant*, 20, 63.
Crow, R.A. et al (1986) A study of patients with an indwelling urethral catheter and related nursing practice. Nursing Practice Research Unit, University of Surrey.
Edwards, L.E. et al (1983) Post-Catheterisation urethral strictures – a clinical and experimental study. *British Journal of Urology*, 55, 53–56.
Kennedy, A.P. et al (1983) Factors related to the problems of long-term catheterisation. *Journal of Advanced Nursing*, 8, 207–12.
McGill, S. (1982) Catheter management: It's the size that's important. *Nursing Mirror*, 154, 48–49.
Molsey, C.V. and Williams, L.A. (1980) Self-retained catheters – a safe method for removal. *British Journal of Urology*, 52, 67.
Studer, U.E. et al (1983) How to fill silicone catheter balloons. *Urology*, 22, 300–02.

47

A tube to suit all NG needs? Evaluation of fine bore nasogastric tubes

Helen Fawcett, RGN
Nutrition Nurse Specialist, The Royal London Hospital, Whitechapel

Claire Yeoman, BSc, SRD
Former Chief Dietitian, The Royal London Hospital, Whitechapel

Fine bore nasogastric (NG) tubes are now widely used in hospitals and by patients at home for the administration of commercially made feeds. These tubes have replaced the wide bore Ryles tubes which were traditionally used, but which caused patient discomfort, oesophagitis and gastric reflux due to their size. Being made of PVC, Ryles tubes could also only be used for a week before they hardened and often cracked. Ryles tubes are, however, indicated where gastric emptying is impaired, and should be reserved for postoperative aspiration and gastric lavage only.

A wide selection of fine bore NG tubes are available on the market and these vary in quality and cost from 80 pence to £11.00 (retail price at the end of 1990). To ensure the tubes chosen are best suited to patient needs, nurses need to know the properties of each and to establish a criteria for selection. To be cost-effective, tubes must be long-lasting, comfortable *in situ* and well secured with adhesive tape to avoid slippage. The NNS in conjunction with ward and endoscopy staff and dietitians at the Royal London Hospital organised a trial to determine which tubes best fulfilled the criteria for nasogastric administration of feed. This chapter charts the progress of the trial and records the results.

The trial first established the criteria fine bore NG tubes must meet to achieve effective administration of commercially made feeds. The criteria identified by discussion between NNS, ward nurses and dietitians to ensure nursing care best fulfils patient needs is listed below:

- All tubes must conform to British Standards.

- Nasogastric tubes must be no greater than FG size eight to prevent nasal trauma and oesophageal discomfort.

- Tubes must be compatible with the feeding equipment used on the ward to avoid both leakage and unnecessary use and expense of different connections and adaptors.

- Tubes must be easy to pass and to aspirate. Confirmation of position by aspiration and then testing with litmus paper, avoids the need for post-insertion X-ray.

- Tubes should be soft and, preferably, made from polyurethane to prevent cracking after prolonged use - polyurethane tubes can be left *in situ* for three months.

- Radio-opaque tubes enable X-rays to be taken clarifying the tube position, if required.

- Wide internal diameter is required to prevent blockage of NG tubes.

- A cap situated at the proximal end of the nasogastric tube to prevent contamination and blockage.

- Tubes must be comfortable for the patient, and, where appropriate, it should be easy for fluids to be swallowed around them.

- Tubes must be cost-effective to avoid overspending on the nutritional support budget.

Study sample

Six fine bore NG tubes which fulfilled the necessary criteria and were widely and easily available were chosen for the trial. These were:
- Fresenius 'Freka' (CH8).
- Merck 'Silk' (CH6).
- Abbott 'Flexiflow' (CH6).
- Cow and Gate 'Flocare' (CH8).
- Viomedex 'Swallow' (CH7/8).
- Portex tubing (cut to the required size) with adaptor (used in the endoscopy unit) (CH6).

Table 1 lists the characteristics of each tube; 10 tubes of each type were tested. They were randomly distributed among patients on the wards and in the endoscopy unit. A good representative sample of patients (60) requiring   nutritional support was used; indications for placement included anorexia (17 patients); CA oesophagus (16 patients); orofacial and ENT surgery (9 patients); neurological disorders such as scleroderma and cerebral problems (10 patients) and inability to swallow - CVA and unconscious patients (8 patients). There was random selection of patients although those having endoscopically placed tubes had portex tubes.

A questionnaire was issued with each tube used in the trial, and nurses were required to complete and return it to the nutrition nurse specialist (NNS). The questionnaires asked nurses to record specific advantages and disadvantages of the tubes, and the results were collated to provide a rating for the equipment used.

Name of tube	1990 price (retail)	Material and size	Internal and external diameter	Distal end shape	Proximal end (cap etc)	Radio-opaque	Tube length	Comments
Fresenius' 'Freka' tube	£4.15	Polyurethane CH8	Ext. 2.8mm Int. 2.1mm	Two, large round side holes	A fitted cap compatible with feeding equipment	Yes	120 cm	Soft, flexible tube, well designed introducer, Easy to pass. Easy to aspirate. Securing tape in patient and 'cigar' connection. Needs a cigar shaped connectionfor flushing with syringes.
Merck 'Silk' tube	£11.00	Polyurethane CH6	Ext. 2.18mm Int. 1.37mm	Scooped spoon end	Fitted cap not compatible with feed equipment without connection	Yes	92 cm	Very soft and flexible. Easy to pass and particularly suitable when tube passage is dififcilt ie, ENT patients. Expensive in comparison to other tube. Needs male/male connection for feeding equipment. Securing tape in packet.
Abbott 'Flexiflow' (now with-drawn from sale)	£2.95	Polymeric PVC CH6	Ext. 2.0mm Int. 1.0mm with two	Round closed end with feed side holes	No cap compatible with feed equipment	Yes	85 cm	No cap. Easy to pass. Tendency to block. Proximal end sometimes cracks.
Viomedex 'Swallow' tube	£5.46	Polyurethane 7/8FG	Ext. 2.5mm Int. 1.7mm	Round closed end. Two large outlet holes	Cap compatible with feed equipment	Yes	80 cm	Slightly stiff tube. Good size outlet holes. Difficult to aspirate due to poor seal on connection. Well packaged with a tray for water and a glove.
Cow & Gate 'Flocare' tube	£3.70	Polyurethane 8FG	Ext. diameter measurements not avaialble Int. 1.5mm	Open ended. Small side holes	No cap. Compatible with feed equipment	Yes	110 cm	No cap. End sometimes kinks as tube is passed.
Portex tubing (with adaptor)		Size 6FG	Ext. 2.0mm Int. 1.0mm	Open ended. No side holes	No cap. Requires adaptor to connect to tube.	Yes	As required cut to size	Cheap. Difficult to aspirate. Tendency to block.

Table 1. Characteristics of each tube.

The study

The tubes were passed by the NNS or qualified nursing staff in accordance with hospital policy, and marked with indelible ink at the nasal exit site so that any slippage could be recorded. All patients on the trial received pump assisted feeding of commercially made feeds, and where there was any risk of perforating the oesophagus (for example, patients with cancer, oesophageal varicies or stricture), tubes were placed by a gastroenterologist in the endoscopy unit. Patients were studied for ten days, and if their tube was changed during the trial, the same type was used.

The questionnaires identified the main nursing requirements for NG administration, and nurses were asked to record the progress of individual patients. Questions included:

• Which type of NG tube was used?

• Was intubation easy or difficult?

• Did any blockages occur? If so, why?

• Was the tube compatible with the feeding equipment?

• Was the tube comfortable (a rating score of 1-5 was given)?

•Were any specific problems encountered with the tube ?

• Why was the tube was removed?

The staff were confident the answers would provide a clear understanding of which fine bore NG tubes best met patients' needs.

Results of the survey

The questionnaire highlighted the main problems affecting the management of patients receiving NG feeding. Tube blockage relating to the size of the internal diameter of the tube was cited as a common problem (14 occurrences). Wider internal tube diameter was shown to reduce the incidence of blockages; Portex tubes (internal diameter 1.0mm), for example, saw most blockages (six) and Fresenius tubes (internal diameter 2.1mm) least (none). Difficulty also occurred in passage of some tubes due to swallowing difficulties, tubes kinking (Cow and Gate two kinked), and tube slippage due to poor adhesive taping (13 occurrences). Incompatible connections with the feed equipment caused delay and extra expense where new connections had to be found, and tubes which could be easily removed by patients were noted as a cause for concern (this happened four times during the trial). The full list of results is given in Table 2.

Tube	Number of tubes	Days in studies	Blockages	Slippages	Removed by patient
Fresenius	10	14	0	1	0
Merk	10	14	2	2	0
Abbott	10	14	3	2	1
Viomdexe	10	14	0	2	2
Cow & Gate	10	14	3	3	1
Portex	10	14	6	3	0

Table 2. Results of the questionnaires.

The results of the questionnaire prove that the design of NG tube is important for the effective management of patients requiring nutritional support. Blockage is always a potential problem, and tubes with wide internal diameters were shown to reduce the risk. Nasogastric tubes require a secure adhesive to prevent slippage, and this was achieved by 'Freka' (Fresenius) and 'Silk' (Merck) tubes. Both tubes were shown in the trial to provide the most effective all-round administration, fulfilling the criteria set in the trial to find a tube which best fulfilled patients' needs.

Bibliography
Taylor, S.J. (1988) A guide to nasogastric feeding equipment. *Professional Nurse*, 4, 2, 91-94.
Neohane, P.P. *et al* (1983) Limitations and drawbacks of 'fine bore' nasogastric tubes. *Clinical Nutrition*, 2, 85-86.
Hobbs, P. (1989) Enteral feeds. *Nursing Times*, 85, 9, 71-73.
Pritchard, A. (Ed.) The Royal Marsden Hospital manual of clinical nursing procedures, (2nd edition).

Acknowledgements
The authors wish to thank the ward nursing staff; the endoscopy unit nursing staff; Dr P. Swain and Dr N. van Someren (for placement of NG tubes in the Endoscopy Unit).

48

How are you supporting your patients? A review of pressure relieving equipment

Carol Dealey, SRN, RCNT
Clinical Nurse Specialist, Tissue Viability, Moseley Hall Hospital and Queen Elizabeth Hospital, Birmingham

In recent years, pressure sores have 'come out of the closet'. Nurses are no longer automatically given the blame when they occur (Anthony, 1989), and as a result, there is much more interest in their management and prevention. There have also been cases of litigation over the development of pressure sores: Livesley and Simpson (1989) state that lack of adequate equipment to provide pressure relief is negligence in the eyes of the law. It is the responsibility of health authorities to provide reasonable facilities for their patients (Tingle, 1990) so it is nurses' responsibility to alert management to the needs of their patients.

The most common places for pressure sores are the sacrum, buttocks and heels (Locket, 1983). They may arise from lying or sitting for long periods on hard surfaces, such as trolleys, operating tables, X-ray tables, worn out mattresses and inappropriate chairs. Nothing lasts forever and all hospitals need to establish regular review and replacement programmes. Where there is no such policy, nurses can instigate a review of equipment, producing evidence of the need for change.

The Department of Health recommends standard hospital mattresses have a life-span of four years. It should be remembered that the covers only remain water resistant if cleaned with soap and water, and that spraying with alcohol damages them. All mattresses should be at least 130mm in depth - the foam in shallower mattresses has been found to collapse after a short time, and once this has happened, the patient is resting on the metal bed base.

To ensure mattresses are replaced at the appropriate time, nurses can instigate a check and replacement programme. Mattresses can be checked by placing both hands on the centre and pressing down. If the metal base can be felt, the mattress needs replacing. All mattresses should be tested annually, and their check date should then be marked on them. As new mattresses arrive, they should also be marked with the date they come into use.

Pressure relief

There is a huge range of pressure relief equipment available, ranging from highly sophisticated beds to heel pads, and this can be confusing when trying to determine what to use and when. Hibbs (1988) has suggested the requirements for a district general hospital. Ward-based nurses may wish to calculate the requirements for their wards, and this can be done by taking a weekly audit of all the patients. On a set day each week, all patients are assessed using a risk assessment scoring system such as Norton (1975) or Waterlow (1985). Those patients with pressure sores are indicated, as is any pressure relieving equipment being used. According to their score, all patients can be identified as falling into no risk, low, medium or high risk categories: the Waterlow score lends itself nicely to this. Over a period of time, a pattern will emerge indicating the average numbers of patients in each category and, thus, the requirements of the ward. Ideally there should be an adequate supply of equipment so that each patient has what is suitable to his or her needs. Table 1 gives appropriate suggestions, which are discussed in more detail in the text.

Low-risk patients
• Sheepskins
• Hollow core fibre pads
• Bead overlays
• Foam overlays
• Gel pads

Medium-risk patients
• Foam overlays
• Foam replacement mattresses
• Combination foam/water mattresses
• Combination foam/gel mattresses
• Alternating air pads
• Water beds
• Double layer alternating air pads

High-risk patients
• Double layer alternating air pads
• Air floatation pads
• Dynamic air floatation mattress
• Air wave mattress
• Low air loss bed
• Air fluidised bed

Table 1. The range of pressure relieving

Low-risk patients
The standard hospital mattress can be used in conjunction with various overlays.

Sheepskins   Probably readily available in most areas, sheepskins have several limitations. They do not provide pressure relief, although they do prevent friction, and while they absorb moisture, such as perspiration, some patients find them too hot. Many sheepskins become lumpy after frequent laundering, and this can actually cause pressure problems.

Hollow core fibre pads   These are also widely used, and many frail and emaciated patients find they provide great comfort. The recent development of vapour-permeable (VP), water resistant covers has made them easier to use with incontinent patients. They can also reduce the frequency of washing, as the cover can easily be washed between patients. A major problem with these mattresses is that many hospital laundries reduce their life-span by washing them at too high a temperature. Some mattresses have the fibre in individual bolsters inside an outer cover. This can be useful in the community, as several bolsters can be washed together in an ordinary washing machine.

Bead overlays   These are made with beads of polystyrene, which help to spread the pressure, and although they are quite thin, they can be amazingly comfortable. Bead overlays are best used with lighter weight patients, as very heavy patients can squash the beads. VP water resistant covers are available.

Foam overlays   These have recently become popular, probably since the provision of VP water resistant covers. An overlay should be between 70-100mm in depth, and most are partly cut through in cube or egg crate shapes, which provides additional pressure relief. While many patients find these overlays comfortable, they raise the height of the bed, which can be a particular problem in fixed height beds, as it can make it difficult for the patient to get in and out of bed.

Gel pads   These help to disperse pressure because of their density. They can be used on trolleys, X-ray tables and operating tables, as they are not radio-opaque. The major disadvantage is that they are rather heavy and cumbersome to move about.

Medium-risk patients
It is possible to use some of the support systems in this category as a replacement mattress. Others may be used on top of a standard mattress.

Foam overlays   May also be suitable for medium-risk patients providing they are at least 100mm in depth.

Foam replacement mattresses   These are being used to replace standard mattresses in some areas. They are made of different densities of foam put together in such a way as to provide extra pressure relief. Usually fairly firm, they are very popular in orthopaedic and spinal injury units. The expected life-span is double that of standard mattresses (Lowthian, 1989), which can be a useful selling point to management.

Combination foam/water mattresses Made up of cells of water set in a foam surround, these may also have a foam layer over the cells. Some are deep enough to be a replacement mattress, and they provide the advantages of water floatation without the disadvantages found with water beds. However, some patients feel 'sea sick' on them or find it more difficult to move. They are inappropriate for patients being rehabilitated as it is difficult to sit on the edge of the bed and push up to standing, and are best used for light patients who are bedfast.

Combination gel/foam mattresses Similar to the above, these are quite heavy to move around as the gel cell remains intact, unlike the water cell, which can be emptied.

Alternating air pads Commonly referred to as ripple mattresses. The original small-cell ripple mattress was unreliable and actually caused pressure problems, but the types now commonly used either have bubble shaped cells or large horizontal cells. The motor causes the cells to alternately inflate and deflate. Care is needed to avoid pucturing the cells, and this equipment should be regularly maintained to avoid breakdown.

Water beds These provide true floatation and pressure relief, but there are several disadvantages in their use. The beds are extremely heavy and must be placed where the floor will carry the weight. This is often near a wall and may cause the patient to feel isolated. It is also not very easy moving patients on a water bed. Some beds are lower than standard beds which puts added strain on the nurses' backs. They are no longer widely used.

Double layer alternating air pads Usually in the form of two layers of alternating air cells. The two layers may work in unison or the bottom layer may be static. A maintenance programme needs to be established for these mattresses.

High-risk patients
Equipment appropriate for these types of patients is of the more sophisticated variety, although some of the support systems from the previous group, such as the double layer alternating air pads, may still be appropriate.

Air floatation pads Designed so that the patient lies 'in' them rather than 'on' them, these are made up of interconnecting cells which are pumped up with air. The pads should not be pumped up too hard, or the pressures will be high. For some patients these pads are an excellent form of pressure relief, but others may find the rubber from which they are made too hot for comfort.

Dynamic air floatation mattress These have figure-of-eight shaped cells which alternately inflate and deflate. The pressures are automatically adjusted according to the weight and position of the patient, and the motor can also be set on static mode, when the pressures remain constant throughout the cells. These mattresses are useful for a range of patients.

Air wave mattress Made up of two layers of air cells which work together as one; the cells work in a sequence of inflation, partial deflation and deflation. The motor is able to regulate the amount of pressure in the cells according to the weight of the patient. An appropriate support system for those patients who cannot be turned.

Low air loss beds These have a mattress composed of a series of air sacs which lie on edge crossways across the bed. The pressures in the sacs can be adjusted either individually or according to the position on the bed, for example, the pressures for the sacs under the patient's buttocks can be set to be different to those under the chest. The bed can be put in a variety of positions by means of electrical controls, which may be used by patients, giving them some control over their immediate environment. These beds can be particularly useful for very heavy patients who are difficult to move or those with contractures who have limited range of positions.

Air fluidised bed Composed of a large tank which is filled with silicone coated beads. The motor causes the beads to aggitate, producing a fluidising effect. The pressures created are lower than capillary pressure and so do not cause ischaemia by capillary closure, while body fluids such as sweat pass from around the patient's skin into the beads and sink to a sieve at the bottom of the tank. These beds are extremely heavy, and should only be used where the floor can carry the weight. They are mainly used in ITU and burns units for critically ill patients.

Seating

For many excellent reasons, patients are 'mobilised' as soon as possible. Unfortuately, this often results in them being left in chairs for long periods, and often, little or no attention is paid to pressure relief on the grounds that the patient is now 'up'. At this stage in their recovery, many patients lack energy and the desire to move about, and are still likely to be at risk of pressure sore development - considerable pressure may be exerted over the ischial tuberosities when seated. Lowry (1989) considered the principles of good seating.

In the hospital setting it is difficult to cater for the many differing needs of patients. Hospital armchairs often fail to promote good posture, but allow the patient to sit in a slumped position. Not only is the patient likely to slide down the chair, increasing the risk of shearing, but it is also more difficult to rise to standing from this position.

Another fairly common sight is that of a patient sitting with legs dangling a few inches from the floor. There is no way this patient can easily help him- or herself to stand, and this may slow down the process of rehabilitation. Finding suitable chairs for tall men can also be a problem, as the seat may not be deep enough, front to back, as well as the chair being too low.

---

1. Instigate a mattress checking and replacement programme in your ward/unit. Encourage management support by warning of the dangers of litigation!

2. Identify all at-risk patients by means of a risk assessment score and then instigate a plan of care. Remember, once the risk has been identified the responsible nurse is accountable for any lack of care.

3. Ensure that turning regimes include regular pressure relief for patients when sitting out of bed.

4. Liaise with the physiotherapist to identify chairs which provide good posture.

5. Weekly audits can be used to identify the average degree of dependency in a patient population as well as the numbers of pressure sores. This provides objective evidence for the equipment requirements for the area and is a useful bargaining tool.

6. Establish contact with local charity, who will often help with the purchase of equipment.

7. Set up teaching programmes for staff and patients to improve understanding in the causes and prevention of pressure sores. Include the medical staff so they understand their responsibilities.

8. Continue to evaluate the progress being made. This provides encouragement and possible justification for further expenditure.

Table 2. Guidelines for preventing pressure sores.

Apart from the fact that many chairs are generally inappropriate, little attention has been paid to developing maintenance or replacement programmes. One hospital survey (Dealey *et al*, 1990) showed that many armchairs were in need of repair and/or the foam in the seat cushions had collapsed. Many hospitals are writing standards of care for their patients, and it should be possible, within the structure component, to cover armchair maintenance programmes as well as mattress checking.

Another aspect of seating which is often neglected is that of wheelchairs, which are extremely important for moving patients from place to place as well as increasing the mobility of those with disabilities. Wheelchairs are often used without a cushion, allowing the canvas base to exert extremely high pressure. Rithalia (1989) stressed the importance of wheelchair cushions, having found mean pressures of 226.1mm/Hg when testing the base alone. Such high pressures would cause sores in a very short time, and time can pass almost unnoticed as a patient waits for an X-ray, a test or to be seen in casualty or outpatients.

Other forms of pressure relief

Unfortunately not all nurses have easy access to adequate pressure relieving equipment, so other strategies need to be employed. The most widely used is a regular regime for turning patients, and this should be extended to standing or lifting patients when they are sitting out of bed. Preston (1988) highlighted the advantages of using the 30 degree tilt position to reduce pressure even on a standard mattress, while judicious placing of pillows or padding can help protect bony prominences such as heels or elbows. Regular checking of all pressure areas can identify other vulnerable spots.

It is easy to feel intimidated by the huge range of equipment regularly advertised in the nursing press, and by the cost of many items. However several simple aims can be set which will improve the quality of patient care and help to reduce the suffering caused by pressure sores. Table 2 gives guidelines for practice. Although pressure sores may not be seen as a 'glamorous' topic, it is a rewarding one. It can also become addictive - you have been warned!

References
Anthony, D. (1989) The pressure sore debate. *Nursing Times* , **85**, 26,74.
Dealey, C., Eden, L., Earwacker, T. (1990) Are your patients sitting comfortably? *Care of the Elderly*, in press.
Hibbs, P. (1988) Action against pressure sores. *Nursing Times* , **84**, 13, 68-73.
Livesley, B. and Simpson, G. (1989) Hard cost of soft sores. *Health Service Journal*, **99**, 5138, 231.
Locket, B. (1983) Prevalence and Incidence. Pressure Sore Disease. Symposium at Royal Hospital and Home for Incurables, London.
Lowry, M. (1989) Are you sitting comfortably? *Professional Nurse*, **5**, 3, 162-64.
Lowthian, P. (1989) Pressure sore prevention. *Nursing*, **3**, 34, 17-23.
Norton, D., McLaren, R., Exton-Smith, A. N. (1975) An Investigation of Geriatric Nursing Problems in Hospital. Churchill Livingstone, Edinburgh.
Preston, K.W. (1988) Positioning for comfort and pressure relief: The 30 degree alternative. *Care - Science and Practice*, **6**, 4, 116-19.
Rithalia, S.V.S. (1989) Comparison of pressure distribution in wheelchair cushions. *Care - Science and Practice*, **7**, 4, 87-92.
Tingle, J. (1990) The important case of Bull. *Nursing Standard*, **4**, 37, 54-55.
Waterlow, J. (1985) A risk assessment card. *Nursing Times*, **81**, 48, 49-55.

49

Back-up for the venous pump: compression hosiery

Jacqueline J. Dale, MSc, SRN, RCNT, DipN
Area Nursing Officer, Lothian Health Board, Edinburgh

Barbara Gibson, SRBM SCN
Leg Ulcer Specialist Sister, Falkirk Royal Infirmary

Pressure has been part of the medical armoury for so long that we tend to take it for granted. However, it is worth going back to first principles and thinking about why compression therapy is used for some diseases of the leg and what effect it has.

The most common reasons for prescribing elastic stockings are: treatment and prevention of varicose veins; treatment and prevention of leg ulcers; control of oedema and prevention of postoperative deep venous thrombosis (DVT). The effect on the leg is to increase blood flow velocity, counteract raised venous pressure and prevent oedema.

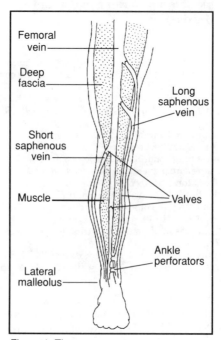

Figure 1. The venous pump.

Leg veins

The venous system of the leg consists of three parts: the deep veins (femoral, popliteal and tibial), which are surrounded and supported by muscle and lie *within* the tough muscle sheath known as the deep fascia; the superficial veins (long and short saphenous) which lie *outside* the fascia and the short connecting veins, known as perforators because they *perforate* the fascia (Figure 1).

Venous pressures

The hydrostatic pressure in the veins is that resulting from the weight of the blood itself, and is highest at the lowest point. When someone is standing upright and motionless the pressure is approximately 90mmHg in the veins of the foot. The superficial veins, however, are protected from such high pressures and are normally maintained, during exercise, by the venous pump at only about 15mmHg. Capillary pressures are a little higher than this at about 25mmHg (Brakee and Kuiper, 1988).

The venous pump

When someone has been standing still for some time, the blood tends to pool in the legs because the venous pump has not been operating. During exercise, blood is propelled upwards towards the heart from the foot by the massaging effect of muscle contraction. The process is usually illustrated by describing the way in which the calf muscles contract and relax during exercise. When a muscle contracts it becomes shorter and thicker and blood is squeezed out of that segment of the vein. When the muscle relaxes the segment is refilled. The cycle is repeated with every movement. The direction of blood flow upwards towards the heart is maintained by a series of pocket-like non-return valves, present in all leg veins. The veins, muscles and valves combine together to act as a pump whose power is supplied by movements of the leg.

The valves are crucial to the efficiency of the pump – if they are missing (some unfortunate people are born without them) or damaged as a result of injury, infection or an episode of DVT, there are serious long-term consequences. The valves in the perforators are the most important, because when they are incompetent, the high pressure in the deep veins is transmitted to the weaker, unsupported superficial veins. These become stretched and tortuous, painful and unsightly (varicose veins). Capillary pressure is increased and fluids including plasma proteins and haemoglobin are forced out into the extravascular space. If neglected, the disease progresses to the condition known as chronic venous insufficiency, which is characterised by oedema, pigmentation, eczema, induration and finally ulceration of the leg.

Recently Gardner and Fox (1984) have used videoradiography techniques to identify and demonstrate other venous pumps which are *independent* of muscle action. The medial plantar veins of the foot contract and empty instantly when pressure is applied to the sole, as in walking. The effect is seen even in a paralysed limb and the pressure achieved is sufficient to overcome a cuff inflated to 100mmHg. It follows, therefore, that the effect of a compression stocking is greatly enhanced by exercise and that walking is more effective than ankle and calf movements alone as an exercise to improve the venous return.

Graduated compression

If firm stockings are applied, the pressure on the skin and underlying tissues gives support to the superficial veins and counteracts the raised capillary pressure, thus preventing oedema. Ideally, for maximum comfort, the external pressure should be no higher than is required to prevent the excessive capillary leakage. The amount depends on the severity of the disease and the size of the leg. Too much pressure is uncomfortable and might result in the patient rejecting the stockings.

An American engineer, Conrad Jobst, who suffered from painful varicose veins himself, understood the haemodynamics and set out to design an elastic stocking in which he would feel as comfortable as when he was standing up to his waist in a swimming pool (Beninson, 1961). He realised the pressure would have to be reduced gradually from the ankle upwards to achieve the same supporting effect as the water.

Research, particularly in the development of the anti-embolism stocking, has shown Jobst's ideas were correct. Several studies have demonstrated that blood velocity is increased when there is a pressure gradient from ankle to knee (Lawrence and Kakkar, 1980; Sigel *et al*, 1975, Cornwall *et al*, 1987).

Types of compression stockings

Although there has been a variety of effective graduated compression stockings on the market for many years, the choice available for prescription on the NHS Drug Tariff was limited until recently. In April 1988 a great step forward was taken when the specifications for inclusion were changed. Instead of basing eligibility solely on the construction of the garment, the rules now take account of the performance of the stocking. The British Standards Institution (BSI) specifies a range of maximum pressures at the ankle and the pressure gradients at calf and thigh (Figure 2). Standard methods for batch testing are laid down and durability is seen as an important attribute. The stockings are required to maintain 85 per cent of the initial pressure after completing 30 washes in accordance with the manufacturers' instructions (BSI, 1985). Synthetic materials are permissible, and the stockings tend to be lighter, easier to put on and more acceptable in appearance. Some are supplied in a range of colours and there are socks of ordinary appearance for men.

Stockings are divided into three classes. The pressures quoted below are as measured by the BSI-approved HATRA method. European manufacturers use different tests which tend to give higher readings. The European equivalents are shown in brackets.

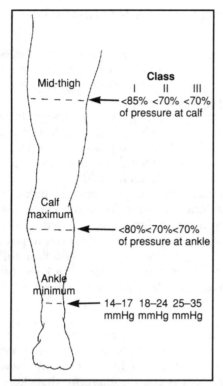

Figure 2. Drug Tariff requirements for pressure gradients in graduated compression hosiery.

Class I These are the lightest, producing pressures of 14-18 (23-28) mmHg at the ankle. Used to treat mild varicose veins and those occurring during pregnancy.

Class II These give medium support in the range of 18-24 (30-40) mmHg at the ankle. Useful for more severe varicosities and venous ulcer prevention in smaller, lighter patients.

Class III These provide 25-35 (40-60) mmHg at the ankle. Prescribed for severe chronic venous insufficiency, severe varicose veins and for ulcer prevention in patients with large, heavy legs.

It is important not to confuse the two sets of measurements when comparing British and Continental products – some manufacturers give both in their accompanying literature. The tests are carried out in a laboratory on a standard former, and it is by no means certain that these pressures will be achieved in actual wear, considering the variability in the size and shape of the human leg. Cornwall *et al* (1987) demonstrated major departures from the expected pressure ranges in a number of brands of stockings but this was before the specifications were changed.

More similar research is now needed to test the new products.

Prescribing

The prescription must specify the class of compression, the type of garment (eg, thigh length or below knee), and the number of pairs to be issued. Suspender belts are available on prescription, but tights are not included in the Drug Tariff.

By no means everyone requiring stockings belongs to a group exempted from prescription charges, and each item prescribed attracts a prescription charge. Normally, two pairs of stockings are needed (one on and one in the wash), so a patient is faced with four prescription charges – more if she also needs a suspender belt.

Some women prefer the appearance of tights or stockings, but compression is seldom necessary above the knee unless there is severe post-phlebitic syndrome or lymphoedema with swelling in the thigh (Ruckley, 1988). Below-knee stockings are easier to put on and remove so patients are more likely to wear them. In addition, full length garments sometimes tend to gather in folds behind the knee, causing constricting bands which impede blood flow and negate the effect of the treatment.

The stockings

Toes   Stockings may have open or closed toes. Open toes are easier to put on correctly and avoid uncomfortable and potentially damaging pressure on the toes. Ordinary tights or socks are usually worn over the top. If the stocking foot is complete, ensure that there is some slack by gently pulling at the toes after the stocking is applied.

Fitting   Support stockings will not be successful unless they fit properly. In many hospitals a trained fitter measures the leg and ensures a good fit, but most stockings are supplied by the local pharmacist using measurements taken by the GP or practice nurse. The required measurements, in centimetres, are: the leg circumference at the thinnest part of the ankle, the fattest part of the calf and for full length stockings, the middle of the thigh. Patients may be given a chart to record their own measurements but they must be taken accurately to ensure a good fit.

Sometimes compression therapy is so successful in reducing oedema that the leg is considerably smaller in size after a few weeks. When replacing the stockings for the first time it is, therefore, advisable to measure the leg again.

Stocking care and application   Putting on elastic stockings may present problems, especially for those with arthritic hips or hands. The aids obtainable for applying ordinary stockings are not suitable for this purpose, and sometimes it is necessary to find a relative or friend who can help elderly patients with these disabilities. If one stocking is applied over another the pressure exerted is cumulative, and in some cases it is advisable to recommend two pairs of Class I stockings, which are much easier to put on and as effective as a Class III stocking (Fentem, 1986).

Illustrated instructions are supplied with most stockings, and it is worth going over them with all new patients and any others who are having difficulties. The garment should be turned inside out as far as the heel. Insert the thumbs into the sides of the foot and slip on the stocking until the heel is correctly placed, then gather up the fabric, ease it over the ankle and up the leg keeping the thumbs inside and spreading it as evenly as possible until it just reaches the knee or thigh. Tight bands or unevenness should be gently smoothed away with the palm of the hand. If the stocking has been pulled up too high, the unwanted length should never be folded over, as this would cause a band of constriction and negate the effect of the pressure gradient. Instead, the garment should be taken all the way back to the ankle and be reapplied more sparingly.

Open-toed stockings are easier to apply if a silky socklet, supplied by some manufacturers, is first slipped over the forefoot and pulled out when the stocking is in place. Sprinkling the leg with talcum powder, and using the lower part of a nylon stocking over the bare leg may also help, while wearing a pair of fine rubber gloves will both protect the fabric from damage by sharp fingernails and rough skin, and make handling easier. A visit to a chiropodist is advisable if hard skin on the feet and rough toenails are likely to cause damage.

Stockings should be taken off at night and put on again in the morning immediately on rising, before any oedema has been allowed to collect.

Washing Frequent washing, preferably daily, improves performance by restoring the shape and removing damaging skin oils prolongs the life of the stocking. A choice of washing procedures is laid down by the BSI and the manufacturers are required to supply their recommended instructions. Patients should be encouraged to read them and follow the advice, which is typically "wash gently by hand in warm soapy water. Do not wring. Dry away from direct heat or sunlight". Washing in water hotter than about 50°C will denature the fibres and make the garment stiffer and less extensible (Fentem, 1986). A machine wash is, therefore, inadvisable. With care, good quality stockings will still give adequate pressure after three or four months, but should then be replaced.

Low pressure is better than no pressure

Too much pressure may be counterproductive. Sigel *et al* (1975) showed that pressures of 18mmHg at the ankle, graduated to 8mmHg at the upper thigh, gave the maximum consistent increase in blood velocity in recumbent patients. Above that level, the flow rate actually decreased in some individuals. Struckmann *et al* (1986) have demonstrated that even low pressures increase the effectiveness of the venous pump and improve the symptoms of venous disease. Those patients who, in spite of the improvements in the new stockings, find they are unable to tolerate the higher grade of compression, might find that they can wear a Class I stocking with some advantage.

Anti-embolism stockings

It is now standard practice in many hospitals for patients with a high risk of developing DVT, who are undergoing surgery or who are on prolonged bed rest, to be fitted with lightweight graduated compression stockings. They should be worn pre- and postoperatively at all times while the patient is in hospital, except when bathing. Nurses in the wards are often responsible for taking the measurements, so it is necessary to ensure that all new staff are familiar with the techniques, that they understand the purpose of the stockings and how they should be worn and that they are able to explain these things to the patients. The full range of sizes must be kept in stock at all times to avoid the problems associated with a poor fit.

The hazards of compression

It hardly needs to be said that compression should never be applied if there is severe arterial disease of the leg, but a salutary report of a survey among surgeons in Scotland (Callam *et al*, 1987) revealed that ulcers or necrosis had been observed in 147 patients. Of these, 73 had been caused by bandages, 36 by compression stockings and 38 by anti-embolism stockings. The damage had necessitated reconstruction of the arteries in seven cases and amputation in 12. Foot pulses should be checked in all patients and if there is any doubt about their presence or strength, further investigation with Doppler ultrasound is essential.

Compliance is all

There are 20 or more brands of compression hosiery now available, and more choice makes it more difficult to keep up-to-date in order to help the patients choose the stockings that will suit them best. In a highly competitive market, the manufacturers provide information and well-illustrated literature about their products, and nurses are advised to study this. The most important contribution nurses can make is to encourage patients to go on wearing their stockings for as long as they are required. In most cases this means for life.

References
Beninson, J. (1960) Six years of pressure-gradient therapy. *Angiololgy*, **12**, 38-45.
Brakee, A.J.M. and Kuiper, J.P. (1988) The influecne of compressive stockings on the haemodynamics in the lower extremities. *Phlebology*, **3**, 147-53.
BSI (1985) British standard specification for graduated compression hosiery. British Standards Institute (BS 86612), London.
Callam, M.J., Ruckley, C.V., Dale, J.J., Harper, D.R. (1986) Hazards of compression treatment of the leg: an estimate from Scottish surgeons. *British Medical Journal*, **295**, 1382.

Cornwall, J.V., Dore, C.J., Lewis, J.D. (1987) Graduated compression and its relation to venous refilling time. *British Medical Journal*, **295**, 1087-90.

Fentem, P.H. (1986) Elastic hosiery. *Pharmacy Update*, **5**, 200-05.

Gardner, A.M.N. and Fox, R.H. (1984) The return to blood to the heart against the force of gravity. In: Negus, D. and Jantet, G. (Eds) Phlebology '85. Libby, London.

Lawrence, D. and Kakkar, V.V. (1980) Graduated external compression of the lower limb: a physiological assessment. *British Journal of Surgery*, **67**, 119-21.

Ruckley, C.V. (1988) Surgical Management of Venous Disease. Wolfe Medical, London.

Sigel, B. *et al* (1975) Type of compression for reducing venous stasis: a study of lower extremities during inactive recumbency. *Archives of Surgery*, **110**, 171-75.

Struckman, J. *et al* (1986) Venous muscle pump improvement by low compression elastic stockings. *Phlebology*, **1**, 97-103.

50
Using modern dressings to effect debridement

Sue Bale, BA, RGN, NDN, HV, DipN
Director Nursing Research, Wound Healing Research Unit, University of Wales College of Medicine, Cardiff

Keith G. Harding, MB, ChB, MRCGP
Director, Wound Healing Research Unit, University of Wales College of Medicine, Cardiff

Traditionally, debridement concerns the removal of slough and necrotic tissue from a wound surface. It is a difficult task requiring intensive nursing management, but in recent years, some of the modern wound management materials have been shown to have a gentle yet effective debriding action. This chapter aims to clarify the use of modern materials for debridement without the need for harsher chemicals.

Why debride?
Let's take a pressure sore with hard, black eschar; this tissue is dead and there is probably extensive tissue loss underneath the eschar. Only when it has been removed, together with any necrotic tissue and slough, will the full extent of the wound be realised. Tissue repair cannot begin until the wound has been fully debrided – then granulation tissue can form and healing by secondary intension will proceed.

Now let's take another pressure sore, this time with sloughy material on the wound surface. Although this is a less difficult problem to deal with, again healing cannot proceed until this material has been removed.

Traditional methods of removal
Surgical   Surgical debridement under either a general or spinal anaesthetic (and occasionally at the patient's bedside) is an extremely skilled procedure, usually undertaken by surgeons. Where tissue damage is extensive and debridement must be effected rapidly, surgery is the method of choice. The necrotic tissue is removed instantly, and the importance of the use of surgery should not be forgotten. Nurses who undertake debridement at the patient's bedside should proceed with great caution. Nerves may be present, and these could be damaged when excising necrotic/sloughy tissue. Blood vessels may also be encountered in the depths of such wounds, and if these are accidentally severed they bleed heavily. In short, unless the tissue is superficial or hanging loose, nurses would be best advised to leave surgery to the surgeon.

Chemical   Hypochlorite agents, such as Eusol. Chloramin T and Milton, and hydrogen peroxide are typical agents used to debride wounds. With hard black eschars these agents often cannot penetrate, fail to rehydrate the eschar and succeed only in damaging the surrounding skin. With softer slough, removal with these substances is more effective, but again the surrounding skin is susceptible, and any granulation tissue present is also damaged.

Prolonged use of hypochlorites can cause renal problems (Johnson, 1986) and air emboli have been caused in deeper wounds when using hydrogen peroxide irrigations (Sleigh and Winter, 1985). Masceration and bleaching of the skin surrounding the wound is extremely common. Having said this, many nurses (and their medical colleagues) find these agents useful in the short-term (3-5 days) to remove soft slough.

Debriding preparations   eg, Aserbine, Malatex. These agents act on necrotic tissue and slough without harming viable tissue. They are often difficult to handle and messy, and may irritate the surrounding skin causing masceration. They are at their most effective on soft slough.

Enzymatic agents   eg, Varidase. Streptokinase dissolves necrotic tissue and slough. It needs to be gently mixed according with the enclosed instructions which should be followed to the letter. It is introduced into an eschar either by injecting it directly into or on top by scoring it with a scalpel before application. In unskilled hands it can be messy and fiddly to use and is expensive.

Modern wound management materials

These products have been designed to provide a good environment for wound healing to proceed (Turner, 1985). As well as fulfilling this function, the polysaccharide, hydrogel and hydrocolloid groups in particular are also able to effectively debride both necrotic and sloughy wounds without traumatising healthy tissue or damaging the skin surrounding the wound. The moist environment they provide allows the necrotic tissue to rehydrate, and once this process has been completed, separation of damaged from healthy tissue quickly ensues. The result is a healthy granulating wound which is undamaged by harsh chemicals.

This action was initially noted by Thomas (1986) when using the granular starch gel Scherisorb and by Johnson (1988a) when using Granuflex, the hydrocolloid material. Debrisan and Iodosorb were designed as cleaning agents, but their application technique has been modified to also deal with harder slough and eschars. These beads can be mixed with saline, and Debrisan plaste is used specifically for this situation. A new product, Iodosorb ointment, can be directly applied and is valuable in removing soft, sloughy material. The following practical tips may assist and encourage nurses to use these materials instead of the traditional treatments to effect debridement.

Polysaccharide paste   When applied to necrotic/sloughy areas, this paste will remove dead tissue without harming the underlying tissue and the surrounding skin. To assist in maintaining the moist environment necessary, Johnson (1988b) recommends using Lyofoam, a polyurethane foam to successfully achieve this. Alternatively, a semipermeable membrane, such as OpSite, also maintains moisture.

Hydrocolloid materials   eg, Granuflex, Biofilm, Comfeel Ulcus. Where some moisture is present at the wound surface, these materials maintain such an environment to allow sloughy/necrotic tissue to separate from viable tissue. They work best with wet sloughy wounds.

It is important to use a sufficiently large sheet of the chosen material to avoid premature leakage and so initiate a dressing change earlier than necessary. The longer the dressing stays in contact with the wound surface in this situation, the better it can perform. The strong odour normally associated with using hydrocolloid materials is even more pronounced when using them in this situation, as the liquifying necrotic tissue produces a very unpleasant odour. This should not be considered unhealthy if debridement is progressing and the necrotic matter is separating from the wound surface, but the patient should be made aware of the reasons for such an unpleasant odour and be reassured that it is both an expected and necessary part of the treatment. Supplementary dressing pads will probably be needed, in case leakage occurs, as the malodorous discharge in this situation could damage clothing (this is not normally necessary when using hydrocolloid materials to dress other types of wounds). At dressing changes the resultant wound exudate should not come into contact with the patient's clothing, bedding or carpets, as it is extremely offensive.

Hydrogels
The most effective of this group is the granular starch gel; Scherisorb. It is effective in the most difficult cases of hard necrotic eschars which fail to respond to conventional treatments. The gel is applied to the necrotic surface with a tongue depressor and a semipermeable film is then used on top, both to keep the gel in place and keep the area moist to allow the necrotic tissue to liquify and separate. A sufficiently large film needs to be applied to cut down the risk of leakage. As with the hydrocolloid materials, odour at dressing changes is extremely unpleasant but should be expected as part of the treatment. Supplementary dressing pads will be needed to absorb any leakage which most commonly occurs when the tissue starts to liquify. During this stage, more frequent (ie daily) dressing changes are often needed. Rapid progress is generally made at this stage and the full extent of the damage becomes apparent. At this time the nurse may become alarmed that the wound is enlarging too quickly, but it should be remembered that the tissue damage has already been done, and up to now all that has been visible is the tip of the

iceberg. Only when full debridement is completed can the extent of the original damage be realised. Nurses regularly blame the dressing or treatment for making the wound bigger when in fact debridement is still continuing and therefore should be encouraged.

A patient has spina bifida and is confined to a wheelchair. A pressure sore on his left knee developed as a result of his right leg lying on top of it in bed during the night. Although adequate pressure relief was quickly obtained, the necrotic area over his knee indicated that extensive tissue damage had occurred. The patient has renal failure, and this, coupled with his loss of sensation in the lower limbs and resultant immobility meant the rate of healing would inevitably be slow.

Following two weeks' treatment with Scherisorb (applied daily and held in place with a semipermeable film), the eschar began to separate and the necrotic tissue liquified. Three weeks later the wound is clean and the granulation tissue begins to form. Treatment continues for 16 weeks and healing is almost complete.

Which debriding agent?

The hypochlorite group and hydrogen peroxide, traditionally used as debriding agents are often ineffective on hard black eschars, due to their failure to penetrate the surface. With softer slough these agents may be effective but easily cause damage to the surrounding skin and can have a deleterious systemic effect. In short, the disadvantages far outweigh the advantages when using these agents.

Enzymatic agents can be difficult to use – the instructions need to be followed so precisely as overmixing can damage the agent. When they are used it is best to seek advice from someone with previous experience, or a pharmacist before use, as mistakes can be expensive. The debriding lotions and creams (Aserbine, Malatex) can be difficult to apply and can also irritate the skin surrounding the wound.

The modern wound management products described, particularly the hydrocolloid and hydrogel products, are effective treatments (in that they quickly allow debridement to take place) but do not harm viable tissue, the skin surrounding the wound or affect the patient systemically. Hopefully they will become more widely used to effect debridement in necrotic and sloughy wounds in the future.

References

Johnson, A. (1986) Cleansing infected wounds. *Nursing Times*, **82**, 37, 30-34.

Johnson, A. (1988a) The case against hypochlorites in the treatment of open wounds. *Care – Science and Practice*, **6**, 3, 86-87.

Johnson, A. (1988b) Standard protocols for treating open wounds. *The Professional Nurse*, **3**, 12, 498-501.

Sleigh, J.W. and Linter, S.P.K. (1985) Hazards of hydrogen peroxide. *British Medical Journal*, **291**, 6510, 1,706.

Thomas, S. (1986) Pressure points. *Community Outlook: Nursing Times*, October, 20-22.

Turner, T. (1985) Semi occlusive and occlusive dressings: In Ryan, T. (Ed.) An environment for healing: the role of occlusion. Royal Society of Medicine Congress, Series No. 88, London.

Index